Child Health Nursing

Reviews & Rationales

Mary Ann Hogan, RN, CS, MSN

Clinical Assistant Professor
University of Massachusetts, Amherst

Judy E. White, RNC, MA, MSN

Director of Nursing
Vital Care, Inc.
Meridian, Mississippi

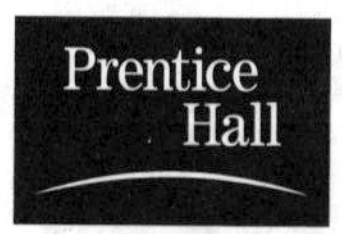

Upper Saddle River, New Jersey 07458

Publisher: Julie Levin Alexander
Executive Editor: Maura Connor
Managing Development Editor: Marilyn Meserve
Development Editor: Jeanne Allison
Director of Production and Manufacturing: Bruce Johnson
Managing Production Editor: Patrick Walsh
Production Liaison: Danielle Newhouse
Production Editor: Jessica Balch, Pine Tree Composition
Manufacturing Buyer: Pat Brown
Design Director: Cheryl Asherman
Design Coordinator: Maria Guglielmo
Interior Designer: Jill Little
Cover Designer: Joseph DePinho
Electronic Art Creation: Precision Graphics
Marketing Manager: Nicole Benson
Production Information Manager: Rachele Triano
Media Editor: Sarah Hayday
New Media Manager: Amy Peltier
New Media Project Manager: Stephen Hartner
Composition: Pine Tree Composition, Inc.
Printer/Binder: Courier/Westford

Pearson Education Ltd., *London*
Pearson Education Australia Pty. Limited, *Sydney*
Pearson Education Singapore, Pte. Ltd.
Pearson Education North Asia Ltd., *Hong Kong*
Pearson Education Canada, Ltd., *Toronto*
Pearson Educaiόn de Mexico, S.A. de C.V.
Pearson Education—Japan, *Tokyo*
Pearson Education Malaysia, Pte. Ltd.
Pearson Education, Upper Saddle River, New Jersey

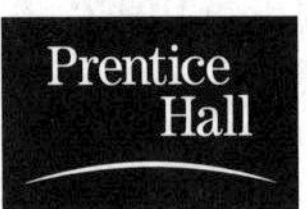

10 9 8 7 6 5 4 3 2 1
ISBN 0-13-030452-2

Contents

Preface

Introduction

Welcome to the new Prentice Hall Reviews and Rationales Series! This 9-book series has been specifically designed to provide a clear and concentrated review of important nursing knowledge in the following content areas:

- Child Health Nursing
- Maternal-Newborn Nursing
- Mental Health Nursing
- Medical-Surgical Nursing
- Pathophysiology
- Pharmacology
- Fundamentals and Skills
- Nutrition and Diet Therapy
- Fluid, Electrolyte, & Acid-Base Balance

The books in this series have been designed for use either by current nursing students as a study aid for nursing course work or NCLEX-RN licensing exam preparation, or by practicing nurses seeking a comprehensive yet concise review of a nursing specialty or subject area.

This series is truly unique. One of its most special features is that it has been authored by a large team of nurse educators from across the United States and Canada to ensure that each chapter is written by a nurse expert in the content area under study. Prentice Hall Health representatives from across North America submitted names of nurse educators and/or clinicians who excel in their respective fields, and these authors were then invited to write a chapter in one or more books. The consulting editor for each book, who is also an expert in that specialty area, then reviewed all chapters submitted for comprehensiveness and accuracy. The series editor designed the overall series in collaboration with a core Prentice Hall team to take full advantage of Prentice Hall's cutting edge technology, and also reviewed the chapters in each book.

All books in the series are identical in their overall design for your convenience (further details follow at the end of this section). As an added value, each book comes with a comprehensive support package, including free CD-ROM, free companion website access, and a Nursing Notes card for quick clinical reference.

STUDY TIPS

Use of this review book should help simplify your study. To make the most of your valuable study time, also follow these simple but important suggestions:

- Use a weekly calendar to schedule study sessions.
  - Outline the timeframes for all of your activities (home, school, appointments, etc.) on a weekly calendar.
  - Find the "holes" in your calendar—the times in which you can plan to study. Add study sessions to the calendar at times when you can expect to be mentally alert and follow it!
- Create the optimal study environment.
  - Eliminate external sources of distraction, such as television, telephone, etc.
  - Eliminate internal sources of distraction, such as hunger, thirst, or dwelling on items or problems that cannot be worked on at the moment.
  - Take a break for 10 minutes or so after each hour of concentrated study both as a reward and an incentive to keep studying.
- Use pre-reading strategies to increase comprehension of chapter material.
  - Skim the headings in the chapter (because they identify chapter content).
  - Read the definitions of key terms, which will help you learn new words to comprehend chapter information.
  - Review all graphic aids (figures, tables, boxes) because they are often used to explain important points in the chapter.
- Read the chapter thoroughly but at a reasonable speed.
  - Comprehension and retention are actually enhanced by not reading too slowly.
  - Do take the time to reread any section that is unclear to you.
- Summarize what you have learned.
  - Use questions supplied with this book, CD-ROM, and companion website to test your recall of chapter content.
  - Review again any sections that correspond to questions you answered incorrectly or incompletely.

TEST TAKING STRATEGIES

Use the following strategies to increase your success on multiple-choice nursing tests or examinations:

- Get sufficient sleep and have something to eat before taking a test. Take deep breaths during the test as needed. Remember, the brain requires oxygen and glucose as fuel. Avoid concentrated sweets before a test, however, to avoid rapid upward and then downward surges in blood glucose levels.
- Read each question carefully, identifying the stem, the four options, and any key words or phrases in either the stem or options.
  - Key words in the stem such as "most important" indicate the need to set priorities, since more than one option is likely to contain a statement that is technically correct.
  - Remember that the presence of absolute words such as "never" or "only" in an option is more likely to make that option incorrect.

- Determine who is the client in the question; often this is the person with the health problem, but it may also be a significant other, relative, friend, or another nurse.
- Decide whether the stem is a true response stem or a false response stem. With a true response stem, the correct answer will be a true statement, and vice-versa.
- Determine what the question is really asking, sometimes referred to as the issue of the question. Evaluate all answer options in relation to this issue, and not strictly to the "correctness" of the statement in each individual option.
- Eliminate options that are obviously incorrect, then go back and reread the stem. Evaluate the remaining options against the stem once more.
- If two answers seem similar and correct, try to decide whether one of them is more global or comprehensive. If the global option includes the alternative option within it, it is likely that the more global response is the correct answer.

The NCLEX-RN Licensing Examination

The NCLEX-RN licensing examination is a Computer Adaptive Test (CAT) that ranges in length from 75 to 265 individual (stand-alone) test items, depending on individual performance during the examination. Upon graduation from a nursing program, successful completion of this exam is the gateway to your professional nursing practice. The blueprint for the exam is reviewed and revised every three years by the National Council of State Boards of Nursing according to the results of a job analysis study of new graduate nurses (practicing within the first six months after graduation). Each question on the exam is coded to one *Client Need Category* and one or more *Integrated Concepts and Processes.*

Client Need Categories

There are 4 categories of client needs, and each exam will contain a minimum and maximum percent of questions from each category. Each major category has subcategories within it. The *Client Need* categories according to the NCLEX-RN Test Plan effective April 2001 are as follows:

- Safe, Effective Care Environment
  - Management of Care (7–13%)
  - Safety and Infection Control (5–11%)
- Health Promotion and Maintenance
  - Growth and Development Throughout the Lifespan (7–13%)
  - Prevention and Early Detection of Disease (5–11%)
- Psychosocial Integrity
  - Coping and Adaptation (5–11%)
  - Psychosocial Adaptation (5–11%)
- Physiological Integrity
  - Basic Care and Comfort (7–13%)
  - Pharmacological and Parenteral Therapies (5–11%)
  - Reduction of Risk Potential (12–18%)
  - Physiological Adaptation (12–18%)

Integrated Concepts and Processes

The integrated concepts and processes identified on the NCLEX-RN Test Plan effective April 2001, with condensed definitions, are as follows:

- Nursing Process: a scientific problem-solving approach used in nursing practice; consisting of assessment, analysis, planning, implementation, and evaluation.

- Caring: client-nurse interaction(s) characterized by mutual respect and trust and directed toward achieving desired client outcomes.
- Communication and Documentation: verbal and/or nonverbal interactions between nurse and others (client, family, health care team); a written or electronic recording of activities or events that occur during client care.
- Cultural Awareness: knowledge and sensitivity to the client's beliefs/values and how these might impact on the client's healthcare experience.
- Self-Care: assisting clients to meet their health care needs, which may include maintaining health or restoring function.
- Teaching/Learning: facilitating client's acquisition of knowledge, skills, and attitudes that lead to behavior change.

More detailed information about this examination may be obtained by visiting the National Council of State Boards of Nursing website at http://www.ncsbn.org and viewing the *NCLEX-RN Examination Test Plan for the National Council Licensure Examination for Registered Nurses.**

How to Get the Most Out of This Book

Chapter Organization

Each chapter has the following elements to guide you during review and study:

- Chapter Objectives: describe what you will be able to know or do after learning the material covered in the chapter.

Objectives

- Review basic principles of growth and development.
- Describe major physical expectations for each developmental age group.
- Identify developmental milestones for various age groups.
- Discuss the reactions to illness and hospitalization for children at various stages of development.

- Review at a Glance: contains a glossary of key terms used in the chapter, with definitions provided up-front and available at your fingertips, to help you stay focused and make the best use of your study time.

Review at a Glance

anticipatory guidance *the process of understanding upcoming developmental needs and then teaching caregivers to meet those needs*

cephalocaudal development *the process by which development proceeds from the head downward through the body and towards the feet*

chronological age *age in years*

critical periods *times when an individual is especially responsive to certain environmental effects, sometimes called sensitive periods*

development *an increase in capability or function; a more complex concept that is a continuous, orderly series of conditions that lead to activities, new motives for activities; and eventual patterns of behavior*

developmental age *age based on functional behavior and ability to adapt to the environment; does not necessarily correspond to chronological age*

- Pretest: this 10-question multiple choice test provides a sample overview of content covered in the chapter and helps you decide what areas need the most—or the least—review.

Pretest

1 The nurse discusses dental care with the parents of a 3-year-old. The nurse explains that by the age of 3, their child should have:

(1) 5 "temporary" teeth.
(2) 10 "temporary" teeth.
(3) 15 "temporary" teeth.
(4) 20 "temporary" teeth.

2 The mother of a 6-month-old infant is concerned that the infant's anterior fontanel is still open. The nurse would inform the mother that further evaluation is needed if the anterior fontanel is open after:

(1) 6 months.
(2) 10 months.
(3) 18 months.
(4) 24 months.

- Practice to Pass questions: these are open-ended questions that stimulate critical thinking and reinforce mastery of the chapter content.

Practice to Pass

What would you explain as normal motor development for a 10-month old infant?

- NCLEX Alerts: the NCLEX icon identifies information or concepts that are likely to be tested on the NCLEX licensing examination. Be sure to learn the information flagged by this type of icon.

NCLEX!

- Case Study: found at the end of the chapter, it provides an opportunity for you to use your critical thinking and clinical reasoning skills to "put it all together;" it describes a true-to-life client case situation and asks you open-ended questions about how you would provide care for that client and/or family.

Case Study

A 6-month-old female infant is brought into the pediatric clinic for a well-baby visit. You as the pediatric nurse will be assigned to care for this family.

1. Identify the primary growth and development expectations for a 6-month-old.
2. What type common behavior is expected of this 6-month-old towards the nurse?
3. What immunization(s) are recommended at this age to maintain health and wellness?

For suggested responses, see page 406.

- Posttest: a 10-question multiple-choice test at the end of the chapter provides new questions that are representative of chapter content, and provide you with feedback about mastery of that content following review and study. All pretest and posttest questions contain rationales for the correct answer, and are coded according to the phase of the nursing process used and the NCLEX category of client need (called the Test Plan). The Test plan codes are PHYS (Physiological Integrity), PSYC (Psychosocial Integrity), SECE (Safe Effective Care Environment), and HPM (Health Promotion and Maintenance).

Posttest

1 When using the otoscope to examine the ears of a 2-year-old child, the nurse should:

(1) Pull the pinna up and back.
(2) Pull the pinna down and back.
(3) Hold the pinna gently but firmly in its normal position.
(4) Hold the pinna against the skull.

2 To assess the height of an 18-month-old child who is brought to the clinic for routine examination, the nurse should:

(1) Measure arm span to estimate adult height.
(2) Use a tape measure.
(3) Use a horizontal measuring board.
(4) Have the child stand on an upright scale and use the measuring arm.

CD-ROM

For those who want to practice taking tests on a computer, the CD-ROM that accompanies the book contains the pretest and posttest questions found in all chapters of the book. In addition, it contains 10 NEW questions for each chapter to help you further evaluate your knowledge base and hone your test-taking skills. In several chapters, one of the questions will have embedded art to use in answering the question. Some of the newly developed NCLEX test items are also designed in this way, so these items will give you valuable practice with this type of question.

Companion Website (CW)

The companion website is a "virtual" reference for virtually all your needs! The CW contains the following:

- 50 NCLEX-style questions: 10 pretest, 10 posttest, 10 CD-ROM, and 20 additional new questions
- Definitions of key terms: the glossary is also stored on the companion website for ease of reference
- In Depth With NCLEX: features drawings or photos that are each accompanied by a one- to two-paragraph explanation. These are especially useful when describing something that is complex, technical (such as equipment), or difficult to mentally visualize.
- Suggested Answers to Practice to Pass and Case Study Questions: easily located on the website, these allow for timely feedback for those who answer chapter questions on the web.

Nursing Notes Clinical Reference Card

This laminated card provides a reference for frequently used facts and information related to the subject matter of the book. These are designed to be useful in the clinical setting, when quick and easy access to information is so important!

About the Child Health Nursing Book

Chapters in this book cover "need-to-know" information about child health nursing, including pediatric growth and development and care of the child with respiratory, cardiac, neurological, renal, gastrointestinal, musculoskeletal, and other health problems. The final chapter focuses on special situations, including autism, child abuse, poisoning, suicide, and others. The term *parent* or *parents* has been used in this book to indicate the primary caregiver(s) for the child. The authors understand and appreciate that there are a variety of family configurations in which a child can grow and thrive.

Acknowledgments

This book is a monumental effort of collaboration. Without the contributions of many individuals, this first edition of *Child Health Nursing: Reviews and Rationales* would not have been possible. We gratefully acknowledge all the contributors who devoted their time and talents to this book. Their chapters will surely assist both students and practicing nurses alike to extend their knowledge in the area of child health.

We owe a special debt of gratitude to the wonderful team at Prentice Hall Health for their enthusiasm for this project, as well as their good humor, expertise, and encouragement as the series developed. Maura Connor, Executive Editor for Nursing, was unending in her creativity, support, encouragement, and belief in the need for this series. Marilyn Meserve, Senior Managing Editor for Nursing, devoted many long hours to coordinating different facets of this project, and tirelessly and cheerfully encouraged our efforts as well. Her high standards and attention to detail contributed greatly to the final "look" of this series. Jeanne Allison, Developmental Editor, actively kept in communication with the different writers in this book, and also facilitated getting the book itself into production. Editorial assistants, including Beth Ann Romph, Sladjana Repic, and others, helped to keep the project moving forward on a day-to-day basis, and we are grateful for their efforts as well. A very special thank you goes to the designers of the book and the production team, led by Danielle Newhouse, who brought our ideas and manuscript into final form.

Thank you to the team at Pine Tree Composition, led by Project Coordinator Jessica Balch, for the detail-oriented work of creating this book. We greatly appreciate their hard work, attention to detail, and spirit of collaboration. A special thanks also goes to Yesenia Kopperman, Assistant Editor for Nursing at Prentice Hall, and to Carlos Cooper, Lisa Donovan, and staff at the Pearson Education Development Group for designing and producing the *Nursing Notes* clinical reference card that accompanies this book.

Finally, both Judy White and Mary Ann Hogan acknowledge and gratefully thank our families, who sacrificed hours of time that would have been spent with them, to bring this book to publication. Their love and support kept us energized, motivated, and at times, even sane. We love you!

---

*Reference: National Council of State Boards of Nursing, Inc. *NCLEX Examination Test Plan for National Council Licensure Examination for Registered Nurses.* Effective April, 2001. Retrieved from the World Wide Web September 5, 2001 at http://www.ncsbn.org/public/resources/res/NCSBNRNTestPlanBooklet.pdf.

Contributors

Jacqueline B. Arnett, RN, BSN
Instructor of Nursing
North Seattle Community College
Seattle, Washington
Chapter 7

J. Mari Beth Barr, PhD, RNC
Assistant Professor
Missouri Southern State College
Department of Nursing
Joplin, Missouri
Chapter 3

Jennifer Jeames Coleman, MSN, RN
Assistant Professor of Nursing
Ida V. Moffet School of Nursing
Samford University
Birmingham, Alabama
Chapter 4 & Chapter 13

Donna Miles Curry, RN, PhD
Associate Professor of Nursing
College of Nursing & Health
Wright State University
Dayton, Ohio
Chapter 6

Vera Dauffenbach, MSN, EdD, RN
Associate Professor
Bellin College of Nursing
Green Bay, Wisconsin
Chapter 2 & Chapter 10

Joseann Helmes DeWitt, MSN, RN, C, CLNC
Assistant Professor
Department of Baccalaureate Nursing
Alcorn State University School of Nursing
Natchez, Mississippi
Chapter 15

Leona M. Florek, MS, RN
Professor of Nursing
Holyoke Community College
Holyoke, Massachusetts
Chapter 12

Gwendolyn T. Martin, MS, RN, CNS, CPN
Assistant Clinical Professor
Texas Woman's University
Dallas, Texas
Chapter 14

Gina M. Orta, MS, RN
Clinical Instructor
Texas Woman's University
Dallas, Texas
Chapter 13

Kathleen Peterson-Sweeney, MS, RN, CPNP
Associate Professor of Nursing
SUNY, College at Brockport
Brockport, New York
Chapter 9

Kimberly A. Serroka, MSN, RN
Assistant Professor
Youngstown State University
Youngstown, Ohio
Chapter 1

Nancy H. Wagner, MSN, RN
Instructor of Nursing
Youngstown State University
Youngstown, Ohio
Chapter 8

Marilyn L. Weitzel, MSN, RN, Doctoral Candidate
Clinical Assistant Professor of Nursing
University of South Alabama
College of Nursing
Mobile, Alabama
Chapter 5 & Chapter 11

Judy E. White, RNC, MA, MSN
Director of Nursing
Vital Care, Inc.
Meridian, Mississippi
Chapter 11

Reviewers

Eva Caldwell, RN, EdD
Assistant Professor
Armstrong Atlantic State University
Savannah, Georgia

Dawn M. Pope, MS, RN, CS-PNP
Clinical Assistant Professor
University of Wisconsin–Oshkosh, College of Nursing
Oshkosh, Wisconsin

Deborah A. Redd-Terrell, RN, MS, CS, CFNP
Assistant Professor
Harry S. Truman College
Flossmoor, Illinois

Gwendolyn P. Taylor, RN, MSN
Practical Nurse Instructor
Augusta Technical College
Thomson, Georgia

Rosemarie C. Westberg, RN, MSN, CPN
Professor & Clinical Coordinator, Nursing
Northern Virginia Community College
Annandale, Virginia

Sharon A. Wilkerson, PhD, RN
Associate Professor of Nursing
Purdue University, School of Nursing
West Lafayette, Indiana

Beatrice Crofts Yorker, JD, RN, MS, CS, FAAN
Professor & Director
San Francisco State University, School of Nursing
San Francisco, California

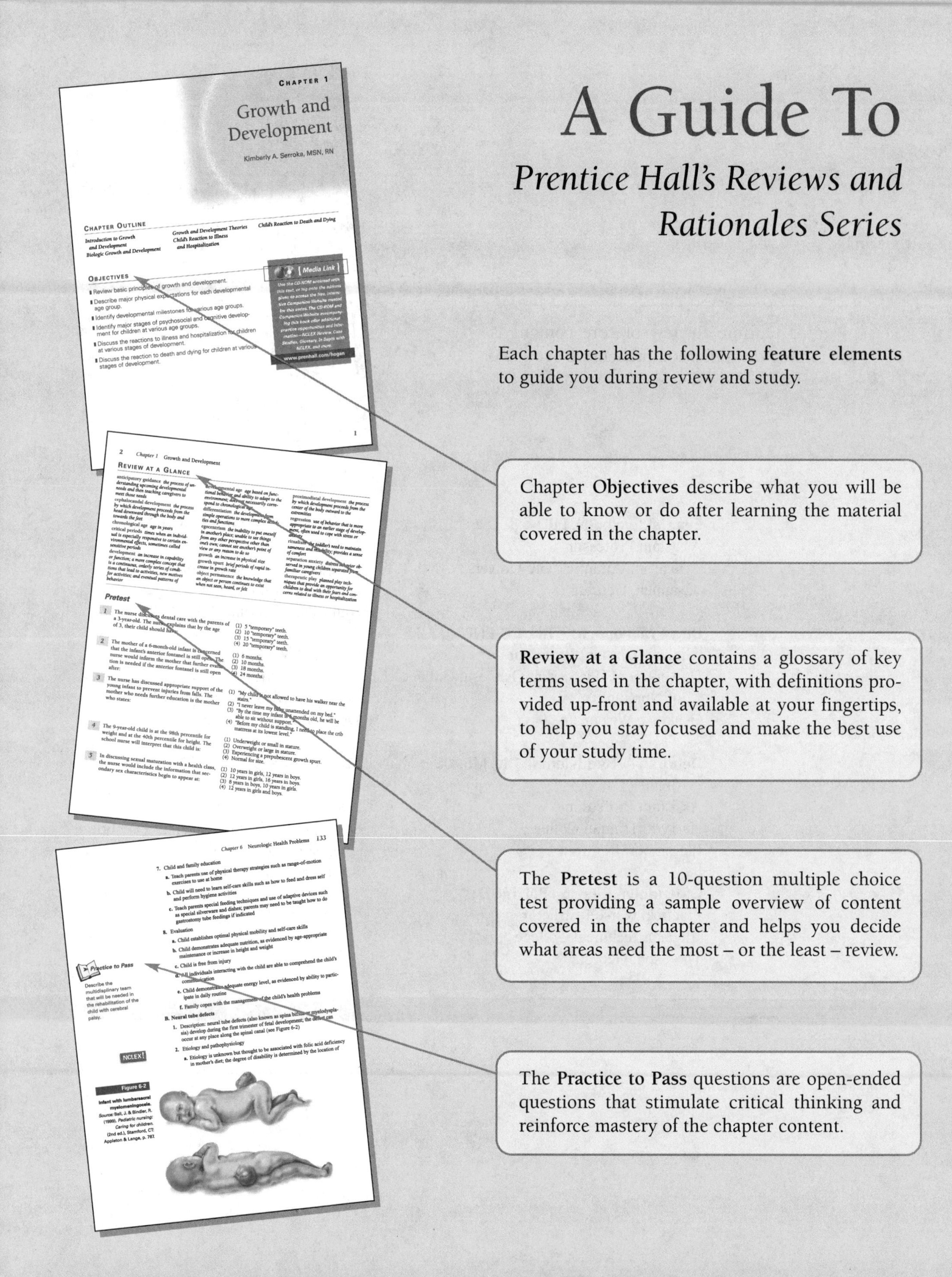

A Guide To

Prentice Hall's Reviews and Rationales Series

Each chapter has the following **feature elements** to guide you during review and study.

Chapter **Objectives** describe what you will be able to know or do after learning the material covered in the chapter.

Review at a Glance contains a glossary of key terms used in the chapter, with definitions provided up-front and available at your fingertips, to help you stay focused and make the best use of your study time.

The **Pretest** is a 10-question multiple choice test providing a sample overview of content covered in the chapter and helps you decide what areas need the most – or the least – review.

The **Practice to Pass** questions are open-ended questions that stimulate critical thinking and reinforce mastery of the chapter content.

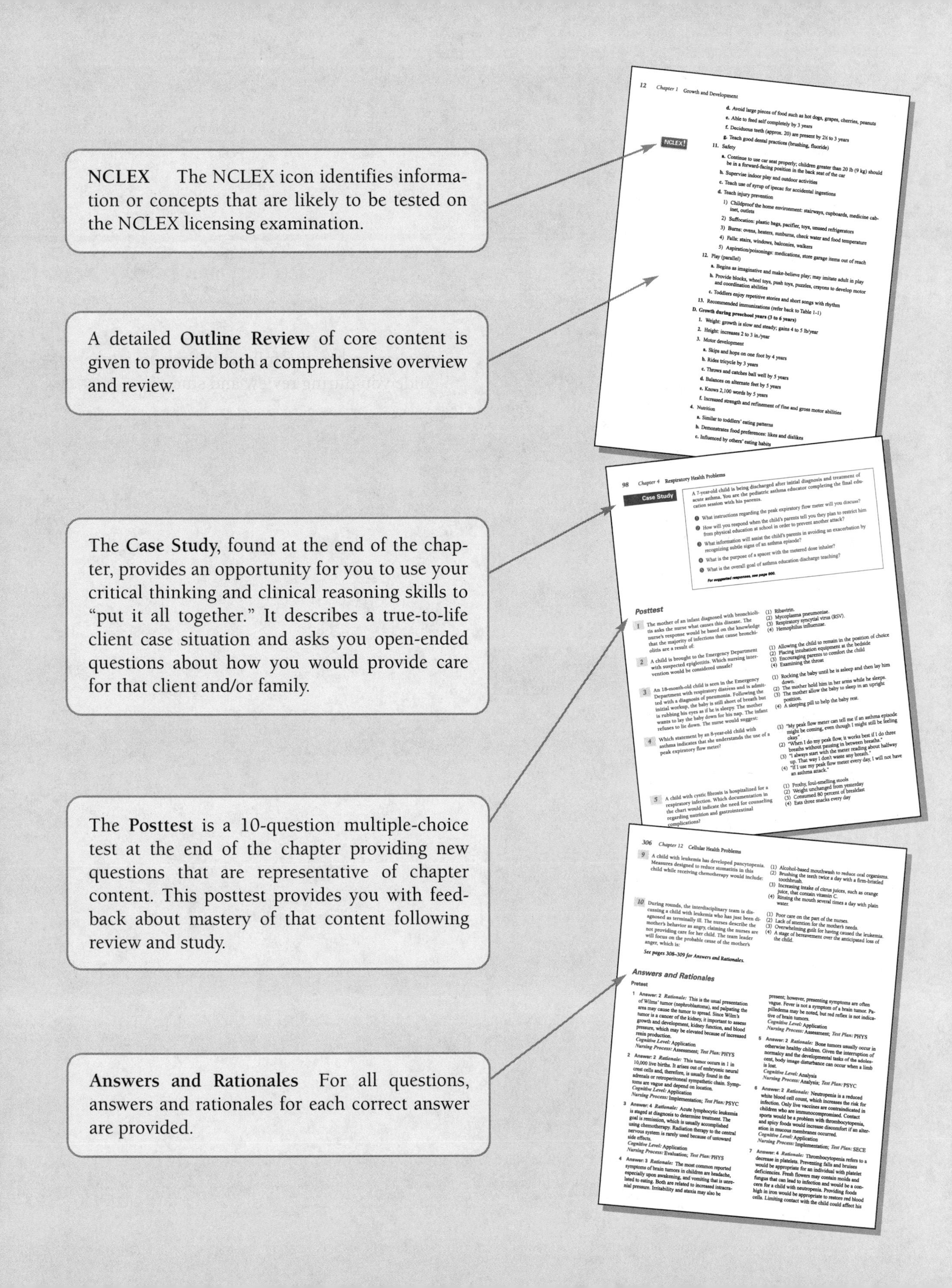
NCLEX The NCLEX icon identifies information or concepts that are likely to be tested on the NCLEX licensing examination.
A detailed Outline Review of core content is given to provide both a comprehensive overview and review.
The Case Study, found at the end of the chapter, provides an opportunity for you to use your critical thinking and clinical reasoning skills to "put it all together." It describes a true-to-life client case situation and asks you open-ended questions about how you would provide care for that client and/or family.
The Posttest is a 10-question multiple-choice test at the end of the chapter providing new questions that are representative of chapter content. This posttest provides you with feedback about mastery of that content following review and study.
Answers and Rationales For all questions, answers and rationales for each correct answer are provided.

Chapter 1

Growth and Development

Kimberly A. Serroka, MSN, RN

Chapter Outline

Objectives

- Review basic principles of growth and development.
- Describe major physical expectations for each developmental age group.
- Identify developmental milestones for various age groups.
- Identify major stages of psychosocial and cognitive development for children at various age groups.
- Discuss the reactions to illness and hospitalization for children at various stages of development.
- Discuss the reaction to death and dying for children at various stages of development.

[Media Link]

Use the CD-ROM enclosed with this text, or log onto the address given to access the free, interactive Companion Website created for this series. The CD-ROM and Companion Website accompanying this book offer additional practice opportunities and information—NCLEX Review, Case Studies, Glossary, In Depth with NCLEX, and more.

www.prenhall.com/hogan

Review at a Glance

anticipatory guidance *the process of understanding upcoming developmental needs and then teaching caregivers to meet those needs*

cephalocaudal development *the process by which development proceeds from the head downward through the body and towards the feet*

chronological age *age in years*

critical periods *times when an individual is especially responsive to certain environmental effects, sometimes called sensitive periods*

development *an increase in capability or function; a more complex concept that is a continuous, orderly series of conditions that lead to activities, new motives for activities; and eventual patterns of behavior*

developmental age *age based on functional behavior and ability to adapt to the environment; does not necessarily correspond to chronological age*

differentiation *the development from simple operations to more complex activities and functions*

egocentrism *the inability to put oneself in another's place; unable to see things from any other perspective other than one's own; cannot see another's point of view or any reason to do so*

growth *an increase in physical size*

growth spurt *brief periods of rapid increase in growth rate*

object permanence *the knowledge that an object or person continues to exist when not seen, heard, or felt*

proximodistal development *the process by which development proceeds from the center of the body outward to the extremities*

regression *use of behavior that is more appropriate to an earlier stage of development, often used to cope with stress or anxiety*

ritualism *the toddler's need to maintain sameness and reliability; provides a sense of comfort*

separation anxiety *distress behavior observed in young children separated from familiar caregivers*

therapeutic play *planned play techniques that provide an opportunity for children to deal with their fears and concerns related to illness or hospitalization*

Pretest

1 The nurse discusses dental care with the parents of a 3-year-old. The nurse explains that by the age of 3, their child should have:

(1) 5 "temporary" teeth.
(2) 10 "temporary" teeth.
(3) 15 "temporary" teeth.
(4) 20 "temporary" teeth.

2 The mother of a 6-month-old infant is concerned that the infant's anterior fontanel is still open. The nurse would inform the mother that further evaluation is needed if the anterior fontanel is still open after:

(1) 6 months.
(2) 10 months.
(3) 18 months.
(4) 24 months.

3 The nurse has discussed appropriate support of the young infant to prevent injuries from falls. The mother who needs further education is the mother who states:

(1) "My child is not allowed to have his walker near the stairs."
(2) "I never leave my baby unattended on my bed."
(3) "By the time my infant is 6 months old, he will be able to sit without support."
(4) "Before my child is standing, I need to place the crib mattress at its lowest level."

4 The 9-year-old child is at the 98th percentile for weight and at the 40th percentile for height. The school nurse will interpret that this child is:

(1) Underweight or small in stature.
(2) Overweight or large in stature.
(3) Experiencing a prepubescent growth spurt.
(4) Normal for size.

5 In discussing sexual maturation with a health class, the nurse would include the information that secondary sex characteristics begin to appear at:

(1) 10 years in girls, 12 years in boys.
(2) 12 years in girls, 16 years in boys.
(3) 8 years in boys, 10 years in girls.
(4) 12 years in girls and boys.

6 A recently hospitalized 2-year-old client screams and shouts that he wants a "bottle." His parents are puzzled, and state that he has drank from a cup for the past year. The nurse explains that:

(1) Irritability is exhibited in all age groups.
(2) Temper tantrums often represent the child's need for parental attention.
(3) Various forms of punishment are necessary when such behaviors occur.
(4) Regression to an earlier behavior often helps the child cope with stress and anxiety.

7 A friend is shopping for a toy to give to her nephew. The friend knows nothing about children and asks what would be the most appropriate toy to give an 18-month-old child. Based on growth and developmental skills, the nurse recommends a:

(1) Tricycle.
(2) Large ball.
(3) Pull toy.
(4) Stuffed animal.

8 The nurse is preparing an 8-year-old child for a procedure. What is the most appropriate nursing intervention?

(1) Provide visual aids, such as dolls, puppets, and diagrams in the explanation.
(2) Provide a written pamphlet for the child to review prior to the procedure.
(3) Discourage any display of emotional outbursts.
(4) Request that parents wait outside while the nurse provides instructions to the child.

9 The nurse explains that the American Academy of Pediatrics recommends formula be continued in a child's dietary intake up until what age?

(1) 6 months
(2) 12 months
(3) 18 months
(4) 24 months

10 Piaget identifies that the 2- to 7-year-old child is in a preoperational stage. The nurse observes a toddler taking a toy from another. The nurse recognizes the child unable to put him- or herself in the place of another is displaying:

(1) Centration.
(2) Negativism.
(3) Egocentrism.
(4) Selfishness.

See page 24 for Answers and Rationales.

I. Introduction to Growth and Development

A. Definition of terms

1. The terms "growth" and "development" are often used interchangeably but have specific meanings
    - a. **Growth:** an increase in the physical size of a whole or any of its parts
    - b. **Development:** continuous, orderly series of conditions that lead to activities, new motives for activities, and eventual patterns of behavior
2. The term **chronological age** is defined as age in years, which differs from **developmental age,** which refers to age based on functional behavior and ability to adapt to the environment

B. Patterns of growth and development

1. Each child displays definite predictable patterns of growth and development

2. These patterns of growth and development are universal and basic to all human beings
3. Individual differences: although the sequence is predictable, rates of growth vary, and individual variation exists in the age at which developmental milestones are reached
4. Directional trends: growth and development follow a specific pattern
   a. **Cephalocaudal development:** (head to tail) the process by which development proceeds from the head downward through the body towards the feet
   b. **Proximodistal development:** (near to far) the process by which development proceeds from the center of the body outward to the extremities
   c. **Differentiation:** the development from simple operations to more complex activities and functions
5. Sequential trends: an orderly sequence; each child normally passes through every stage
   a. Each stage is affected by the preceding stage and affects those stages that follow
   b. **Critical periods:** time period in which the child is especially responsive to certain environmental effects; sometimes called sensitive periods
   c. Positive and negative stimuli enhance or defer the achievement of a skill or function

C. Factors influencing development

1. Genetics: a family history of diseases may be inherited by unique genes that are linked to specific disorders; chromosomes carry genes that determine physical characteristics, intellectual potential, and personality
2. Nutrition: the greatest influence on physical growth and intellectual development; adequate nutrition provides essentials for physiologic needs, which promote health and prevent illness
3. Prenatal and environmental factors: beginning with the nutrition from the mother to exposures in utero such as alcohol, smoking, infections, drugs; environmental exposures, such as radiation and chemicals, influence growth and development of the developing child
4. Family and community: a stimulating environment from the family helps a child reach his or her potential; family structure and community support services influence the environment in the process of growth and development of the child
5. Cultural factors: customs, traditions, and attitudes of cultural groups influence the child's growth and development regarding physical health, social interaction, and assumed roles

D. Developmental stages

1. Prenatal period
   a. Germinal: conception to 2 weeks
   b. Embryonic: 2 weeks to 8 weeks
   c. Fetal: 8 weeks to 40 weeks (birth)

2. Infancy period
    a. Neonatal: birth to 28 days
    b. Infancy: 1 to 12 months
3. Early childhood period
    a. Toddler: 1 to 3 years
    b. Preschooler: 3 to 6 years
4. Middle childhood period: the "school age" period from 6 to 12 years
5. Later childhood period: 13 to 18 years
    a. Prepubertal: 10 to 13 years
    b. Adolescence: 13 to 18 years

E. Importance of anticipatory guidance

1. **Anticipatory guidance** is the process of understanding upcoming developmental needs and then teaching caregivers to meet those needs
2. Information on what parents are to expect in each developmental stage includes:
    a. Health habits
    b. Prevention of illness and injury
    c. Prevention of poisonings
    d. Nutrition
    e. Dental care
    f. Sexuality
3. Health promotion guidance also helps to develop strategies to enhance social development, family and community relationships, school and vocational achievement

II. Biologic Growth and Development

A. Neonatal period (birth to 1 month)

1. General appearance: newborn's head is one-quarter of the body length; the child is top heavy with short lower extremities
2. Weight: 6 to 8 lb; gains 5 to 7 oz (142 to 198 g) weekly for first 6 months
3. Height: 20 in. (50 cm); grows 1 in. (2.5 cm) monthly for first 6 months
4. Head circumference: 33 to 35 cm (13 to 14 in.); head circumference is greater than chest circumference

B. Growth during infancy (1 to 12 months)

1. Weight: doubles birth weight in 6 months; triples birth weight in 1 year
2. Height: increases 50 percent by 1 year
3. Head growth is rapid; brain increases in weight 2.5 times by 1 year

a. Head circumference exceeds chest circumference

b. Posterior fontanel closes at 2 to 3 months

c. Anterior fontanel closes by 12 to 18 months

4. Reflexes present at birth

a. Moro: startle reflex elicited by loud noise or sudden change in position

b. Tonic neck: elicted when infant lies supine and head is turned to one side; the infant will assume a "fencing position"

c. Gag, cough, blink, pupillary: protective reflexes

d. Grasp: the infant's hands and feet will grasp when the hand or foot is stimulated

e. Rooting: elicited when side of mouth is touched, causing the child to turn to that side

f. Babinski: fanning of the toes when sole of foot is stroked upward

5. Reflexes that appear during infancy

a. Parachute: involves extension of arms when suspended in prone position and lowered suddenly

b. Landau: when the infant is suspended horizontally, the head is raised

c. Labyrinth righting: provides orientation of the head in space

d. Body righting: when you turn the hips to the side, the body follows

6. Gross motor development: developmental maturation in posture, head balance, sitting, creeping, standing, and walking

a. Gains head control by 4 months

b. Rolls from back to side by 4 months

c. Rolls from abdomen to back by 5 months

d. Rolls from back to abdomen by 6 months

e. Sits alone without support by 8 months

f. Stands holding furniture by 9 months

g. Crawls (may go backward initially) by 10 months

h. Creeps with abdomen off floor by 11 months

i. Cruises (walking upright while holding furniture) by 10–12 months

j. Can sit down from upright position by 10–12 months

k. Walks well with one hand held by 12 months

7. Fine motor development: use of hands and fingers to grasp objects

a. Hand predominantly closed at 1 month

b. Desires to grasp at 3 months

c. Two-handed, voluntary grasp at 5 months

   d. Holds bottle, grasps feet at 6 months
   e. Transfers from hand to hand by 7 months
   f. Pincer grasp established by 10 months
   g. Neat pincer grasp (e.g., picks up raisin) with thumb and finger by 12 months

8. Sensory development
   a. Hearing and touch well developed at birth
   b. Sight not fully developed until 6 years; differentiates light and dark at birth; prefers human face; smiles at 2 months
   c. Usually searches and turns head to locate sounds by 2 months
   d. Has taste preferences by 6 months
   e. Responds to own name by 7 months
   f. Able to follow moving objects; visual acuity 20/50 or better; amblyopia may develop by 12 months
   g. Can vocalize four words by 1 year

Box 1-1

Introduction of Solid Foods in Infancy

Recommendation	Rationale
Introduce rice cereal at 6 months.	Rice cereal is easy to digest, has low allergenic potential, and contains iron.
Introduce fruits or vegetables at 6–8 months.	Fruits and vegetables provide needed vitamins.
Introduce meats at 8–10 months.	Meats are harder to digest, have high protein load, and should not be fed until close to 1 year of age.
Use single-food prepared baby foods rather than combination meals.	Combination meals usually contain more sugar, salt, and fillers.
Introduce one new food at a time, waiting at least 3 days to introduce another.	If a food allergy develops, it will be easy to identify.
Avoid carrots, beets, and spinach before 4 months of age.	Their nitrates can be converted to nitrite by yount infants, causing methemoglobinemia.
Infants can be fed mashed portions of table foods such as carrots, rice, and potatoes.	This is a less expensive alternative to jars of commercially prepared baby food; it allows parents of various cultural groups to feed ethnic foods to infants.
Avoid adding sugar, salt, spices when mixing own baby foods.	Infants need not become accustomed to these flavors; they may get too much sodium from salt or develop gastric distress from some spices.
Avoid honey until at least 1 year of age.	Infants cannot detoxify *Clostridium botulinum* spores sometimes present in honey and can develop botulism.

Source: Ball, J. & Bindler, R. (1999). *Pediatric nursing: Caring for children* (2nd ed.). Stamford, CT: Appleton & Lange.

9. Nutrition
   a. Human breast milk is the most complete and easily digested
   b. Commercially prepared iron-fortified formulas used for bottle feeding closely resemble the nutritional content of human milk; recommended for first 12 months
   c. Solids are introduced no sooner than 6 months to avoid exposure to allergens
   d. Iron-fortified rice cereal is introduced first because of its low allergenic potential
   e. Eruption of deciduous "baby" teeth by 5 to 6 months; lateral incisors erupt first; increase in drooling and saliva; slight elevated temperature may be associated with teething
   f. Gradual weaning from breast to bottle to cup during second 6 months of infancy
   g. Juices may be introduced, diluted 1:1 at 6 months; preferably given by a cup
   h. Introduction of fruits, vegetables, and meats (one food each week is recommended to identify any allergy)
   i. Junior foods or chopped table foods introduced by 12 months
   j. No more than 32 oz formula per 24 hours should be given to infants, to avoid iron-deficiency anemia

NCLEX!

10. Safety
    a. Infants up to 20 lb (9 kg) should be restrained in a rear-facing car seat in the middle of the back seat of the car
    b. Keep siderails of crib up
    c. Never leave infant unattended on table, bed, bathtub
    d. Check temperature of bath water, formula, foods
    e. Avoid giving bottles at naps or bedtime (may cause dental caries)
    f. Teach injury prevention
       1) Aspiration of foreign objects (buttons, toys, peanuts, hotdogs)
       2) Suffocation (plastic bags, strangulation)
       3) Falls
       4) Poisonings
       5) Burns (electric cords, wall outlets, radiators, pots and pans on stoves)
11. Play (solitary)
    a. Provide black/white contrasts for premature and newborn infants
    b. Hang mobile 8 to 10 inches from infant's face
    c. Provide sensory stimuli (bath water) and tactile stimuli (feel of various shapes of objects), large toys, balls (see Box 1-2)
    d. Expose to environmental sounds: rattles, musical toys

Box 1-2

Favorite Toys and Activities in Infancy

Birth to 2 months

- Mobiles, black-and-white patterns, mirrors
- Music boxes, singing, tape players, soft voices
- Rocking and cuddling
- Moving legs and arms while listening to singing and talking
- Varying stimuli—different rooms, sounds, visual images

3 to 6 months

- Rattles
- Stuffed animals
- Soft toys with contrasting colors
- Noise-making objects that are easily grasped

6 to 12 months

- Large blocks
- Teething toys
- Toys that pop apart and back together
- Nesting cups and other objects that fit into one another or stack
- Surprise toys such as jack-in-the-box
- Social interaction with adults and other children
- Games such as peek-a-boo
- Soft balls
- Push and pull toys

Source: Ball, J. & Bindler, R. (1999). *Pediatric nursing: Caring for children* (2nd ed.). Stamford, CT: Appleton & Lange.

e. Use variety of primary-colored objects during infancy

f. Place unbreakable mirror in crib for infants to focus on their face

g. Provide toys that let infants practice skills to grasp manipulate objects

h. Vocalization provides pleasure in relationships with people (smiling, cooing, laughing)

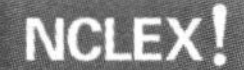

12. Recommended immunization schedule (Figure 1-1)

a. Hepatitis B: 1st (0 to 2 months), 2nd (1 to 4 months), 3rd (6 to 18 months)

b. Diphtheria-tetanus-acellular pertussis (DTaP): 1st (2 months), 2nd (4 months), 3rd (6 months), 4th (15 to 18 months), 5th (4 to 6 years)

c. *Haemophilus influenzae* type B (Hib): 1st (2 months), 2nd (4 months), 3rd (6 months), 4th (12 to 18 months)

d. Inactivated poliovirus vaccine (IPV): 1st (2 months), 2nd (4 months), 3rd (6 to 18 months), 4th (4 to 6 years)

e. Heptavalent conjugant pneumococcal vaccine (PCV): 1st (2 months), 2nd (4 months), 3rd (6 months), 4th (12 to 15 months)

Figure 1-1

Recommended Childhood Immunization Schedule in the United States

Source: Recommended Childhood Immunization Schedule United States. January–December, 2001. http://www.cdc.gov/nip/recs/child-schedule.PDF (February 2, 2001).

Recommended Childhood Immunization Schedule United States, January - December 2001

Vaccines[1] are listed under routinely recommended ages. Bars indicate range of recommended ages for immunization. Any dose not given at the recommended age should be given as a "catch-up" immunization at any subsequent visit when indicated and feasible. Ovals indicate vaccines to be given if previously recommended doses were missed or given earlier than the recommended minimum age.

Age ▶ / Vaccine ▼	Birth	1 mo	2 mos	4 mos	6 mos	12 mos	15 mos	18 mos	24 mos	4-6 yrs	11-12 yrs	14-18 yrs
Hepatitis B[2]	Hep B #1											
		Hep B #2			Hep B #3						(Hep B[2])	
Diphtheria, Tetanus, Pertussis[3]			DTaP	DTaP	DTaP		DTaP[3]			DTaP	Td	
H. influenzae type b[4]			Hib	Hib	Hib	Hib						
Inactivated Polio[5]			IPV	IPV	IPV[5]					IPV[5]		
Pneumococcal Conjugate[6]			PCV	PCV	PCV	PCV						
Measles, Mumps, Rubella[7]						MMR				MMR[7]	(MMR[7])	
Varicella[8]						Var					(Var[8])	
Hepatitis A[9]									Hep A — in selected areas[9]			

Approved by the Advisory Committee on Immunization Practices (ACIP), the American Academy of Pediatrics (AAP), and the American Academy of Family Physicians (AAFP).

1. This schedule indicates the recommended ages for routine administration of currently licensed childhood vaccines, as of 11/1/00, for children through 18 years of age. Additional vaccines may be licensed and recommended during the year. Licensed combination vaccines may be used whenever any components of the combination are indicated and its other components are not contraindicated. Providers should consult the manufacturers' package inserts for detailed recommendations.

2. Infants born to HBsAg-negative mothers should receive the 1st dose of hepatitis B (Hep B) vaccine by age 2 months. The 2nd dose should be at least one month after the 1st dose. The 3rd dose should be administered at least 4 months after the 1st dose and at least 2 months after the 2nd dose, but not before 6 months of age for infants.
Infants born to HBsAg-positive mothers should receive hepatitis B vaccine and 0.5 mL hepatitis B immune globulin (HBIG) within 12 hours of birth at separate sites. The 2nd dose is recommended at 1-2 months of age and the 3rd dose at 6 months of age.
Infants born to mothers whose HBsAg status is unknown should receive hepatitis B vaccine within 12 hours of birth. Maternal blood should be drawn at the time of delivery to determine the mother's HBsAg status; if the HBsAg test is positive, the infant should receive HBIG as soon as possible (no later than 1 week of age).
All children and adolescents who have not been immunized against hepatitis B should begin the series during any visit. Special efforts should be made to immunize children who were born in or whose parents were born in areas of the world with moderate or high endemicity of hepatitis B virus infection.

3. The 4th dose of DTaP (diphtheria and tetanus toxoids and acellular pertussis vaccine) may be administered as early as 12 months of age, provided 6 months have elapsed since the 3rd dose and the child is unlikely to return at age 15-18 months. Td (tetanus and diphtheria toxoids) is recommended at 11-12 years of age if at least 5 years have elapsed since the last dose of DTP, DTaP or DT. Subsequent routine Td boosters are recommended every 10 years.

4. Three *Haemophilus influenzae* type b (Hib) conjugate vaccines are licensed for infant use. If PRP-OMP (PedvaxHIBÆ or ComVaxÆ [Merck]) is administered at 2 and 4 months of age, a dose at 6 months is not required. Because clinical studies in infants have demonstrated that using some combination products may induce a lower immune response to the Hib vaccine component, DTaP/Hib combination products should not be used for primary immunization in infants at 2, 4 or 6 months of age, unless FDA-approved for these ages.

5. An all-IPV schedule is recommended for routine childhood polio vaccination in the United States. All children should receive four doses of IPV at 2 months, 4 months, 6-18 months, and 4-6 years of age. Oral polio vaccine (OPV) should be used only in selected circumstances. (See MMWR May 19, 2000/49(RR-5);1-22).

6. The heptavalent conjugate pneumococcal vaccine (PCV) is recommended for all children 2-23 months of age. It also is recommended for certain children 24-59 months of age. (See MMWR Oct. 6, 2000/49(RR-9);1-35).

7. The 2nd dose of measles, mumps, and rubella (MMR) vaccine is recommended routinely at 4-6 years of age but may be administered during any visit, provided at least 4 weeks have elapsed since receipt of the 1st dose and that both doses are administered beginning at or after 12 months of age. Those who have not previously received the second dose should complete the schedule by the 11-12 year old visit.

8. Varicella (Var) vaccine is recommended at any visit on or after the first birthday for susceptible children, i.e. those who lack a reliable history of chickenpox (as judged by a health care provider) and who have not been immunized. Susceptible persons 13 years of age or older should receive 2 doses, given at least 4 weeks apart.

9. Hepatitis A (Hep A) is shaded to indicate its recommended use in selected states and/or regions, and for certain high risk groups; consult your local public health authority. (See MMWR Oct. 1, 1999/48(RR-12); 1-37).

For additional information about the vaccines listed above, please visit the National Immunization Program Home Page at http://www.cdc.gov/nip/ or call the National Immunization Hotline at 800-232-2522 (English) or 800-232-0233 (Spanish).

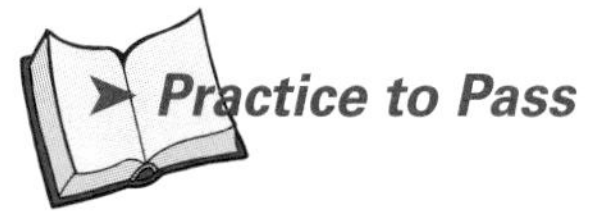

What would you explain as normal motor development for a 10-month old infant?

f. Measles-mumps-rubella (MMR): 1st (15 to 18 months), 2nd (4 to 6 years)

g. Varicella: (15 to 18 months)

C. Growth during the toddler years (1 to 3 years)

1. Weight: growth rate slows considerably; weight is four times the birth rate by 2½ years

2. Height: at 2 years height is 50 percent of future adult height

3. Head circumference: 19½ to 20 in. (49 to 50 cm) by 2 years; increases only 3 cm in second year; achieves 90 percent of adult-size brain by 2 years

4. Anterior fontanel closes by 18 months

5. Gross motor development: still clumsy at this age

a. Walks without help (usually by 15 months)

b. Jumps in place by 18 months

c. Goes up stairs (with 2 feet on each step) by 24 months

d. Runs fairly well (wide stance) by 24 months

6. Fine motor development

a. Uses cup well by 15 months

b. Builds a tower of two cubes by 15 months

c. Holds crayon with fingers by 24 to 30 months

d. Good hand-finger coordination by 30 months

e. Copies a circle by 3 years

7. Sensory development

a. Binocular vision well developed by 15 months

b. Knows own name by 12 months; refers to self

c. Follows simple directions by 2 years

d. Identifies geometric forms by 18 months

e. Uses short sentences by 18 months to 2 years

f. Remembers and repeats 3 numbers by 3 years

g. Able to speak 300 words by 2 years

8. **Object permanence** is the knowledge that an object or person continues to exist when not seen, heard, or felt

9. Ritualistic behavior is exhibited during the toddler period; **ritualism** is the toddler's need to maintain sameness and reliability; provides sense of comfort

10. Nutrition

a. Growth slows at age 12 to 18 months; thus appetite and need for intake decrease

b. Toddlers are picky, ritualistic eaters

c. Avoid more than 32 oz formula/day to prevent iron-deficiency anemia

d. Avoid large pieces of food such as hot dogs, grapes, cherries, peanuts

e. Able to feed self completely by 3 years

f. Deciduous teeth (approx. 20) are present by 2½ to 3 years

g. Teach good dental practices (brushing, fluoride)

NCLEX!

11. Safety

a. Continue to use car seat properly; children greater than 20 lb (9 kg) should be in a forward-facing position in the back seat of the car

b. Supervise indoor play and outdoor activities

c. Teach use of syrup of ipecac for accidental ingestions

d. Teach injury prevention

1) Childproof the home environment: stairways, cupboards, medicine cabinet, outlets

2) Suffocation: plastic bags, pacifier, toys, unused refrigerators

3) Burns: ovens, heaters, sunburns, check water and food temperature

4) Falls: stairs, windows, balconies, walkers

5) Aspiration/poisonings: medications, store garage items out of reach

12. Play (parallel)

a. Begins as imaginative and make-believe play; may imitate adult in play

b. Provide blocks, wheel toys, push toys, puzzles, crayons to develop motor and coordination abilities

c. Toddlers enjoy repetitive stories and short songs with rhythm

13. Recommended immunizations (refer back to Figure 1-1)

D. Growth during preschool years (3 to 6 years)

1. Weight: growth is slow and steady; gains 4 to 5 lb/year

2. Height: increases 2 to 3 in./year

3. Motor development

a. Skips and hops on one foot by 4 years

b. Rides tricycle by 3 years

c. Throws and catches ball well by 5 years

d. Balances on alternate feet by 5 years

e. Knows 2,100 words by 5 years

f. Increased strength and refinement of fine and gross motor abilities

4. Nutrition

a. Similar to toddlers' eating patterns

b. Demonstrates food preferences: likes and dislikes

c. Influenced by others' eating habits

d. Caloric requirement: 90 kcal/kg/day

e. Reinforce good dental hygiene: regular exams, brushing, fluoride, less concentrated sugar

5. Safety

a. Car seat belt can provide safety when child reaches either 40 lb or 4 years or 40 inches

b. Able to learn safety habits

c. Teach injury prevention

1) Traffic safety

2) Strangers

3) Fire prevention/safety

4) Water safety; drowning

6. Play (associative)

a. Enjoys imitative and dramatic play

b. Imitates same-sex role in play

c. Provide toys to develop motor and coordination skills (tricycle, clay, paints, swings, sliding board)

d. Parental supervision of television

e. Enjoys "sing-along" songs with rhythm

7. Recommended immunizations (refer back to Figure 1-1)

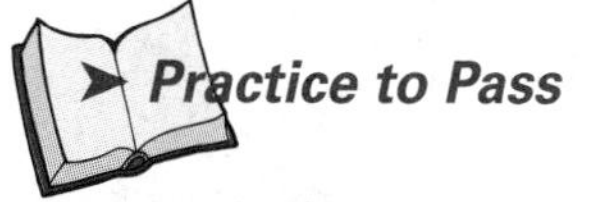

The mother of a 2½-year-old tells you that her child is into everything. What safety precautions will you discuss with her today?

a. Review necessary immunizations prior to entering kindergarten

b. Boosters

1) 5th DTaP (4 to 6 years)

2) 4th IPV (4 to 6 years)

3) 2nd MMR (4 to 6 years)

c. Hepatitis A (4 to 18 years): in selected areas

E. Growth during school-age years (6 to 12 years)

1. Weight: steady, slow growth; gains approximately 5 lb/yr

2. Height: increases 1 to 2 in./year; boys and girls differ little at first, but by end of this period girls will gain more weight and height compared to boys

3. Motor/sensory development

a. Bone growth faster than muscle and ligament development

b. Susceptible to greenstick fractures

c. Movements become more limber, graceful, and coordinated

d. Have greater stamina and energy

e. Vision 20/20 by 6 to 7 years; myopia may appear by 8 years

4. Nutrition

a. Risk of obesity in this age group

b. Identify those falling above 95th percentile and below 5th percentile in weight and height on plotted growth charts

c. Requirement of 85 kcal/kg/day

d. Tendency to eat "junk" foods, empty calories

e. Secondary sex characteristics begin at 10 years in girls; 12 years in boys

f. Loses first deciduous teeth at age 6; by age 12 has all permanent teeth, except final molars

5. Safety

a. Incidence of accidents/injuries less likely

b. Teach proper use of sports equipment

c. Discourage risk-taking behaviors (smoking, alcohol, drugs, sex)

d. Introduce sex education

e. Teach injury prevention

1) Bicycle safety

2) Firearms

3) Smoking education

4) Hobbies/handicrafts

6. Play (cooperative)

a. Comprehends rules and rituals of games

b. Enjoys team play; helps learn values and develop sense of accomplishment

c. Enjoys athletic activities such as swimming, soccer, hiking, bicycling, basketball, baseball, football

d. Provide construction toys: puzzles, erector sets, Legos™

e. Good eye/hand coordination: interested in video and computer games (needs monitoring and time limits with this activity)

f. Enjoys music, adventure stories, competitive activities

7. Recommended immunizations (refer back to Figure 1-1)

a. Recheck records to identify any missed immunizations

b. Tetanus and diphtheria (Td) recommended every 10 years

c. If child has not received 2nd MMR, administer prior to 7th grade (11 to 12 years)

d. If child has never received Varicella immunization, administer at 11 to 12 years

e. Hepatitis A—in selected areas

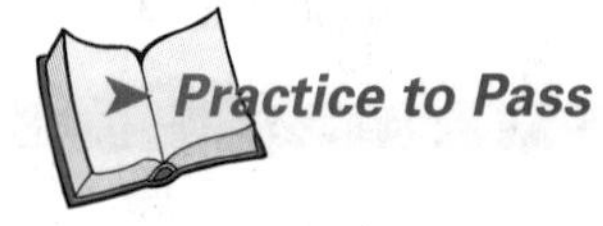

A 6-year-old child will enter kindergarten this fall. List all immunizations that he/she is required to have received.

F. Growth during adolescence (13 to 18 years)

1. Weight: rapid period of growth causes anxiety; girls gain 15 to 55 lb (7 to 25 kg); boys gain 15 to 65 lb (7 to 29 kg)
2. Height: attain final 20 percent of mature height; girls: height increases approximately 3 in./year, slows at menarche, stops at 16 years; boys: increases 4 in./year, growth spurt approximately at 13 years, slows in late teens
3. Puberty
   a. Related to hormonal changes
   b. Apocrine glands become active, may develop body odor
   c. Appearance of acne on face, back, trunk
   d. Development of secondary sex characteristics: girls experience breast development, menarche (average age 12½ yrs), pubic hair; boys experience enlargement of testes (13 years), increase in scrotum and penis size, nocturnal emission, pubic hair, vocal changes, possibly gynecomastia
4. Nutrition
   a. **Growth spurt:** brief period of rapid increase in growth
   b. "Hollow leg stage": appetite increases
   c. Nutrition requirements: 60 to 80 kcal/kg/day—1,500 to 3,000 kcal/day (11 to 14 yrs); 2,100 to 3,900 kcal/day (15 to 18 years)
   d. At risk for fad diets; food choices influenced by peers
   e. Require increased calcium for skeletal growth
   f. Continue emphasis on prevention of caries and good dental hygiene
   g. Final molars erupt at end of adolescent period; orthodontia common dental need

NCLEX!

5. Safety
   a. Accidents are leading cause of death: motor vehicle accidents (MVA), sports, firearms
   b. Provide drug and alcohol education
   c. Provide sex education
   d. Discourage risk-taking activities
   e. Adolescents may display lack of impulse control, reckless behaviors, sense of invulnerability
   f. Teach health promotion: breast self-exams (BSE), self-testicular exams
   g. Teach injury prevention
      1) Proper use of sports equipment (protective gear)
      2) Diving, drowning
      3) Provide driver's education
      4) Use of seat belts

5) Violence prevention

6) Crisis intervention (stress, depression, eating disorders)

7) Provide information about the risks of body piercing

h. Reinforce rules when necessary

6. Play/activities

a. Enjoys sports, school activities, peer group activities (movies, dances, eating out, music, videos, computers)

b. Interest in heterosexual relationships common

7. Recommended immunizations (see Figure 1-1 again)

a. Review records for any missed immunizations

b. Td recommended every 10 years; hepatitis A in selected areas

III. Growth and Development Theories

A. Stages of Piaget's theory of cognitive development

1. Sensorimotor (birth to 2 years)

a. An infant learns about the world through the senses and motor activity

b. Progresses from reflex activity through simple repetitive behaviors to imitative behaviors

c. Develops a sense of "cause and effect"

d. Language enables the child to better understand the world

e. Curiosity, experimentation, and exploration result in the learning process

f. Object permanence is fully developed

2. Preoperational (2 to 7 years)

a. Forms symbolic thought

b. Exhibits **egocentrism**—unable to put oneself in the place of another

c. Unable to understand conservation (e.g., clay shapes, glasses of liquid)

d. Increasing ability to use language

e. Play becomes more socialized

f. Can concentrate on only one characteristic of an object at a time (centration)

3. Concrete operational (7 to 11 years)

a. Thoughts become increasingly logical and coherent

b. Able to shift attention from one perceptual attribute to another (decentration)

c. Concrete thinkers: view things as "black or white," right or wrong, no in between or "gray areas"

d. Able to classify and sort facts, do problem-solving

e. Acquires conservation skills

Practice to Pass

The nurse observes a 2-year-old child having a tantrum. What should the response to the parents be?

4. Formal operations (11 years to death)

a. Able to logically manipulate abstract and unobservable concepts

b. Adaptable and flexible

c. Able to deal with contradictions

d. Uses scientific approach to problem-solve

e. Able to conceive the distant future

B. Stages of Erickson's theory of psychosocial development

1. Trust vs. mistrust (birth to 1 year)

a. The task of the first year of life is to establish trust in the people providing care

b. Mistrust develops if basic needs are inconsistently or inadequately met

2. Autonomy vs. shame and doubt (1 to 3 years)

a. Increased ability to control self and environment

b. Practices and attains new physical skills, developing autonomy

c. Symbolizes independence by controlling body secretions, saying "no" when asked to do something, and directing motor activity

d. If successful, develops self-confidence and willpower; if criticized or unsuccessful develops a sense of shame and doubt about his or her abilities

3. Initiative vs. guilt (3 to 6 years)

a. A child explores the physical world with all the senses, initiates new activities, and considers new ideas

b. Initiative is demonstrated when the child is able to formulate and carry out a plan of action

c. Develops a conscience

d. If successful, develops direction and purpose; if criticized, leads to feelings of guilt and a lack of purpose

4. Industry vs. inferiority (6 to 12 years)

a. Middle years of childhood displays development of new interests and involvement in activities

b. Learns to follow rules

c. Acquires reading, writing, math, and social skills

d. If successful, develops confidence and enjoys learning about new things; if compared to others, may develop feeling of inadequacy; inferiority may develop if too much is expected

5. Identity vs. role confusion (12 to 18 years)

a. Rapid and marked physical changes

b. Preoccupation with physical appearance

c. Examines and redefines self, family, peer group, and community

d. Experiments with different roles

e. Peer group very important

f. If successful, develops confidence in self-identity and optimism; if unable to establish meaningful definition of self, develops role confusion

IV. Child's Reaction to Illness and Hospitalization

A. Infants and toddlers

1. Parent–child relationship is disturbed

2. Unpredictable routine of the hospital promotes feelings of distrust

3. Infants and toddlers experience **separation anxiety,** which is distress behavior that is observed in young children, between the ages of 6 and 30 months, when separated from familiar caregivers; separation anxiety reaches its peak around 15 months

a. Stages of separation anxiety

1) Protest: child appears sad, agitated, angry, inconsolable, watches desperately for parents to return

2) Despair: child appears sad, hopeless, withdrawn; acts ambivalent when parents return

3) Detachment: child appears happy, interested in environment, becomes attached to staff members; may ignore parents

NCLEX!

b. Nursing interventions related to separation anxiety

1) Goal is to preserve child's trust

2) Reassure child that parents will return

3) Provide "rooming in" to encourage parent–child attachment

4) Have parents leave a personal article, picture, or favorite toy with child

5) Maintain usual routine and rituals, whenever possible

6) Allow choices, whenever possible, to return control to parent and child

NCLEX!

4. Responses to pain

a. Infants will have increases in blood pressure and heart rate and decrease in arterial oxygen saturation

b. Harsh, tense, or loud crying

c. Facial grimacing, flinching, thrashing of extremities

d. Toddlers will verbally indicate discomfort ("no," "ouch," "hurts")

e. Generalized restlessness, uncooperative, clings to family member

5. **Regression:** use of behavior that is more appropriate to an earlier stage of development, often used to cope with stress or anxiety

a. Result is lack of control, toddler may become frustrated, returns to bottle, temper tantrums, incontinence

b. Help parents to understand changes in behavior; avoid punishment

B. Preschoolers

1. Major fears
   a. Mutilation: has general lack of understanding of body integrity
   b. Intrusive procedures: will misinterpret words, has active imagination
2. Very egocentric and present-oriented
3. Perceives illness as punishment; associates own actions with disease; may believe hospitalization is punishment for bad behavior
4. Some degree of separation anxiety still exists; may become uncooperative, develop nightmares, become withdrawn or aggressive
5. Nursing interventions
   a. Encourage parents to participate in child care
   b. Allow child to express feelings
   c. Give simple explanations; avoid medical terminology
   d. Provide **therapeutic play** (planned play techniques that provide an opportunity for children to deal with their fears and concerns related to illness or hospitalization)
   e. Allow child to manipulate and play with equipment
   f. Maintain trusting relationship with parents and child; allow time for questions
   g. Praise the child, focus on the desired behavior, give rewards (stickers)
6. May show signs of regression, like the toddler (loss of bowel and bladder control)

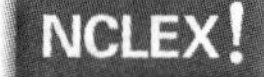

7. Response to pain
   a. All children have a major fear of needles; preschoolers will deny pain to avoid an injection
   b. Restlessness, irritability, cries, kicks with experiences of pain
   c. Able to describe the location and intensity of pain

C. School-age children

1. Major fears
   a. Pain and bodily injury
   b. Loss of control
   c. Fears often related to school, peers, and family
2. Ask relevant questions, want to know reasons for procedures, tests
3. Have a more realistic understanding of their disease
4. Become distressed over separation from family and peers

NCLEX!

5. Nursing interventions
   a. Communicate openly and honestly; explain rules
   b. Clarify any misconceptions

c. Encourage child's participation in care to maintain sense of control and independence

d. Provide visiting for siblings and peers

e. Use age-appropriate therapeutic play to provide an opportunity for children to deal with their fears and concerns related to illness or hospitalization

f. Art therapy to assist child to express feelings

g. Provide explanations; use visual aids such as diagrams, models, and body outlines

h. Praise the child; focus on the desired behavior

NCLEX!

6. Response to pain

a. Able to describe pain, concerned with disability and death

b. Girls express pain more than boys

c. Demonstrate overt behaviors: biting, kicking, crying, and bargaining

d. Cues to pain: facial expression, silence, false sense of being "okay"

D. Adolescents

1. Major fears

a. Loss of independence

b. Loss of identity

c. Body image disturbance

d. Rejection by others

2. Separation from peers is a source of anxiety

3. Physical appearance has major importance to how adolescents perceive themselves

4. Behavior exhibited by loss of control: anger, withdrawal, uncooperativeness, power struggles

5. Reluctant to ask questions; questions competency of others, will verify answers from more than one individual to determine if others are being truthful

6. Often believe they are invincible, nothing can hurt them; resulting in risk-taking and noncompliant behaviors

NCLEX!

7. Nursing interventions

a. Involve adolescent in plan of care

b. Support relationships with family and peers

c. Provide consistent and truthful explanations; can use abstract terms

d. Accept emotional outburts

e. Promote communication between adolescents and their parents

NCLEX!

8. Response to pain

a. Associates pain with being different from peers

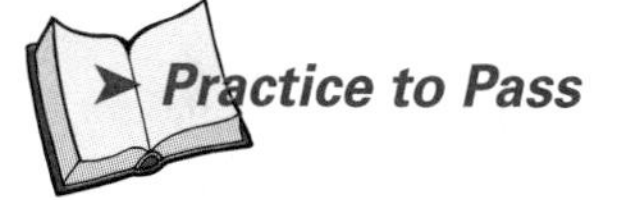

The nurse is to start an IV infusion on a 5-year-old child. What interventions can be used to decrease anxiety of this intrusive procedure?

b. May exhibit projected confidence, conceited attitude, withdraws, rejects others

c. Increase muscle tension and body control

d. Understands cause and effect; able to describe pain

E. Nursing diagnoses for the hospitalized child

1. Altered nutrition: Less than body requirements related to unfamiliar foods, separation from caregiver, strange environment, or disease process
2. Ineffective individual coping related to anxiety of hospitalization and procedures
3. Diversional activity deficit related to separation from normal activities and peers
4. Altered family processes related to hospitalization
5. Self-care deficit related to physical disability, change in environment, and regression
6. Sleep pattern disturbance related to unfamiliar environment, separation from caregiver, or discomfort
7. Pain related to disease process or specific injury

V. Child's Reaction to Death and Dying

A. Infants and toddlers

1. Both lack an understanding of the concept of death
2. Infants react to loss of the caregiver with behaviors such as crying, sleeping more, and eating less
3. Aware someone is missing, may experience separation anxiety
4. Toddlers may develop fearfulness, become more attached to remaining parent, cease walking and talking

B. Preschoolers

1. View death as temporary and reversible
2. Magical thinking and egocentricity lead to the belief that the dead person will come back
3. View death as a punishment; believe bad thoughts and actions cause death
4. First exposure to death is frequently the death of a pet
5. Common behaviors: nightmares, bowel and bladder problems, crying, anger, out-of-control behaviors
6. Preschoolers will ask a lot of questions, may display fascination with death

C. School-age children

1. View death as irreversible, but not necessarily inevitable
2. By age 10, understand death is universal and will happen to them
3. May believe death serves as a punishment for wrongdoing

4. May deny sadness, attempt to act like an adult
5. Common behaviors: difficulty with concentration in school, psychosomatic complaints, acting-out behaviors

D. Adolescents

1. View death as irreversible, universal, and inevitable
2. Seen as a personal but distant event
3. Develop a better understanding between illness and death
4. Sense of invincibility conflicts fear of death
5. Common behaviors: feelings of loneliness, sadness, fear, depression; acting out behaviors may include risk-taking, delinquency, suicide attempts, promiscuity

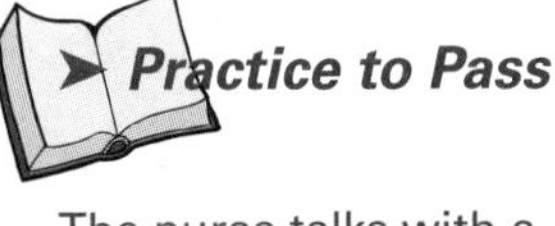

The nurse talks with a 15-year-old student about the sudden death of a grandparent. What are the expected reactions of adolescents to death and dying?

E. Nursing diagnoses for the child experiencing death and dying

1. Anticipatory grieving related to impending death of a child/parent
2. Anxiety elated to diagnosis and/or impending death
3. Ineffective coping related to death of a child/parent
4. Sleep pattern disturbance related to grieving, anxiety, sadness, feelings of depression

Case Study

A 6-month-old female infant is brought into the pediatric clinic for a well-baby visit. You as the pediatric nurse will be assigned to care for this family.

❶ Identify the primary growth and development expectations for a 6-month-old.

❷ What type common behavior is expected of this 6-month-old towards the nurse?

❸ What immunization(s) are recommended at this age to maintain health and wellness?

❹ Identify what types of toys would be appropriate for play for this 6-month-old child.

❺ What information would you give these parents regarding anticipatory guidance?

For suggested responses, see page 407.

Posttest

1 A mother asks the pediatric nurse about what she should begin to feed her 6-month-old infant. The correct response is:

(1) Egg whites are the least allergenic food to be introduced into the baby's diet.
(2) Rice cereal is the first solid introduced that is least allergenic of the cereals.
(3) Formula is the only source of nutrition given for the first year.
(4) Fruits and vegetables are good sources of iron.

2 A 1-year-old male child is scheduled for a routine exam at the pediatric clinic. The child's birth weight was 8 lbs, 2 oz. The child now weighs 18 lbs, 4 oz. The nurse knows that this weight is:

(1) Below the expected weight.
(2) Appropriate for the child's age.
(3) Above the expected weight.
(4) Individualized and thus unpredictable.

3 The nurse provides anticipatory guidance to parents of a 3-year-old child. Instructions should include:

(1) To restrain the child in the car seat facing rear in the back seat of the car.
(2) The use of syrup of ipecac for accidental poisonings.
(3) Drug and alcohol education.
(4) The proper use of sports equipment.

4 A school nurse prepares a lecture on puberty for 5th- and 6th-grade girls. She asks the group, "What is the first sign of puberty?" A student correctly replies:

(1) "The appearance of breast buds."
(2) "An increase in energy and appetite."
(3) "The occurrence of the first menarche."
(4) "Appearance of body odor."

5 The mother discusses with the nurse that her toddler asks every night for a bedtime story. The mother asks why the child does this. The nurse would explain that this behavior demonstrates:

(1) Ritualism.
(2) Object permanence.
(3) Dependency.
(4) Conservation.

6 Whenever the parents of a 10-month-old leave their hospitalized child for short periods, he begins to cry and scream. The nurse explains that this behavior demonstrates that the child:

(1) Needs to remain with his parents at all times.
(2) Is experiencing separation anxiety.
(3) Is experiencing discomfort.
(4) Is extremely spoiled.

7 A teenager refuses to wear the clothes his mother bought for him. He states he wants to look like the other kids at school and wear clothes like they wear. The nurse explains this behavior is an example of teenage rebellion related to internal conflicts of:

(1) Autonomy vs. shame and doubt.
(2) Trust vs. mistrust.
(3) Identity vs. role confusion.
(4) Initiative vs. inferiority.

8 In providing her 8-month-old child's medical history, the mother states the child has received one MMR vaccine. The nurse taking the history should:

(1) Ask the mother if the child has received the MMR booster.
(2) Plan to administer the MMR booster.
(3) Explain that one MMR vaccine is all that is required.
(4) Plan to administer another MMR vaccine after the child is 1 year old.

9 The mother of a 5-year-old expresses concern about her child who believes that "Grandma is still alive" 3 months after the grandmother's death. The nurse explains that:

(1) Magical thinking often accounts for a preschooler who believes that dead people will come back.
(2) There is a need for psychological counseling for this child and family.
(3) This is a form of regression exhibited by the preschooler.
(4) The child is in denial regarding Grandma's death.

10 Hospitalization of a child results in disturbance of the dynamics in family life. The most appropriate nursing diagnosis is:

(1) Diversional activity deficit related to separations from siblings and peers.
(2) Sleep pattern disturbance related to unfamiliar surroundings.
(3) Altered family processes related to hospitalization.
(4) Ineffective individual coping related to procedures.

See pages 25–26 for Answers and Rationales.

Answers and Rationales

Pretest

1 **Answer: 4** ***Rationale:*** Children have 20 deciduous teeth that erupt between 6 months and 24 months of age. The deciduous teeth are lost beginning at age 6 through age 12, and they are replaced by permanent teeth. The other choices are incorrect.
Cognitive Level: Application
Nursing Process: Assessment; ***Test Plan:*** HPM

2 **Answer: 3** ***Rationale:*** Fontanels are inspected and palpated for size, tenseness, and pulsation. The anterior fontanel should be soft, flat, and pulsatile with the child in the sitting position. The anterior fontanel should be completely closed by age 12 to 18 months. If the fontanel is found to be open after 18 months, the child is referred for further evaluation.
Cognitive Level: Application
Nursing Process: Assessment; ***Test Plan:*** HPM

3 **Answer: 3** ***Rationale:*** By age 8 months, infants can sit well while unsupported. Infants can now explore their environment. Avoid walkers near stairs and fence stairways. At age 4 months, the infant rolls over; by age 6 months, the baby sits with support and at 12 months stands, cruises around furniture, and walks with one hand held.
Cognitive Level: Application
Nursing Process: Evaluation; ***Test Plan:*** HPM

4 **Answer: 2** ***Rationale:*** The NCHS growth charts use the 5th and 95th percentiles as criteria for determining those children who fall outside the normal limits for growth. Children whose height and weight are above the 95th percentile are considered overweight or large for stature. Prepubescent growth spurts are between 10 to 12 years for girls and 12 to 14 years for boys. This is not a normal proportion for height and weight for this 9-year-old.
Cognitive Level: Analysis
Nursing Process: Analysis; ***Test Plan:*** HPM

5 **Answer: 1** ***Rationale:*** Secondary sex characteristics begin at 10 to 12 years for girls and 12 to 14 years for boys. The growth in girls is accompanied by an increase in breast size and development of pubic hair, and lastly menstruation. In boys, the growth spurt includes growth in size of the penis and testes and pubic hair development.
Cognitive Level: Application
Nursing Process: Implementation; ***Test Plan:*** HPM

6 **Answer: 4** ***Rationale:*** Regression usually occurs in instances of stress when the child attempts to cope by reverting to patterns of behavior from earlier stages of development. Regression is common in toddlers; it lessens the threat of illness, hospitalization, or separation. A need to revert to use of the bottle, refusal to use the potty, or temper tantrums represent forms of behaviors exhibited as regression. It should be explained to parents that regression is a temporary coping mechanism; the best approach is to ignore it and praise appropriate behavior. Any form of punishment is not advisable.
Cognitive Level: Analysis
Nursing Process: Implementation; ***Test Plan:*** PSYC

7 **Answer: 3** ***Rationale:*** Toddlers enjoy physical skills in play, such as push and pull toys that enhance fine and gross motor abilities. Stuffed animals are favorite toys for the 3- to 6-month-old, but be cautious of buttons and pieces that can easily be aspirated. A large ball is pleasurable for the infant to develop grasp and manipulation. Preschoolers enjoy tricycles and climbing toys, which develop muscles and coordination.
Cognitive Level: Application
Nursing Process: Implementation; ***Test Plan:*** HPM

8 **Answer: 1** ***Rationale:*** Visual aids such as dolls, puppets, and outlines of the body can be used to illustrate the cause and treatment of the child's illness. Use of such equipment provides information for the school-age child to understand and cope with feelings about the procedure. Written pamphlets should be given to the parents to review prior to the procedure. Children should be allowed to cry or verbalize their feelings without guilt as long as they hold still. Parents should be given a choice to accompany their child during the procedure.
Cognitive Level: Application
Nursing Process: Implementation; ***Test Plan:*** PSYC

9 **Answer: 2** ***Rationale:*** The American Academy of Pediatrics (AAP) recommends that all formulas be fortified with iron and continued for the first 12 months. Whole milk should not be introduced to infants until after 1 year of age. Pasteurized cow's milk is deficient in iron, zinc, and vitamin C, and has a high renal solute load. Solid foods are introduced between 4 and 6 months of age.
Cognitive Level: Application
Nursing Process: Implementation; ***Test Plan:*** PHYS

10 **Answer: 3** ***Rationale:*** The child in the preoperational stage is egocentric and is unable to see things

from another's perspective. Logic is not well developed. Magical thinking is common. Centration is focusing on only one particular aspect of a situation. Negativism is a common toddler response of "no" to situations and requests. Selfishness is a negative behavior exhibited by the child who refuses to share with another.
Cognitive Level: Analysis
Nursing Process: Analysis; ***Test Plan:*** HPM

Posttest

1 **Answer: 2** ***Rationale:*** Introduction of solid food is recommended at age 4 to 6 months, when the gastrointestinal system has matured sufficiently to handle complex nutrients. The suck reflex and tongue-thrust reflex diminish at 4 months of age. Rice cereal is the first solid food because it is a rich source of iron and rarely induces allergic reactions. Fruits and vegetables, good sources of vitamins and fiber, are introduced after cereal, one at a time to determine allergic reactions. Egg whites are highly allergenic.
Cognitive Level: Application
Nursing Process: Implementation; ***Test Plan:*** HPM

2 **Answer: 1** ***Rationale:*** The first year of life is one of rapid growth. The birth weight usually doubles by 6 months and triples by the end of the first year. The other choices are incorrect.
Cognitive Level: Analysis
Nursing Process: Assessment; ***Test Plan:*** HPM

3 **Answer: 2** ***Rationale:*** Nurses are instrumental in teaching parents how to make the toddler's environment safe by providing instructions about keeping syrup of ipecac available, having the Poison Control Center number close to the phone, using child-resistant containers and cupboard safety closures, and keeping medicines and other poisonous materials locked away. Infants are to be restrained in rear-facing car seat, school-age children should be taught the proper use of sports equipment, and adolescents should be provided education regarding drug and alcohol abuse.
Cognitive Level: Application
Nursing Process: Implementation; ***Test Plan:*** HPM

4 **Answer: 1** ***Rationale:*** Puberty is a process that brings about the development of secondary sex characteristics, which begin with the appearance of breast buds at 9 to 11 years followed by the growth of pubic hair. Menarche follows approximately 1 year later. Body odor may result later because of an increase in secretions from the apocrine glands.
Cognitive Level: Application
Nursing Process: Evaluation; ***Test Plan:*** HPM

5 **Answer: 1** ***Rationale:*** The toddler insists on sameness (such as a nightly bedtime story). Ritualism allows the toddler to have a sense of control and to feel more secure and confident. The child may experience distress if this routine is not followed. Object permanence is when the infant develops an awareness that objects continue to exist when they are out of sight. Dependency is the need for a caregiver (parent) to provide total care for another (infant). The school-age child masters the concept of conservation; learns that certain properties of objects do not change simply because their form or appearance has changed.
Cognitive Level: Analysis
Nursing Process: Implementation; ***Test Plan:*** HPM

6 **Answer: 2** ***Rationale:*** Infants and toddlers between the ages of 6 months and 30 months experience separation anxiety. There are three stages of separation anxiety. The child who demonstrates crying and rejecting anyone other than the parent is in protest, the first stage of separation anxiety. This behavior does not exhibit spoiling or any indication of discomfort. The second stage is despair. The child expresses hopelessness, appears quiet, and is withdrawn. The third stage is detachment. The child becomes interested in the environment, especially the caregivers. If the parents return, the child ignores them.
Cognitive Level: Analysis
Nursing Process: Assessment; ***Test Plan:*** HPM

7 **Answer: 3** ***Rationale:*** Erikson's theory of psychosocial development states that the child is faced with conflicts that need to be resolved. Erikson identifies stages of personality development. Identity vs. role confusion (12 to 19 years) is a period when adolescents search for answers regarding their future. During this time, the child rejects the identity presented by his parents and attempts to create his own identity. Identity is often based on peers. Positive outcomes result in optimism and confidence. Negative outcomes result in sense of purposelessness or deviance.
Cognitive Level: Application
Nursing Process: Assessment; ***Test Plan:*** HPM

8 **Answer: 4** ***Rationale:*** This mother may have been mistaken about the vaccine. Maternal antibodies interfere with the vaccine when it is given before 12 months of age. Even if the child has had the vaccine, it will need to be repeated. The first measles-mumps-

rubella (MMR) should be administered to the child between the ages 12 to 15 months. The second is given at age 4 to 6 years or 11 to 12 years. Because of outbreaks of measles in preschoolers, school-age children, and college students in the 1980s, a second dose was added to the recommended childhood immunization schedule. The MMR is a vaccine that is not given to infants younger than 12 months old.
Cognitive Level: Application
Nursing Process: Planning; ***Test Plan:*** HPM

9 Answer: 1 ***Rationale:*** The preschooler believes that death is reversible. Their magical thinking and egocentricity often results in their belief that the deceased will come back to life. Preschoolers also often will blame themselves for the death of another.
Cognitive Level: Analysis
Nursing Process: Implementation; ***Test Plan:*** PSYC

10 Answer: 3 ***Rationale:*** Identification of nursing diagnoses that apply to the specific problem(s) of the child and family is an essential step of the nursing process. Family-centered care addresses the needs of the family members, including the child's siblings. The primary goals are to maintain the relationship with the child and siblings during the period of separation while hospitalized and avoid boredom and distress for the hospitalized child.
Cognitive Level: Analysis
Nursing Process: Planning; ***Test Plan:*** PSYC

References

Ashwill, J. W. & Droske, S. C. (1997). *Nursing care of children: Principles and practice.* Philadelphia: W. B. Saunders, pp. 26–201, 221, 258–425.

Ball, J. & Bindler, R. (1999). *Pediatric nursing* (2nd ed.). Stamford, CT: Appleton & Lange, pp. 8–12, 26–91, 178–284, 370–381.

Ball, J. & Bindler, R. (1999). *Quick reference to pediatric clinical skills.* Stamford, CT: Appleton & Lange, pp. 2, 10–11, 17–19.

Bowden, V. R., Dickey, S. B., & Greenberg, C. S. (1998). *Children and their families: The continuum of care.* Philadelphia: W. B. Saunders, pp. 169–342, 370–381, 470–471, 624.

Jarvis, C. (2000). *Physical examination and health assessment* (3rd ed.). Philadelphia: W. B. Saunders, p. 381.

Wong, D., Hockenberry-Eaton, M., Wilson, D., Winkelstein, M., Ahmann, E., & DiVito-Thomas, P. (1999). *Whaley and Wong's nursing care of infants and children* (6th ed.). St. Louis: Mosby, pp. 118–152, 237–242, 297–298, 560–615, 679–688, 706, 880–905.

CHAPTER 2

Nursing Process, Physical Assessment, and Common Laboratory Tests

Vera Dauffenbach, MSN, EdD, RN

CHAPTER OUTLINE

OBJECTIVES

- Discuss the areas of medical history to be included in the assessment of a child.
- Describe the physical assessment of a child.
- Identify the four areas evaluated by the Denver Developmental Screening Test (Denver II).

[Media Link]

Use the CD-ROM enclosed with this text, or log onto the address given to access the free, interactive Companion Website created for this series. The CD-ROM and Companion Website accompanying this book offer additional practice opportunities and information—NCLEX Review, Case Studies, Glossary, In Depth with NCLEX, and more.

www.prenhall.com/hogan

REVIEW AT A GLANCE

amblyopia *visual condition in which the brain suppresses vision in the eye with weaker muscle; also known as "lazy eye"*

cerumen *waxy substance secreted in the outer third of the ear canal; also known as earwax*

facies *the expression and appearance of the face*

fremitus *vibrations of the voice transmitted through the chest wall of a person speaking; can be palpated with hands on the chest or back or auscultated with a stethoscope*

genogram *a family map of three or more generations that records relationships, deaths, occupations, and health and illness history*

lordosis *anterior convex curvature of the lumbar spine*

Mongolian spots *bluish-colored area usually located in the sacral region of newborn Asian, Native American, and African-American infants; usually disappears in childhood*

objective data *information obtained through physical assessment techniques and diagnostic studies*

scoliosis *lateral curvature of the spine*

strabismus *lack of eye muscle coordination caused by one muscle being weaker than the other*

subjective data *information obtained from the child and family using interview techniques*

Pretest

1 **A 7-month-old infant has all of the following abilities. Which skill was most recently acquired?**

(1) Smiling at self in a mirror
(2) Transferring a rattle from one hand to the other
(3) Rolling from back to abdomen
(4) Imitating sounds

2 **The school health nurse is doing vision testing. Visual acuity is assessed using:**

(1) The Snellen eye chart.
(2) An ophthalmoscope.
(3) The cover-uncover test.
(4) The Weber test.

3 **Children are usually brought to the clinic for health care by a parent. At what age is it appropriate for the nurse to question the child about presenting symptoms?**

(1) 3 years
(2) 5 years
(3) 7 years
(4) 9 years

4 **When recording the health history of a child, what information that is uniquely pertinent to children is important for the nurse to obtain?**

(1) Past hospitalizations
(2) Coping strategies
(3) Immunization status
(4) Past accidents

5 **A mother overhears a nurse state that the nurse is going to complete a genogram and asks the nurse what that means. The nurse's reply would be based on knowledge that a genogram is useful for visually showing what information?**

(1) Treatment protocols
(2) Family history
(3) Past history
(4) Immunization status

6 **When plotting a child's height and weight on a growth grid, the nurse understands that which range represents the normal percentile range for children?**

(1) 10th to 90th percentile
(2) 25th to 75th percentile
(3) 50th to 100th percentile
(4) 5th to 95th percentile

7 **When assessing a child who complains of abdominal pain, what is the most appropriate nursing action?**

(1) Palpate the most painful area first.
(2) Palpate for rebound tenderness.
(3) Avoid painful areas until the end of the assessment.
(4) Use deep palpation for abdominal tenderness.

8 **When sharing the purpose of the Denver Development Screening Test (Denver II) with parents of an 18-month-old, the nurse should explain that:**

(1) The Denver II is a test that will predict future intellectual ability.
(2) The Denver II is a screening test used to detect children who may be slow in development.
(3) The Denver II is used for early detection of speech disorders.
(4) The Denver II measures psychological, cognitive, and social development.

9 **What should the nurse do first when preparing to do a physical assessment on a sleeping 8-month-old baby?**

(1) Measure the occipital-frontal head circumference.
(2) Auscultate the heart and lungs.
(3) Check the eyes for the red reflex.
(4) Wake the baby.

10 **When preparing to examine a preschool child, the nurse should:**

(1) Give detailed explanations to alleviate the child's anxiety.
(2) Give reassurance and feedback to the child during the examination.
(3) Suggest that the child act like "the big kids" when he or she is examined.
(4) Say that the shirt is the only clothing that must be removed.

See page 54 for Answers and Rationales.

I. Nursing Process

A. Assessment

1. **Subjective data:** information obtained from the child and family using interview techniques
2. **Objective data:** information obtained through physical assessment techniques and diagnostic studies
3. Provides a basis for identifying problems and serves as a baseline against which to compare further assessments
4. Data should be recorded systematically

B. Nursing diagnosis

1. Statement of actual or potential health problems that can be resolved, diminished, or changed by nursing interventions
2. Standardized labels assigned to specific nursing diagnoses by North American Nursing Diagnosis Association (NANDA)
3. Has three parts: problem statement, etiology, and signs and symptoms

C. Planning

1. Setting outcomes that allow nurses to develop courses of action that will assist the client achieve improved or optimal functioning
2. Includes determination of priorities

3. Requires setting long- and short-term goals
4. Includes selecting interventions that assist the client to achieve goals
5. Becomes part of the client's record

D. Implementation

1. Phase in which the nurse works with the client, family, and healthcare team to perform interventions designated in the care plan
2. Independent functions: carrying out interventions prescribed by the nurse on the care plan that have been initiated without the direction or supervision of another healthcare professional; based on an assessment of the client's needs
3. Dependent functions: carrying out physician-prescribed orders
4. Interdependent functions: actions performed jointly by nurses and other members of the healthcare team (sometimes called collaborative functions)

E. Evaluation

1. Examines the client's progress toward long- and short-term goals
2. Identifies factors that contribute to ability to achieve or not achieve goals
3. Allows for modification or continuance of the care plan

II. Nursing History

NCLEX!

A. Major source of subjective data from family and child

B. Provides opportunity to observe parent-child interactions

C. Communication strategies

1. Provide privacy and comfort
2. Use therapeutic techniques, such as open-ended questions, clarification, and summarizing as appropriate
3. Employ active listening
4. Observe nonverbal behavior for consistency with words and tone of voice
5. Show empathy

D. Demographic and biographical information

1. Child's name, nickname, parents' names
2. Addresses of child and parents
3. Telephone numbers and emergency contacts
4. Ages of child, siblings, parents
5. Ethnic identification and religion

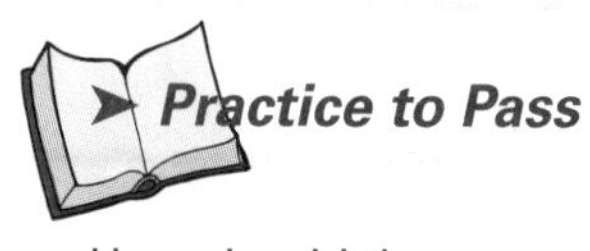

How should the nurse provide a comfortable environment for taking a health history of a young child?

E. Reason for seeking care

1. Sometimes called "chief complaint"
2. May be wellness- or illness-oriented
3. Record in the words of the informant, parent, or child

F. History of present illness

1. Onset and location

a. Date and time

b. Sudden or gradual

c. Generalized or anatomically precise location

d. Sequence of events

2. Quality or character

a. Description of symptoms

b. Worsening, improving, or staying the same

3. Quantity or severity

a. Relates to amounts (vomited, for example)

b. How symptoms interfere with daily activities

4. Duration or timing

5. Aggravating or alleviating factors (that make it worse or better)

6. Perceptions of parent and/or child

7. Associated factors

G. Past medical history

1. Birth history

a. Length of pregnancy

b. Mother's health

c. Access to prenatal care

d. Medications taken during pregnancy

e. Alcohol, tobacco, or street-drug use

f. Duration of labor

g. Type of delivery

h. Apgar scores, if known

i. Birth weight, length, head circumference

j. Postnatal health problems

k. Feeding

1) Formula, including type

2) Breast-feeding, including length of time

2. Past illnesses

3. Hospitalizations, injuries, accidents, or surgeries

4. Allergies

a. Medication

   b. Food

   c. Environmental

5. Immunizations including boosters

6. Habits and behaviors

   a. Sleep

   b. Discipline

   c. Socialization

   d. Exercise or activity

   e. Behavior issues

   f. Wellness behaviors

   g. Use of alcohol, drugs, nicotine, or caffeine

   h. Sexuality issues

7. Medications taken regularly

   a. Prescription

   b. Over-the-counter

   c. Home or folk remedies

8. Developmental data

   a. Age at which child achieved specific developmental milestones, including first held head erect, first rolled over, first sat unsupported, first steps, first used words appropriately, bowel and bladder control

   b. Current developmental performance measured by a screening tool such as Denver II, if known

   c. Academic performance, if in school

9. Nutritional data

   a. Early infancy (birth to 6 months)

   b. Later infancy (6 to 12 months)

   c. Toddler

   d. Preschool

   e. School age

   f. Adolescence

   g. Timing and frequency of meals and snacks

   h. Ethnic or cultural considerations in food choices

   i. Use a 24-hour diet recall or food frequency record to assess adequacy of diet

10. Family history

   NCLEX!

   a. Primarily for the purpose of discovering the potential or actual existence of hereditary or familial diseases in the child or parents

b. Includes a **genogram** (pictorial representation of family "tree") that includes hereditary diseases, ages and causes of death, and chronic conditions (see Figure 2-1)

c. Family structure

1) Family composition: immediate and extended members of the family

2) Previous marriages, divorces, separations, or deaths of spouses

3) Home and community environment: type of dwelling, sleeping arrangements, safety features, relationships with neighbors

4) Occupations and education of family members, including work schedules

5) Cultural and religious traditions, including language spoken at home

d. Family function

1) Family interactions and roles: amount of intimacy and closeness among family members, ways family members relate to one another

2) Power, decision making, and problem solving: maintenance and clarity of boundaries between parents and children, understanding of who makes the rules in the family and what happens when they are broken

3) Communication: clarity and directness of communication among family members, patterns of relating to one another, agreement between verbal and nonverbal communication

4) Expression of feelings and individuality: ability to freely express feelings of anger, joy, sadness, etc., and freedom to grow as an individual

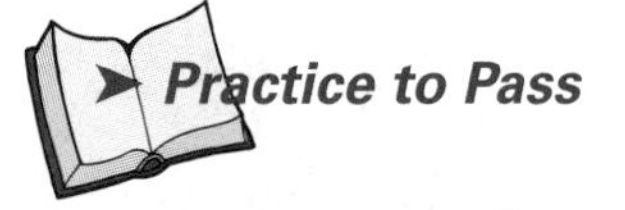

What are some questions the nurse should ask to assess cultural and religious traditions in a child's family?

11. Review of physical systems

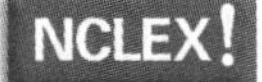

a. Includes a specific review of each body system

b. Begin with a broad question about the child's overall health

Figure 2-1

Sample genogram.

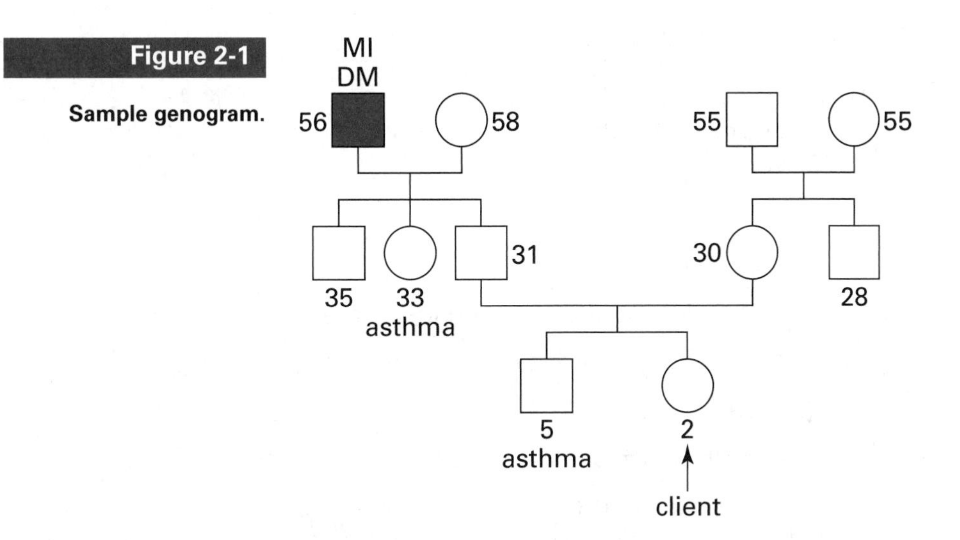

c. Integument

1) Pruritus

2) Rashes, including location

3) Acne

4) Bruising

5) Hair growth or loss

6) Disorders or deformities of nails

d. Head

1) Headaches

2) Dizziness or injuries

e. Eyes

1) Visual problems: bumping into things, squinting, blurred vision, holding books close or sitting close to television or computer

2) Rubbing eyes

3) Eye infections

4) Glasses or contact lenses

f. Ears

1) Earaches: frequency and treatment

2) Evidence of hearing loss, needing to repeat requests, loud voice

3) Previous hearing testing

g. Nose

1) History of nosebleeds

2) Constant or frequent runny or stuffy nose

3) Problems with sense of smell

h. Mouth

1) Mouth breathing

2) Dental visits, child's dentist

3) Tooth-care habits: brushing, flossing

4) Toothaches

i. Throat

1) Sore throats

2) Difficulty swallowing or choking

3) Hoarseness or voice problems

j. Neck

1) Stiffness or problems moving

2) Difficulty in holding head erect

k. Chest

1) Breast enlargement or development

2) Breast self-examination for adolescents

l. Respiratory

1) Frequency of colds

2) Coughing or wheezing

3) Difficulty breathing

4) Sputum production

5) History of pneumonia or tuberculosis (TB)

6) Date of last TB test

m. Cardiovascular

1) Cyanosis or fatigue on exertion

2) History of heart murmurs, anemia, or rheumatic fever

3) Blood type, if known

n. Gastrointestinal

1) Nausea or vomiting

2) Jaundice

3) Change in bowel habits, diarrhea, or constipation

o. Genitourinary

1) Pain on urination

2) Unpleasant odor to urine

3) Enuresis

4) Testicular self-examination, for adolescents

p. Gynecological

1) Date or age of menarche

2) Date of last menstrual period

3) Pain on menstruation

4) Vaginal discharge

5) Last Pap smear, if sexually active

6) Contraception use, if sexually active

q. Musculoskeletal

1) Weakness

2) Clumsiness or lack of coordination

3) Back or joint pain

4) Muscle pain or cramps

5) Abnormal gait or posturing or spasticity
6) History of fractures or sprains
7) Usual activity level

r. Neurological

1) History of seizures
2) Speech problems
3) Nightmares or fears
4) Dizziness or tremors
5) Learning disabilities or problems with attention at home or school

12. Review of psychosocial systems

a. Family composition

1) Family members in the home and their relationship to child
2) Marital status of parents
3) Parents' educational level
4) Persons participating in the care of the child
5) Recent changes or crises in family

b. Financial resources

1) Family members' employment status or occupation
2) Health insurance coverage

c. Home environment

1) Safe play area
2) Well or community water supply
3) Availability of heat, electricity, etc.
4) Transportation arrangements
5) Neighborhood safety issues

d. Child care arrangements

1) Day-care resources needed/available
2) School attended

e. Daily living habits

1) Peer relationships
2) Sleep, rest, activity patterns
3) Social activities
4) Self-esteem and body image

f. Child's temperament

III. Physical Assessment of the Child

A. General considerations

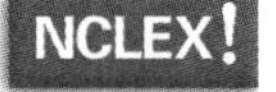

1. Developmental level of the child is the most important consideration for a successful assessment (see Table 2-1)
2. Each healthcare visit becomes a learning experience for child and parents; it becomes an opportunity for positive relationships
3. Use terms understandable to and appropriate for child and parents
4. Allow child to become familiar with examiner prior to beginning examination

NCLEX!

5. Save distressful or intrusive parts of the examination for last
6. Encourage active participation of the child or parents when possible
7. Prepare child and parents for new or painful procedures
8. Examine child in a comfortable and secure position
9. Perform the assessment in an organized sequence
10. Reassure the child throughout the examination
11. Praise cooperation

B. Methods of restraint

1. May be necessary with infants, toddlers, or uncooperative children
2. When examining eyes, ears, nose, or throat, examiner may need to have a parent or other adult hold child supine with arms extended alongside the head

Table 2-1

Age-Specific Approaches to Physical Assessment

Age	Approach
Infant	Child lying flat or held in parent's arms Use distraction with older infant Assess heart, pulse, lungs, respirations while quiet, then head-to-toe Eyes, ears, and mouth near end Check reflexes as body parts are examined Moro reflex last
Toddler	Minimal contact initially Allow to inspect equipment Assess heart and lungs while quiet, then head-to-toe Eyes, ears, and mouth last
Preschool	Allow to handle equipment Head-to-toe if cooperative Same as toddler if uncooperative
School age	Respect privacy Explain procedures Head-to-toe Genitalia last
Adolescent	Explain findings Proceed as for school age child

3. "Hug" method has child sit on parent's lap with the legs to one side and one arm tucked under parent's arm while the parent holds the other arm securely; child's legs may need to be held between parent's legs to prevent kicking
4. Ask another adult if parent is distressed and cannot help

C. Growth measurements

1. Plot results on growth charts; length/height to age, weight to age, length to weight

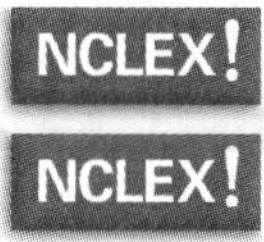

2. Overall pattern of growth is more important than any single measurement
3. Use 5th and 95th percentiles for determining which children are outside normal limits
4. Length/height
    - **a.** Recumbent length (birth to 36 months) with child supine and legs extended
    - **b.** Use crown to heel measurement
    - **c.** Children older than 2 years may stand shoeless as straight as possible
5. Weight
    - **a.** Use appropriately sized beam scale
    - **b.** Weigh naked infant lying or sitting
    - **c.** Weigh older children on upright scale dressed only in underpants or light gown
6. Head circumference

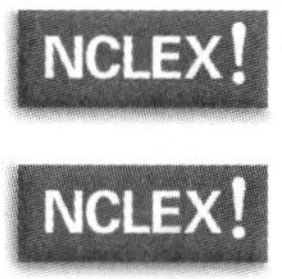

    - **a.** Should be measured at every physical assessment for infants and toddlers under 2 years
    - **b.** Is best indication of brain growth
    - **c.** Place measuring tape over most prominent part of occiput and just above supraorbital ridges (see Figure 2-2)

NCLEX!

    - **d.** Always measure head circumference of child suspected of having a neurological problem or developmental delay
    - **e.** Use paper or nonstretching tape
    - **f.** Make three measurements and take average as number to record
    - **g.** Percentiles should be comparable to child's height and weight
    - **h.** Head circumference exceeds chest circumference until between 1 and 2 years of age
7. Chest circumference
    - **a.** Is usually done at birth and early infancy
    - **b.** Place measuring tape at the level of the nipple with child supine (see Figure 2-2)
    - **c.** Take measurement midway between inspiration and expiration
    - **d.** Head and chest circumference should be approximately equal between 1 and 2 years of age
    - **e.** During childhood, chest circumference exceeds head circumference by 2 to 3 inches

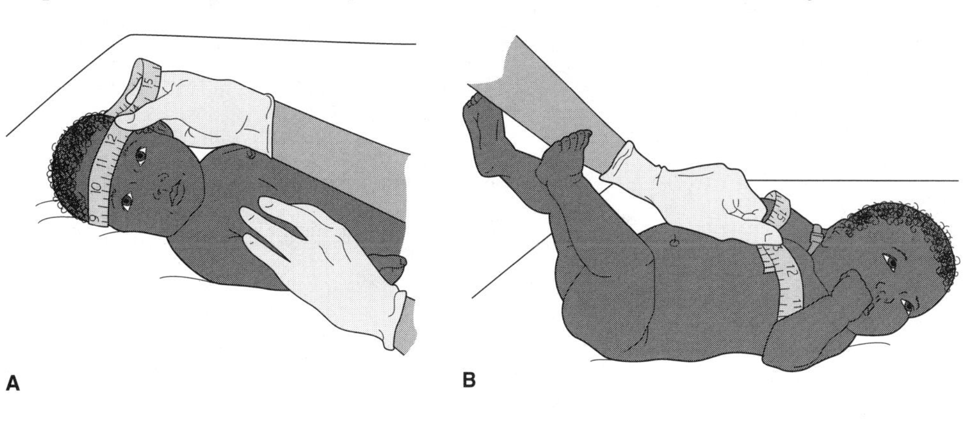

Figure 2-2

Head and chest girth measurements.
Source: Olds, S., et al. (2000). *Maternal newborn nursing* (6th ed.). Upper Saddle River, NJ: Prentice Hall Health, p. 717.

D. Vital signs (see Table 2-2)

1. Temperature
   a. Rectal, axillary, skin, or tympanic when assessing infants
   b. Oral route may be used in children over 4 years of age
   c. Use rectal only when necessary because of discomfort and intrusiveness
   d. May be altered by exercise, crying, stress, or environmental conditions
   e. Record method used, along with results
   f. When using nonmercury thermometers, follow manufacturer's directions carefully regarding instrument placement in mouth or ear

NCLEX!

2. Pulse
   a. Try to take with child at rest, sleeping, or lying quietly
   b. Apical pulse for children younger than 2 years
   c. Count for one full minute
   d. Radial pulse in children over 2 years of age
   e. May be altered by anxiety, activity, pain, crying, medications, or disease
   f. Record rate, rhythm, quality, and amplitude

Table 2-2

Normal Vital Signs for Infants and Children

Age	Average Pulse	Average Respirations	Average Blood Pressure
Newborn	120	35	73/50
1 year	120	30	90/56
2 years	110	25	91/55
4 years	100	25	92/55
6 years	100	22	96/57
10 years	90	20	100/61
14 years			
Female	85	16	114/65
Male	80	16	114/65
18 years			
Female	75	16	121/70
Male	70	16	121/70

3. Respirations
    a. Try to take while child is at rest, sleeping, or lying quietly
    b. Measure in infants and young children by observing abdominal movements
    c. Measure in older children by observing rise and fall of chest
    d. Record rate, rhythm, and quality
    e. May be altered by anxiety, activity, medications, fever, or disease
4. Blood pressure
    a. Measure annually in children over 3 years of age
    b. Select cuff width that covers 75 percent of the length of the upper arm
    c. Cuff should encircle arm circumference without overlapping
    d. Use Doppler or electronic device for infants
    e. May be altered by anxiety, activity, crying, medications, or disease

Practice to Pass

What are several strategies the nurse should use to ensure an adequate physical assessment of a toddler?

E. General appearance

1. Cumulative, subjective impression of a child's physical appearance, nutrition status, behavior, hygiene, personality, posture and body movement, interactions with parents and nurse, speech and development
2. Observe **facies** (facial expression and appearance of child) for clues about illness, pain, fear, etc.

F. Skin, hair, and nails

1. Inspect and palpate
2. Skin: note color, texture, temperature, moisture, turgor, edema, rashes, or lesions
    a. **Mongolian spots:** bluish-colored areas common on buttocks or lower back of dark-skinned infants; they disappear with age
    b. Storkbites, café au lait stains, or port-wine stains are common birthmarks
    c. Bruises in various stages or unusual locations or circular burn areas may indicate child abuse
    d. Acne vulgaris may be present in adolescents
3. Hair: observe for color, distribution, characteristics, quality, infestations, and texture
4. Nails: note color, texture, shape, and condition; clubbing frequently indicates pulmonary disease

G. Head, neck, and cervical lymph nodes

1. Inspect and palpate the head, neck, and lymph nodes
2. Head: note shape and symmetry
    a. Anterior fontanel: closes by 12 to 18 months
    b. Posterior fontanel: closes by 2 months
    c. Infant should be able to hold head erect by 4 months of age

d. Newborn skull may show molding from birth process or flattening from repeated lying in same position

e. Note symmetry by having older child make faces

3. Neck and lymph nodes: note size, mobility, swelling, temperature, and tenderness

a. The thyroid is difficult to palpate in infants because of their thick neck

b. Palpate submaxillary, sublingual, and parotid glands

c. Observe trachea for midline placement

d. Determine mobility of neck

H. Mouth, throat, nose, and sinuses

1. Inspect mouth, nose, and throat, and palpate sinuses

2. Mouth and throat

a. Examine last in young children; it is intrusive and may provoke fear

b. Note tooth eruption, condition of gums, lips, teeth, palates, tonsils, tongue, and buccal mucosa

c. Deciduous teeth erupt by about 6 months of age; all 20 appear by about 2½ years

d. Teeth begin to fall out at about 6 years when permanent teeth erupt; this progresses until all 32 teeth erupt by late adolescence

e. Tonsils may normally be enlarged, atrophying to stable adult size by late adolescence

3. Nose and sinuses

a. Push up tip of nose and shine light into each nostril

b. Note structure, patency of nares, discharge, tenderness, and any color or swelling of turbinates

c. Percuss and palpate sinuses of children over age 3; sinuses of infants and young children not palpable

I. Eyes

1. Inspect external eye

a. Note position, slant, epicanthal folds, eyelid placement, swelling, discharge, color of sclera and conjunctiva, redness, eyebrows, and lashes

b. Epicanthal folds are normal in Asian children, suggestive of Down syndrome in others

c. Outer canthus should be in line with tip of pinna

2. Visual acuity tests (see Table 2-3)

a. Snellen Letter Chart for school-age children

b. Snellen Symbol Chart (E Chart) for preschool age

c. Faye Symbol Chart (pictures) for preschool age

d. Visual acuity difficult to assess in infants; tested by observing infant's ability to fixate and follow objects

e. Should be able to differentiate colors by 5 years

Table 2-3

Visual Acuity by Age

Age	Visual Acuity
Birth	20/300
4–6 months	20/200
12 months	20/100
2 years	20/50–20/40
4–6 years	20/30–20/20
7 years	20/20

3. Extraocular muscle tests

a. Cover-uncover test: Cover one eye and have child look at object; observe uncovered eye for movement; remove cover and observe that eye for movement

b. Eye movement during cover-uncover test may indicate **strabismus** (lack of eye muscle coordination), which can lead to **amblyopia** (blindness caused by weak eye muscle)

c. Hirschberg test: Shine light on cornea while child looks straight ahead; light should reflect symmetrically in center of both pupils

d. Unequal reflection may indicate strabismus

4. Ophthalmoscopic examination

a. Same procedure as for adults

b. Save until last; may require restraint or distraction

c. Red reflex should be present

d. Expected finding: pupils equal, round, and reactive to light and accommodation (PERRLA)

e. Permanent eye color by 9 months

J. Ears

1. Inspect and palpate external ear for placement, discharge, and lesions

2. Inspect internal ear with otoscope

a. Save until last; this usually requires restraint in infants and young children

b. With infants, pull pinna down and back because canal is short and straight

c. With older child, pull pinna up and back like adult

d. Observe for **cerumen** (ear wax), foreign bodies, or discharge

e. Tympanic membrane should be pearly gray to light pink with landmarks visible

f. Tympanic membranes redden during crying

g. Assess mobility of tympanic membrane with pneumatic otoscope

h. Tympanic membrane should move with pressure

3. Hearing acuity

a. Tested in infants by noting reaction to loud noise

b. Newborns exhibit moro (startle) reflex and blink eyes

c. Older children may be tested with whispered voice

d. Audiometry testing of all children should be done prior to entering school

K. Thorax and lungs

1. Inspect shape of thorax and respiratory effort

a. Evaluate respirations for rate, depth (deep or shallow), quality (effortless, difficult, or labored), and rhythm (regular or irregular)

b. Evaluate breath sounds for noise, grunting, snoring, etc.

2. Palpate back or chest for respiratory movement and **fremitus** (conduction of voice sounds through respiratory tract)

3. Percuss lungs

a. Hyperresonance is normal in infants and young children because of the thinness of chest wall

b. Begin with anterior lung from apex to base with child lying or sitting

4. Auscultate lungs

a. Encourage deep breathing in children by having them blow a pinwheel, cotton ball, or other readily available object

b. Breath sounds may seem louder or harsher because of thin chest wall

c. Use both open bell and closed diaphragm of stethoscope

5. Inspect and palpate breasts

a. Newborns may have enlarged or engorged breasts due to influence of maternal hormones

b. Breast exam and teaching of breast self-exam for adolescents

L. Heart

1. Inspect and palpate the precordium for heaves and apical impulse

2. Perform early in exam because quiet environment and child are essential

a. Apical pulse at 4th intercostal space (ICS) until age 7

b. Apical pulse at 5th ICS after age 7

c. Apical pulse to the left of the midclavicular line (MCL) until age 4

d. Apical pulse just lateral to left MCL from 4 to 6 years

e. Apical pulse at left of MCL by age 7

2. Auscultate heart sounds

a. Note rate, which should be regular and same as radial pulse

b. Sinus arrhythmia (rate speeds up with inspiration and slows with expiration) is common in children

c. Evaluate rhythm, which should be even and regular

d. Evaluate quality for clarity as opposed to muffled

e. Note intensity, which should not be heavy or pounding

f. Evaluate for presence of murmurs

g. Sounds are louder and higher pitched and of shorter duration in infants and children

M. Abdomen

NCLEX!

1. To promote relaxation and cooperation, have child place one hand beneath examiner's, use age-appropriate distraction, or use conversation focused on topic of interest to child; inspect shape
   a. Abdomen is prominent when standing and supine in infants and children until age 4
   b. After age 4, abdomen is somewhat prominent when standing but flat when supine
   c. Scaphoid abdomen is indicative of malnutrition or dehydration
   d. Umbilicus should be pink without redness or discharge
   e. Umbilical hernias fairly common, especially in African American children
2. Auscultate bowel sounds the same as for adults
3. Palpate for masses or tenderness
   a. Liver palpable 1 to 2 cm (0.4 to 0.8 inch) below right costal margin in young children
   b. Spleen, kidneys, and bladder palpated same as for adults
   c. Begin with light palpation and progress to deeper
   d. Palpate tender or painful areas last
   e. Palpate for inguinal or femoral hernias

N. Genitalia

NCLEX!

1. Always wear gloves during examination
2. Assess development of secondary sexual characteristics with Tanner's Sexual Maturity Rating scale
3. Male
   a. Inspect penis and urinary meatus
   b. Foreskin should be retractable by 3 months
   c. Redness, discharge, or lacerations in young children may indicate abuse
   d. Inspect and palpate scrotum and testes to determine if both are descended
   e. In young children, testicle may withdraw into inguinal canal because of cremasteric reflex
   f. Block cremasteric reflex in infants by beginning palpation at inguinal ring and moving down to scrotum
   g. Check for inguinal hernias by having child blow or bear down
4. Female
   a. Inspect external genitalia for evidence of discharge or redness which may indicate abuse in young children
   b. Internal examination for sexually active adolescents, or at age 16 to 18

O. Anus and rectum

1. Inspect for patency in infants
2. Skin should be smooth and free of lesions
3. Internal exam not done unless symptoms suggest a problem

P. Musculoskeletal

1. Inspect neck, extremities, hips, and spine for symmetry, increased or decreased mobility, and anatomical defects
   - **a.** Extremities should be warm, mobile, with pulses strong and equal bilaterally
   - **b.** Newborn's feet may be turned in but can be manipulated to normal position without resistance
   - **c.** True deformities do not return to normal position with manipulation
     - 1) *Metatarsus varus:* forefoot turned in
     - 2) *Talipes varus:* adduction of the forefoot and inversion of the entire foot
     - 3) *Talipes equinovarus:* Clubfoot, adduction of the forefoot, inversion of entire foot, and pointing downward of entire foot
     - 4) Medial tibial torsion: entire foot turned in while knee remains straight
     - 5) Medial femoral torsion: entire leg turned in with the foot
2. Assess for congenital hip dislocation
   - **a.** Assessed until about 1 year
   - **b.** Use Ortolani's maneuver
     - 1) With infant supine, flex knees while holding thumbs on mid-thighs and fingers over greater trochanters
     - 2) Abduct legs, moving knees outward and down toward table
   - **c.** Use Barlow's maneuver
     - 1) With infant supine, flex knees while holding thumbs on mid-thighs and fingers over greater trochanters
     - 2) Adduct legs until thumbs touch
   - **d.** Gluteal folds should be equal, hips abduct easily, and legs should be the same length
3. Assess spine and posture
   - **a.** Newborn spine is flexible and rounded
   - **b.** Cervical curve develops by 3 to 4 months
   - **c.** Lumbar curve develops by 12 to 18 months
   - **d.** Normal toddler has **lordosis** (exaggerated curvature of lumbar spine)
   - **e.** Check for **scoliosis** (lateral curvature of the spine) in adolescent girls by looking at spine as child is bent over with knees straight
4. Assess gait, joints, and muscles
   - **a.** Observe unobtrusively during history

b. Toddlers have wide-based gait and are usually bowlegged

c. Children 2 to 7 are often mildly knock-kneed

d. Scissoring gait in which thighs cross over each other with each step is common in cerebral palsy

e. Joints should have full range of motion, and muscles should be equally strong bilaterally

Q. Neurologic

NCLEX!

1. Integrate into overall assessment as much as possible

2. Assess child over 2 years the same as adult

3. Newborn and infant assessment

a. Observe symmetry of spontaneous movements, appearance, positioning, posture, and responsiveness to parents and environment

b. Assess level of consciousness, behavior, adaptation, and speech

4. Autonomic infant reflexes

a. Rooting reflex

1) Touch infant's lip or cheek, and infant should turn head toward stimulation and open mouth

2) Should disappear by 3 to 4 months

b. Sucking reflex

1) Infant should suck vigorously when gloved finger inserted into infant's mouth

2) Disappears by 10 to 12 months

c. Palmar grasp reflex

1) Pressing fingers against palmar surface of infant's hand produces grasp strong enough to pull infant to sitting position

2) Disappears by 3 to 4 months

d. Plantar grasp reflex

1) Touching the ball of the foot causes toes to curl downward tightly

2) Disappears by 8 to 10 months

e. Tonic neck reflex

1) With infant supine, turn head to one side; arm and leg on side to which head is turned will extend and opposite extremities will flex

2) Appears at about 2 months and disappears by 4 to 6 months

f. Moro reflex

1) Also called startle reflex

2) When a loud noise is created, the infant flexes and abducts legs, laterally extends arms, forms a "C" with thumb and forefinger, and fans other fingers

3) Immediately followed by anterior flexion and adduction of arms

4) Disappears by 3 months

g. Babinski reflex

1) While holding the infant's foot, stroke up the lateral edge across the ball

2) Positive reflex is fanning of the toes

3) Some infants have normal adult response of flexion of toes

4) Either response should be symmetrical bilaterally

5) Disappears within 2 years

h. Stepping reflex

1) Holding the infant upright with support under arms, let feet touch a surface and infant appears to take steps in a walking motion

2) Disappears by 2 months

5. Presence of reflexes beyond expected times indicates CNS problem

6. Cranial nerves and deep tendon reflexes are the same as for adults

7. Hand preference develops during preschool years

8. Observe for "soft" neurologic signs

a. The gray area between normal and abnormal, those things which may change with maturation

b. Short attention span, easy distractibility

c. Impulsiveness

d. Poor coordination

e. Language and articulation problems

f. Problems with learning, especially reading, writing, and arithmetic

IV. Common Laboratory Tests

A. Routine blood chemistry tests

1. Red blood count (RBC) or erythrocytes

a. Normal range for children 3.2 to 5.2 million/mm^3

b. Elevated in severe diarrhea or dehydration

c. Decreased in anemias, leukemia, and after hemorrhage

2. Hematocrit (Hct)

a. Normal range for children 30 to 54 percent

b. Elevated in dehydration

c. Decreased in anemias or after blood loss

d. Routine screening of toddlers and young schoolage children desirable

3. Hemoglobin (Hgb)

a. Normal range for children 10.3 to 18 g/dL

b. Increased in polycythemia or chronic obstructive pulmonary disease

c. Decreased in anemias, after blood loss, or excessive fluid intake

d. Routine screening of toddlers and young school-age children desirable

4. Platelet (thrombocyte) count

a. Normal range for children 150,000 to 465,000/mm^3

b. Increased in infections, acute blood loss, and splenectomy

c. Decreased in cancer, renal or liver disease, and aplastic anemia

5. White blood count (WBC) or leukocytes

a. Normal range in children 5,000 to 13,000/mm^3

b. Increased in acute infections, burns, leukemia, and sickle cell anemia

c. Decreased in aplastic anemia and viral infections

B. Serum electrolytes

1. Potassium (K)

a. Normal range in children 3.5 to 5.5 mEq/L

b. Increased (hyperkalemia) in renal failure, severe burns or tissue trauma, or metabolic acidosis

c. Decreased (hypokalemia) in vomiting, diarrhea, dehydration, gastric suctioning, or metabolic alkalosis

2. Sodium (Na)

a. Normal range in children 135 to 145 mEq/L

b. Increased in dehydration, severe vomiting, and diarrhea

c. Decreased in gastric suctioning, burns, or tissue injury

3. Chloride (Cl)

a. Normal range in children 95 to 105 mEq/L

b. Increased in dehydration, high serum Na level, metabolic acidosis

c. Decreased in vomiting, diarrhea, acute infections, burns, or metabolic alkalosis

4. Magnesium (Mg)

a. Normal range in children 1.6 to 2.6 mEq/L

b. Increased in severe dehydration, renal failure, early diabetes mellitus, and leukemia

c. Decreased in protein malnutrition, hypokalemia, or chronic diarrhea

5. Calcium (Ca)

a. Normal range in children 4.4 to 5.8 mEq/L

b. Increased in multiple fractures or hyperparathyroidism

c. Decreased in lack of calcium or vitamin D intake, burns, or diarrhea

C. Lead

1. Accumulates in the body with exposure and can lead to significant health problems
2. Desirable levels are below 9 μg/dL; levels between 10 to 20 μg/dL suggest need for more frequent monitoring; levels above 20 μg/dL usually require pharmacologic treatment
3. Increased in exposure to high levels of lead through heater fumes, lead-based paint, unglazed pottery, or batteries
4. Desirable to screen toddlers and children who are considered at high risk because of possible environmental exposure

D. Glucose

1. Normal range in children 60 to 105 mg/dL
2. Increased in diabetes mellitus, burns, severe infections
3. Deceased in hypoglycemia or malnutrition

E. Cholesterol

1. Normal range in children 130 to 170 mg/dL
2. Increased in hypercholesterolemia or uncontrolled diabetes mellitus
3. Decreased in starvation or hyperthyroidism
4. Screen children and adolescents if positive family history of high cholesterol

F. Triglycerides

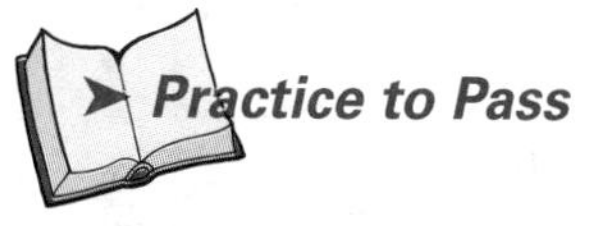

How will the nurse decide which laboratory screening tests would be appropriate for a 7-year-old child?

1. Normal range in children 10 to 140 mg/dL
2. Increased in high-carbohydrate diet, hyperlipoproteinemia, or uncontrolled diabetes mellitus
3. Decreased in protein malnutrition
4. Screen children and adolescents if positive family history of elevated triglycerides

V. Denver Developmental Screening Test II (Denver II)

A. Purpose

1. Detection of potential developmental problems in young children
2. Used to confirm suspicion of developmental delay
3. Can be used to monitor children at risk for developmental delays

B. Description (see Figure 2-3)

NCLEX!

1. Designed to be used on well children between birth and 6 years
2. The test assesses performance on age-appropriate tasks
3. Should not be used in place of diagnostic evaluation or physical assessment
4. Assesses four areas of functioning
   a. Personal–social: getting along with people and caring for personal needs

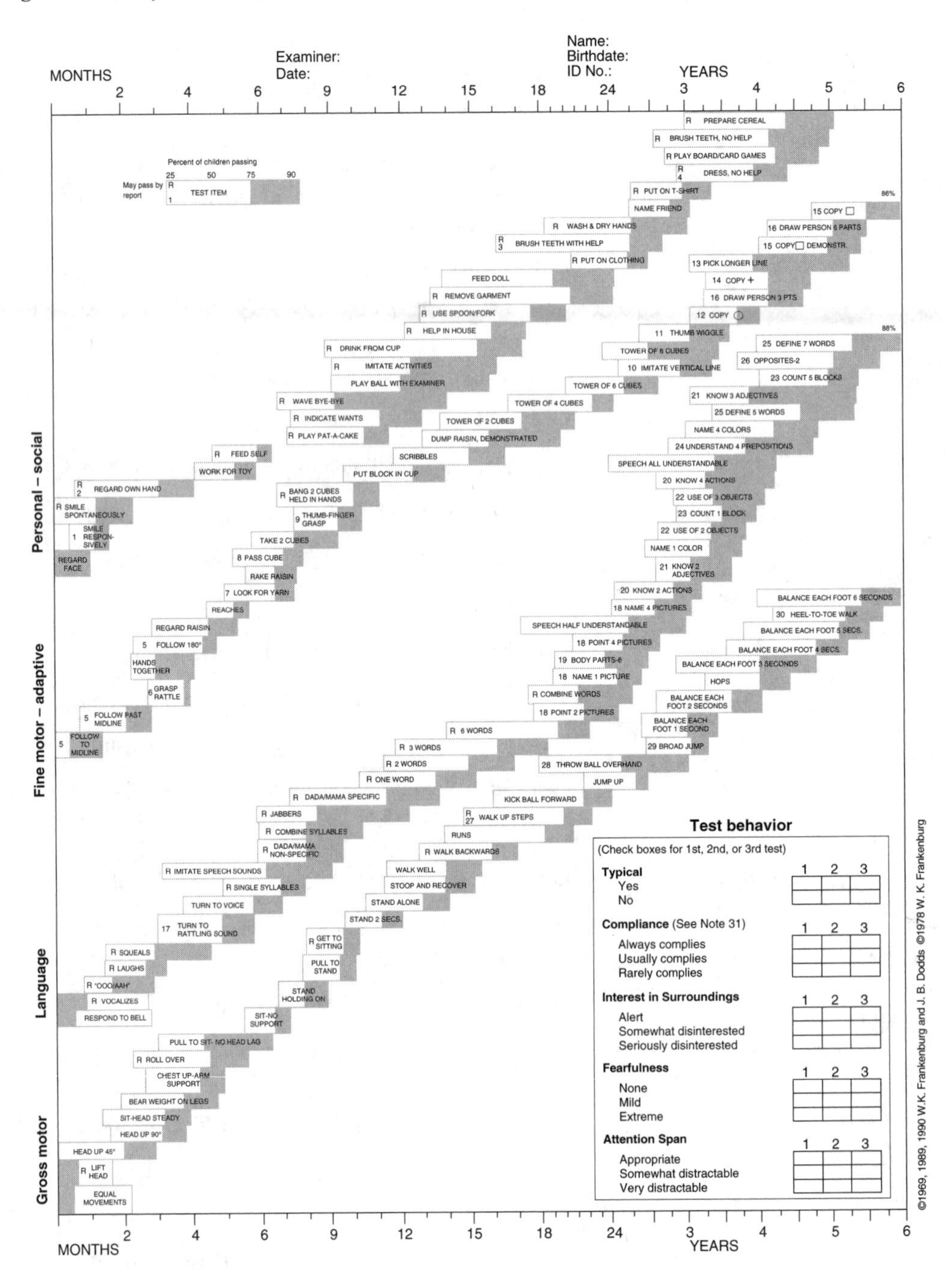

Figure 2-3

Denver Developmental Screening Test II (Denver II).

Source: Ball, J. & Bindler, R. (1999). *Pediatric nursing: Caring for children* (2nd ed.). Stamford, CT: Appleton & Lange, pp. 216–217.

b. Fine motor–adaptive: hand-eye coordination, manipulation of small objects, and problem solving

c. Language: hearing, understanding, and using language

d. Gross motor: sitting, walking, jumping, and large muscle movement

5. "Test behavior" items completed at conclusion of test to rate child's behavior

6. Becomes basis for nursing care plan to provide activities that promote development in weak areas

Figure 2-3

(continued)

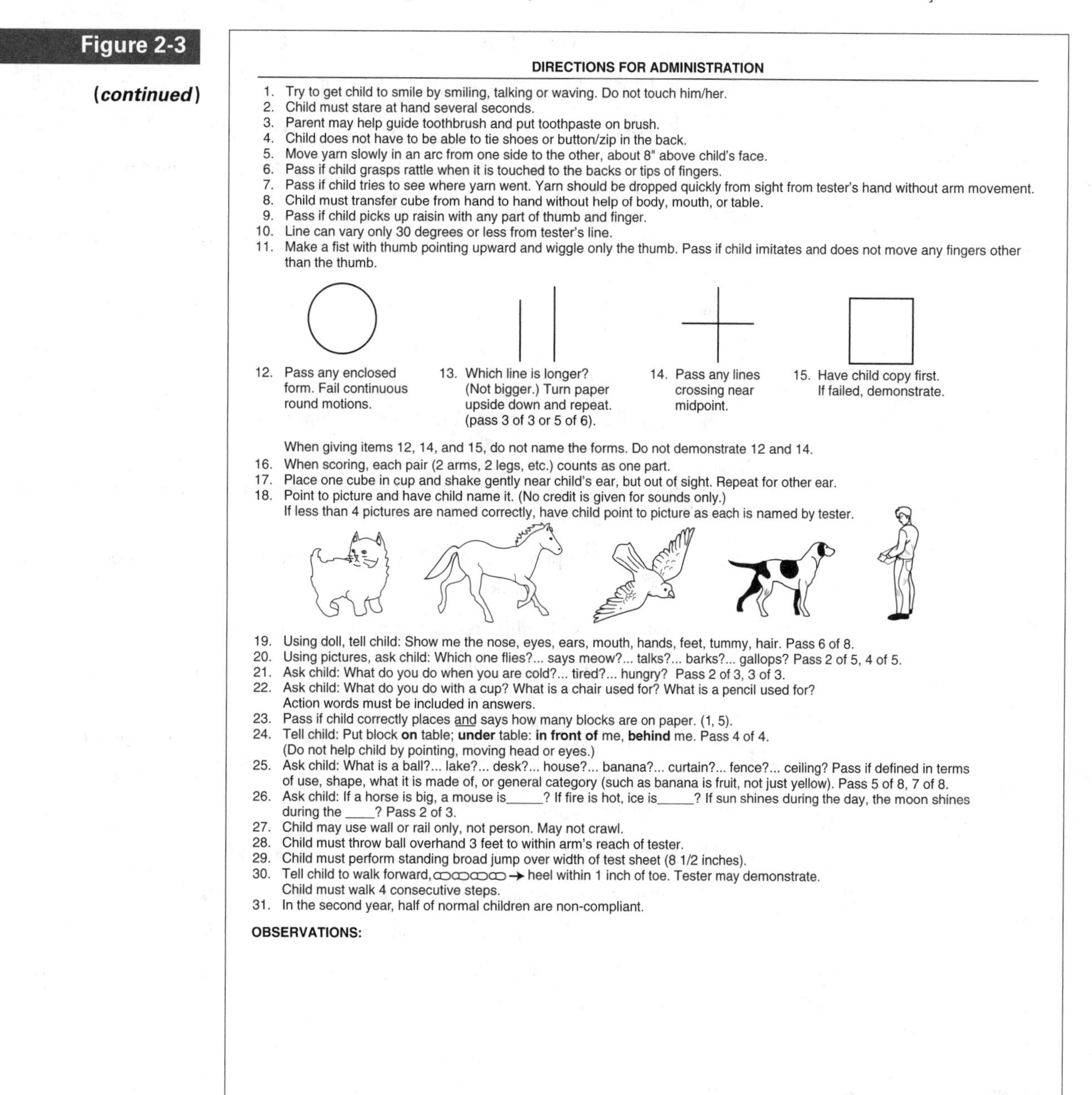

DIRECTIONS FOR ADMINISTRATION

1. Try to get child to smile by smiling, talking or waving. Do not touch him/her.
2. Child must stare at hand several seconds.
3. Parent may help guide toothbrush and put toothpaste on brush.
4. Child does not have to be able to tie shoes or button/zip in the back.
5. Move yarn slowly in an arc from one side to the other, about 8" above child's face.
6. Pass if child grasps rattle when it is touched to the backs or tips of fingers.
7. Pass if child tries to see where yarn went. Yarn should be dropped quickly from sight from tester's hand without arm movement.
8. Child must transfer cube from hand to hand without help of body, mouth, or table.
9. Pass if child picks up raisin with any part of thumb and finger.
10. Line can vary only 30 degrees or less from tester's line.
11. Make a fist with thumb pointing upward and wiggle only the thumb. Pass if child imitates and does not move any fingers other than the thumb.

12. Pass any enclosed form. Fail continuous round motions.
13. Which line is longer? (Not bigger.) Turn paper upside down and repeat. (pass 3 of 3 or 5 of 6).
14. Pass any lines crossing near midpoint.
15. Have child copy first. If failed, demonstrate.

When giving items 12, 14, and 15, do not name the forms. Do not demonstrate 12 and 14.

16. When scoring, each pair (2 arms, 2 legs, etc.) counts as one part.
17. Place one cube in cup and shake gently near child's ear, but out of sight. Repeat for other ear.
18. Point to picture and have child name it. (No credit is given for sounds only.) If less than 4 pictures are named correctly, have child point to picture as each is named by tester.
19. Using doll, tell child: Show me the nose, eyes, ears, mouth, hands, feet, tummy, hair. Pass 6 of 8.
20. Using pictures, ask child: Which one flies?... says meow?... talks?... barks?... gallops? Pass 2 of 5, 4 of 5.
21. Ask child: What do you do when you are cold?... tired?... hungry? Pass 2 of 3, 3 of 3.
22. Ask child: What do you do with a cup? What is a chair used for? What is a pencil used for? Action words must be included in answers.
23. Pass if child correctly places and says how many blocks are on paper. (1, 5).
24. Tell child: Put block **on** table; **under** table: **in front of** me, **behind** me. Pass 4 of 4. (Do not help child by pointing, moving head or eyes.)
25. Ask child: What is a ball?... lake?... desk?... house?... banana?... curtain?... fence?... ceiling? Pass if defined in terms of use, shape, what it is made of, or general category (such as banana is fruit, not just yellow). Pass 5 of 8, 7 of 8.
26. Ask child: If a horse is big, a mouse is_____? If fire is hot, ice is_____? If sun shines during the day, the moon shines during the ____? Pass 2 of 3.
27. Child may use wall or rail only, not person. May not crawl.
28. Child must throw ball overhand 3 feet to within arm's reach of tester.
29. Child must perform standing broad jump over width of test sheet (8 1/2 inches).
30. Tell child to walk forward, → heel within 1 inch of toe. Tester may demonstrate. Child must walk 4 consecutive steps.
31. In the second year, half of normal children are non-compliant.

OBSERVATIONS:

C. Test administration

NCLEX!

1. Age calculation is very important and must be done according to guidelines
2. Age may be adjusted for prematurity between birth and 2 years only
3. Items that require "report" from parent should be scored first
4. Easy tasks are administered first with praise given regardless of pass or fail on that item

5. Materials from test kit (blocks, etc.) should be used next
    a. Only material used for specific testing item should be visible to child
    b. Keep all other materials out of sight until needed
6. For infants, all items that need to be administered with the baby lying down should be done at the same time
7. In each testing area, begin with items to the left of child's age line and move right
8. Generally, administer items to the right of any passes until three failures are recorded
9. Scoring
    a. P (Pass): successful performance of an item, or caregiver reports that child does the item
    b. F (Fail): unsuccessful performance of an item, or caregiver reports that child does not do the item
    c. NO (No opportunity): only used for "report" items; child does not have opportunity to do the item
    d. R (Refused): child refuses to attempt item
    e. C (Caution): when child fails or refuses an item on which the age line falls between 75th and 90th percentile
    f. D (Delayed): when child fails or refuses item that 90 percent of standardized sample passed

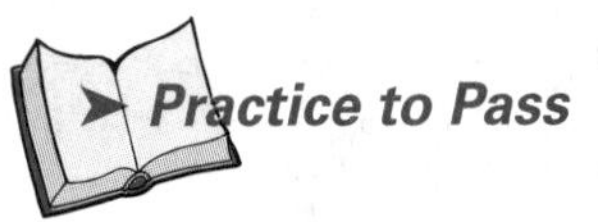

How should the nurse explain the Denver II to an anxious parent?

D. Test interpretation

1. Normal: no delays, maximum of one caution
2. Suspect: two or more cautions, or one or more delays
3. Untestable: refusal on one or more items to left of child's age
4. Referral only after retest is also suspect or untestable and other assessments (physical or history) indicate a need

Case Study

The nurse is preparing to do a health history and physical assessment on a 5-year-old child whose family is new to the area.

❶ Why does the nurse want to establish quickly the reason for the visit?

❷ How can the nurse make the mother and child feel comfortable?

❸ What strategies should the nurse employ to gain the trust and cooperation of the child?

❹ What measures will the nurse use to establish the child's nutritional status?

❺ What laboratory tests might the nurse want to consider ordering for this child?

For suggested responses, see page 407.

Posttest

1 When using the otoscope to examine the ears of a 2-year-old child, the nurse should:

(1) Pull the pinna up and back.
(2) Pull the pinna down and back.
(3) Hold the pinna gently but firmly in its normal position.
(4) Hold the pinna against the skull.

2 To assess the height of an 18-month-old child who is brought to the clinic for routine examination, the nurse should:

(1) Measure arm span to estimate adult height.
(2) Use a tape measure.
(3) Use a horizontal measuring board.
(4) Have the child stand on an upright scale and use the measuring arm.

3 At what age is it appropriate to change the sequence of the examination of the child from that of chest and thorax first to head-to-toe?

(1) Infant
(2) Toddler
(3) Preschool child
(4) Schoolage child

4 The best description of a nursing diagnosis is:

(1) A process used to evaluate the etiology of a disease.
(2) A nursing judgment about the health of an individual.
(3) A problem-oriented description of an actual or potential health problem.
(4) An efficient basis for communicating client data among nurses.

5 Screening for strabismus and amblyopia should be part of the physical assessment of which children?

(1) All children under 18
(2) Infants
(3) Preschool children
(4) Schoolage children

6 In infants, a positive Babinski reflex is:

(1) An indication of a neurological problem.
(2) Dorsiflexion of the toes.
(3) Fanning of the toes.
(4) Withdrawing the foot from the stimulus.

7 The review of systems part of the health history is best described as:

(1) The description of the health problem in the informant's words.
(2) The objective data recorded by the nurse.
(3) The evaluation of the past and present health of each body system.
(4) A general statement about the overall health of the child.

8 The nurse would perform abdominal percussion to assess for:

(1) Tenderness.
(2) Inflammation.
(3) Density of tissues and organs.
(4) Size and placement of liver.

9 When assessing a 4-year-old child with a persistent cough, the nurse would assess respirations by observing which muscle group?

(1) Thoracic
(2) Abdominal
(3) Accessory
(4) Intercostal

10 **When assessing the fontanels of a 6-week-old infant, how soon does the nurse expect the posterior fontanel to close?**

(1) By 3 months
(2) By 6 months
(3) By 12 months
(4) By 18 months

See pages 54–55 for Answers and Rationales.

Answers and Rationales

Pretest

1 **Answer: 2** ***Rationale:*** An infant of 7 months just begins to transfer objects from one hand to the other. Smiling at self begins at about 5 months; imitating sounds and rolling over begin at about 6 months of age.
Cognitive Level: Analysis
Nursing Process: Assessment; ***Test Plan:*** HPM

2 **Answer: 1** ***Rationale:*** The Snellen eye chart measures visual acuity by assessing from a set distance how well a child can see. An ophthalmoscope looks at the internal parts of the eye, the cover-uncover test measures eye muscle coordination, and the Weber test measures hearing.
Cognitive Level: Application
Nursing Process: Assessment; ***Test Plan:*** HPM

3 **Answer: 3** ***Rationale:*** By age 7, most children are able to clearly and in chronological order describe symptoms. Their vocabulary is extensive enough to have words to describe what they are feeling, time of onset, changes from the norm, etc.
Cognitive Level: Analysis
Nursing Process: Assessment; ***Test Plan:*** HPM

4 **Answer: 3** ***Rationale:*** It is important for the nurse to know the immunization record and status for any child. If a child is not up to date with immunizations it is up to the nurse to plan with the family a schedule to get necessary immunizations. Hospitalizations, coping mechanisms, and accidents are important for the nurse, but immunizations are uniquely important for pediatric clients.
Cognitive Level: Analysis
Nursing Process: Assessment; ***Test Plan:*** HPM

5 **Answer: 2** ***Rationale:*** The purpose of a genogram is to have a pictorial representation of a child's family history. It identifies at least three generations by gender, age, health status, cause of death, and family genetic relationships. Past history, treatment, and immunizations are not recorded on a genogram.
Cognitive Level: Analysis
Nursing Process: Implementation; ***Test Plan:*** HPM

6 **Answer: 4** ***Rationale:*** The normal range for most children falls somewhere between the 5th and 95th percentile. The other ranges do not accommodate as many variations in height and weight that are considered normal.
Cognitive Level: Application
Nursing Process: Assessment; ***Test Plan:*** HPM

7 **Answer: 3** ***Rationale:*** Save the painful area for last to avoid abdominal guarding and to gain the child's trust. Always tell the child before touching a tender area.
Cognitive Level: Analysis
Nursing Process: Assessment; ***Test Plan:*** PHYS

8 **Answer: 2** ***Rationale:*** The Denver II is used to screen children for possible developmental delays in the areas of gross-motor skills, language, fine-motor skills, and personal-social development. The Denver II does not measure intelligence, cognitive, or speech difficulties.
Cognitive Level: Application
Nursing Process: Assessment; ***Test Plan:*** HPM

9 **Answer: 2** ***Rationale:*** Auscultation is always easiest in a sleeping or quiet baby. Checking the eyes is considered invasive and should be saved for the end of the examination. There is no need to awaken the child because he or she will begin to stir once the examination begins.
Cognitive Level: Analysis
Nursing Process: Assessment; ***Test Plan:*** HPM

10 **Answer: 2** ***Rationale:*** The preschooler may be somewhat anxious so the nurse should give feedback and reassurance about what will be done. Children do not need detailed explanations nor do they need to be told to act older than they are. Most children at this age are willing to remove clothing.
Cognitive Level: Application
Nursing Process: Assessment; ***Test Plan:*** HPM

Posttest

1 **Answer: 2** ***Rationale:*** The ear canal in infants and young children is shorter, wider, and more horizontally positioned than in older children. To adequately

examine the tympanic membrane in young children the pinna must be pulled back and down.
Cognitive Level: Application
Nursing Process: Assessment; ***Test Plan:*** HPM

2 **Answer: 3** ***Rationale:*** Children younger than 2 or 3 should be measured lying down, preferably on a horizontal measuring board, to get an accurate assessment of height. A tape measure would be used to measure head circumference. An arm-span measure is not an appropriate estimation of adult height.
Cognitive Level: Application
Nursing Process: Assessment; ***Test Plan:*** HPM

3 **Answer: 4** ***Rationale:*** The schoolage years are the first time a child is able to reliably cooperate with the examiner and not squirm, talk, or otherwise interrupt the exam. In younger children, it is essential to begin with the chest and thorax because the child needs to be quiet and at rest.
Cognitive Level: Analysis
Nursing Process: Assessment; ***Test Plan:*** HPM

4 **Answer: 3** ***Rationale:*** A nursing diagnosis is a statement of an actual or potential problem that can be resolved or changed by nursing interventions. It involves the use of common labels established by NANDA. Nursing diagnoses are based on data collected by the nurse but are not related to disease etiology or judgments of the overall health status of a client.
Cognitive Level: Knowledge
Nursing Process: Analysis; ***Test Plan:*** HPM

5 **Answer: 3** ***Rationale:*** Strabismus is detected with the cover-uncover test that can first be reliably administered to children over the age of 2. It is important to detect the problem early to prevent amblyopia. By school age, vision loss would have occurred.
Cognitive Level: Analysis
Nursing Process: Assessment; ***Test Plan:*** HPM

6 **Answer: 3** ***Rationale:*** A positive Babinski in infants is a fanning of the toes when a stimulus is applied to the foot along the lateral edge and across the ball. The response disappears by about age 2.
Cognitive Level: Application
Nursing Process: Assessment; ***Test Plan:*** HPM

7 **Answer: 3** ***Rationale:*** The review of systems is a systematic review of each body system with respect to past and present health problems. It is designed to provide a basis for focusing the physical assessment on problem areas. The statement of the health problem is the reason for seeking care, sometimes called the chief complaint. Objective data is gathered during the physical assessment and from laboratory data.
Cognitive Level: Knowledge
Nursing Process: Assessment; ***Test Plan:*** HPM

8 **Answer: 3** ***Rationale:*** Percussion produces sounds of varying loudness and pitch depending on the organs and tissue density. The nurse assesses the liver with palpation and percussion, but not for placement. Inflammation is assessed with inspection, and tenderness is assessed with palpation.
Cognitive Level: Analysis
Nursing Process: Assessment; ***Test Plan:*** HPM

9 **Answer: 2** ***Rationale:*** Infants and young children use the diaphragm and abdominal muscles for respiration, so the nurse would watch the rise and fall of the abdomen to count respirations. Use of accessory or intercostal muscles may be observed in respiratory distress.
Cognitive Level: Application
Nursing Process: Assessment; ***Test Plan:*** HPM

10 **Answer: 1** ***Rationale:*** The posterior fontanel closes by 3 months of age. The anterior fontanel closes by 18 months.
Cognitive Level: Application
Nursing Process: Assessment; ***Test Plan:*** HPM

References

Ball, J. & Bindler, R. (1999). *Pediatric nursing: Caring for children* (2nd ed.). Stamford, CT: Appleton & Lange, pp. 6–7, 54–119, 133, 147, 169.

Barkauskas, V. H., Stoltenberg-Allen, K., Baumann, L. C. & Darling-Fisher, C. (1998). *Health & physical assessment* (2nd ed.). St. Louis: Mosby, pp. 646–712.

Behrman, R. F., Kliegman, B. M., & Jenson, H. R. (Eds.). (2000). *Nelson's textbook of pediatrics* (16th ed.). St. Louis: Mosby, pp. 30–61.

Bowden, V. R., Dickey, S. B., & Greenberg, C. S. (1998). *Children and their families: The continuum of care.* Philadelphia: W. B. Saunders, pp. 345–385.

Fischbach, F. (2000). *A manual of laboratory and diagnostic tests* (6th ed.). Philadelphia: Lippincott.

Frankenburg, W. K., Dodds, J., Archer, P., Bresnick, B., Maschka, P., Edelman, N., & Shapiro, H. (1992). *Denver II training manual.* Denver: Denver Developmental Materials, Inc., pp. 1–48.

Jarvis, C. (2000). *Physical examination and health assessment* (3rd ed.) Philadelphia: W. B. Saunders.

Kee, J. L. (2001). *Handbook of laboratory and diagnostic tests with nursing implications* (4th ed.). Upper Saddle River, NJ: Prentice Hall, Inc.

Kozier, B., Erb, G., Berman, A. J., & Burke, K. (2000). *Fundamentals of nursing: Concepts, process, and practice* (6th ed.). Upper Saddle River, NJ: Prentice Hall, Inc., pp. 268–340.

Leasia, M. S. & Monahan, F. D. (1997). *A practical guide to health assessment.* Philadelphia: W. B. Saunders, pp. 1–74.

Weber, J. (1997). *Nurses' handbook of health assessment* (3rd ed.). Philadelphia: Lippincott, pp. 356–396.

Weber, J. & Kelley, J. (1998). *Health assessment in nursing.* Philadelphia: Lippincott, pp. 893–1016.

Wong, D., Hockenberry-Eaton, M., Wilson, D., Winkelstein, M., Ahmann, E., & DiVito-Thomas, P. (1999). *Whaley and Wong's nursing care of infants and children* (6th ed.). St. Louis: Mosby, pp. 200–298.

CHAPTER 3

Eye, Ear, Nose, and Throat Problems

J. Mari Beth Barr, PhD, RNC

CHAPTER OUTLINE

Disorders of the Ear
Disorders of the Eye
Disorders of the Throat
Disorders of the Nose

OBJECTIVES

- Identify data essential to the assessment of alterations in health of the sensory organs in a child.
- Discuss the clinical manifestations and pathophysiology of alterations in health of the sensory organs in a child.
- Discuss therapeutic management of a child with alterations in health of the sensory organs.
- Describe nursing management of a child with alterations in health of the sensory organs.

[Media Link]

Use the CD-ROM enclosed with this text, or log onto the address given to access the free, interactive Companion Website created for this series. The CD-ROM and Companion Website accompanying this book offer additional practice opportunities and information—NCLEX Review, Case Studies, Glossary, In Depth with NCLEX, and more.

www.prenhall.com/hogan

REVIEW AT A GLANCE

amblyopia *"lazy eye" results when one eye does not receive sufficient stimulation; can cause eventual loss of vision in the affected eye*

conjunctivitis *inflammation of the conjunctiva, which can result from a variety of causes*

corneal light reflex (Hirschberg test) *a screening test for strabismus and symmetrical alignment of the eyes*

cover-uncover test *a screening test for "lazy eye"*

epistaxis *nosebleed*

otitis media *inflammation of the middle ear*

pharyngitis *inflammation of the pharynx*

sensory impairment *a general term that indicates disability that may range in severity from mild to profound; includes hearing impairment and visual impairment*

strabismus *misalignment of eyes*

tonsillitis *inflammation of the tonsils, resulting in tonsillar enlargement, frequently occurs with pharyngitis*

Pretest

1 The physician orders amoxicillin (Amoxil) 500 mg IVPB q 8 hours for a pediatric client with tonsillitis. What is the appropriate nursing action?

(1) Question the order because the route of administration is incorrect.
(2) Give the medication as ordered.
(3) Question the order because the dosage is too high.
(4) Question the order because the dosing frequency is incorrect.

2 The nurse administers cefprozil (Cefzil) as ordered to a 22-month-old client with bacterial pharyngitis. The nurse notes patches of white on the child's oral mucosa that cannot be removed. Which condition does the nurse suspect?

(1) Allergic reaction to the medication manifested by the development of stomatitis
(2) A herpes simplex virus infection
(3) Oral thrush caused by *Candida albicans*
(4) Mumps

3 A pediatric client has been diagnosed with otitis media. The nurse should place highest priority on teaching the parent:

(1) How to administer ear drops.
(2) The importance of completing the full course of antibiotic therapy.
(3) About myringotomy and tympanostomy tube insertion.
(4) About eliminating environmental allergens.

4 Nursing care of the child who is postoperative for a tonsillectomy should include:

(1) Applying warm, moist compresses to the neck area.
(2) Observing for excessive swallowing.
(3) Maintaining the child in a supine position.
(4) Offering warm liquids with a straw for the child to sip.

5 The nurse is caring for a child with a common cold (nasopharyngitis). The primary goal of nursing care is directed toward:

(1) Preventing injury.
(2) Promoting nutrition.
(3) Relieving symptoms.
(4) Administering antibiotics.

6 The nurse obtains a health history on a pediatric client. A sign alerting the nurse to possible hearing impairment in the child is:

(1) Distractability and short attention span.
(2) Disinterest in reading story books.
(3) Turning up the volume on the family television set.
(4) Temper tantrums.

7 **The nurse is caring for a 1-month-old client who is blind, secondary to retinopathy of prematurity. The nurse is teaching the parents about activities to promote their infant's development. Which of the following statements by the nurse is correct?**

(1) "Infants with visual impairment respond to tactile stimuli rather than auditory stimuli."
(2) "Talking, holding, and singing to your baby are appropriate activities at this age."
(3) "You should expect your baby to smile in response to your voice by 4 months of age."
(4) "Position the baby side-lying in the crib at all times, and avoid loud noises that could startle the infant."

8 **The nurse is assessing a child with conjunctivitis (pink eye). Which of the following would the nurse most likely assess?**

(1) Serous drainage from the affected eye
(2) Severe eye pain
(3) Periorbital edema
(4) Crusting of eyelids and eyelashes

9 **The nurse teaches a child with conjunctivitis measures to prevent the spread of infection. The nurse recognizes that further teaching is needed when the child states the following:**

(1) "I will wash my hands frequently."
(2) "I will use a tissue to clean my eye and then throw the tissue away."
(3) "I will use my own washcloth and towel, and not use my brother's."
(4) "I will carry a handkerchief with me so that I can wipe my eyes during the day."

10 **A 4-month-old infant has severe nasal congestion, nasal mucous drainage and crusting in and around the nares. What is the best way for the nurse to clear the infant's nasal passages?**

(1) Administer vasoconstrictive nose drops every 3 hours.
(2) Place the infant in a mist tent.
(3) Administer saline drops in the nose and suction with bulb syringe.
(4) Instruct the client to blow the nose and keep disposable tissues handy.

See pages 72–73 for Answers and Rationales.

I. Disorders of the Ear

A. *Otitis media*

1. Description

a. Inflammation of the middle ear

b. One of the most common childhood illnesses

2. Etiology and pathophysiology

a. Greatest incidence is between 6 and 36 months of age during winter months

b. Otitis media is related to Eustachian tube dysfunction; the Eustachian tube provides drainage and ventilation of the middle ear; when it is blocked as a result of edema from an upper-respiratory infection, fluid can accumulate in the middle ear; this fluid is a medium for bacterial growth and the development of middle ear infection (see Figure 3-1)

c. Children with facial malformations such as cleft palate and Down syndrome have anatomic variations of their Eustachian tubes, which can make them more vulnerable to otitis media

Figure 3-1

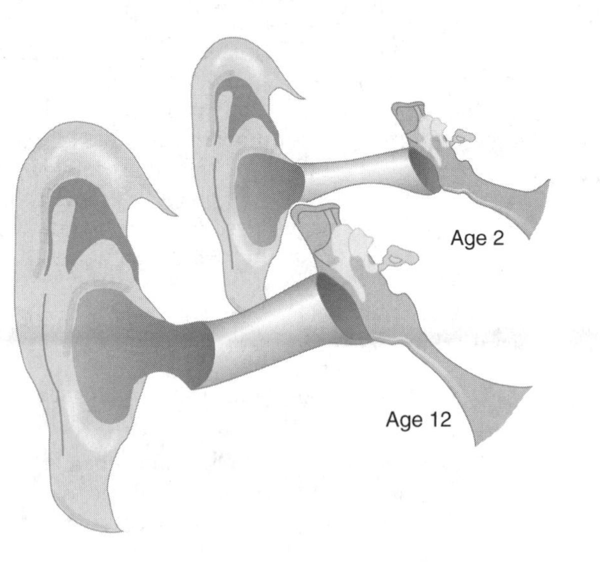

Eustacian tube in a child. *Source:* Ball, J. & Bindler, R. (1999). *Pediatric nursing: Caring for children* (2nd ed.). Stamford, CT: Appleton & Lange, p. 713.

d. Causative organisms: the most common organisms in otitis media are *Streptococcus pneumoniae, Haemophilus influenzae,* and *Neisseria catarrhalis*

3. Assessment

a. Ear pain, irritability, diarrhea, fever and vomiting are common

b. Pulling at the affected ear may be noted; some children are asymptomatic

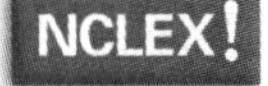

c. Diagnosis is based on an examination of the tympanic membrane using an otoscope; a red, bulging, nonmobile tympanic membrane is indicative of otitis media

4. Priority nursing diagnoses

a. Pain

b. Hyperthermia

c. Risk for injury

5. Planning and implementation

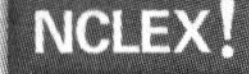

a. Teach parents that as the child grows older, the position of the Eustachian tube changes to facilitate drainage of the middle ear

b. Recurrent infections will eventually cease

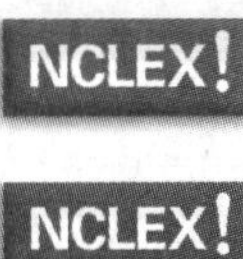

c. Parents should avoid smoking around the child, as exposure to secondhand smoke increases the incidence of otitis media

d. Parents should be taught that otitis media is a bacterial infection and requires a full course of treatment with antibiotics; parents should be cautioned to avoid discontinuing the antibiotic when symptoms subside, but they should be encouraged to complete the full course of antibiotic therapy, usually 10 to 14 days

e. Nursing management of the child with tympanostomy tubes: usually the surgery is accomplished in a day-surgery center, not an inpatient hospital setting

1) Parents should be taught to give acetaminophen (Tylenol) for discomfort following the myringotomy and insertion of tympanostomy tubes

2) Parents should follow their physician's directions for postoperative care of the ear, often eardrops are prescribed

3) Some physicians require parents to insert earplugs for bathing and swimming and avoid water in the ear canal; others do not

4) Parents should be taught that ear tubes will spontaneously extrude and fall out; they may note the presence of the spool-shaped tube in the child's ear canal; ear tubes usually fall out in about 1 year

6. Medication therapy

a. Antibiotic therapy for 10 to 14 days; first-line drugs are amoxicillin (Amoxil), and trimethoprim-sulfamethoxazole (Bactrim, Septra); both drugs are given orally

b. Recurrent or chronic otitis media infections may require prophylactic antibiotic therapy as a 6-month trial

7. Surgical procedures

a. Myringotomy is surgical incision of the tympanic membrane

b. Tympanostomy tubes are used for drainage and ventilation of the middle ear

8. Child and family education

a. Teach parents signs and symptoms of otitis media

b. Explain the need to monitor and treat temperature

NCLEX!

c. Explain how to administer medication safely and effectively (complete full course of antibiotic therapy even if feeling better; give doses on time)

9. Evaluation: child recovers from otitis media without sequelae; parents describe safe and effective medication administration

B. Hearing impairment

1. Description

a. Condition that interferes with the ability to receive auditory communications from the environment

b. There are three types of hearing impairment: conductive hearing loss, sensorineural hearing loss, and mixed hearing loss

c. Hearing impairment is one form of **sensory impairment,** while visual impairment would be another

2. Etiology and pathophysiology

a. Conductive hearing loss: occurs when tympanic membrane cannot vibrate freely, or when sounds cannot reach middle ear; common causes are otitis media, impacted cerumen, and foreign body in the ear canal

NCLEX!

b. Sensorineural hearing loss: occurs with damage to the cochlea or auditory nerve; sensorineural hearing loss may be congenital (as in congenital rubella syndrome) or acquired (ototoxic drugs); the hearing loss may also be genetic in origin, as in the hearing loss of those affected with Tay-Sachs disease

c. Mixed hearing loss: mixed hearing loss involves a combination of conductive and sensorineural hearing losses

NCLEX!

3. Assessment

a. In infants and young children with hearing loss, language development is affected; hearing loss should be diagnosed as early as possible to promote optimal development

b. Signs of hearing impairment in infancy: does not startle to loud noises, arouses to touch and not noise, does not turn head to sounds or localize sounds, little or no babbling or vocalizations

c. Signs of hearing impairment in toddlers and preschoolers: communicates through gestures; little or no speech, unintelligible speech; developmental delay; no response to doorbell, telephone

d. Signs of hearing impairment in school-aged children and adolescents: sits close to speaker or turns up TV volume loudly, poor school performance, speech problems, cannot correctly respond except when able to view speaker's face

e. Diagnosis: the type of hearing loss is diagnosed by otoscopic examination, tympanography, and audiography

4. Priority nursing diagnoses

a. Sensory/perceptual alterations (auditory)

b. Impaired verbal communication

c. Risk for altered growth and development

d. Risk for ineffective family coping

5. Planning and implementation

a. If hearing loss is correctable, treatment of the cause underlying the hearing loss is accomplished, for example, removal of a foreign body in conductive loss

b. If the hearing loss cannot be corrected, a multidisciplinary team consisting of the otolaryngologist, audiologist, pediatrician, nurse, and speech-language pathologist should work with the child and family to obtain appropriate therapies and enhance communication

c. Hearing aids may be prescribed

f. Nurses function in preventing acquired hearing loss through educating others to avoid exposure to loud noises

g. Advocate prompt treatment of otitis media

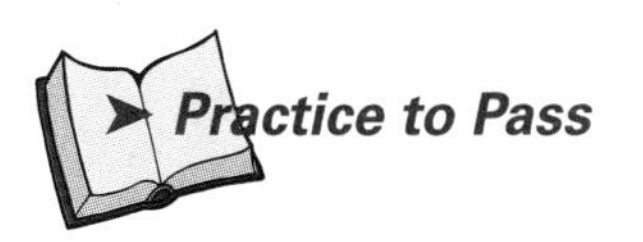

An 18-month-old client with a history of chronic otitis media is scheduled for bilateral myringotomy with placement of tympanostomy tubes. What content will you plan to include in your preoperative and postoperative teaching sessions with the parents?

h. Nurses should be skilled in developmental assessment to aid in early identification of infants and children with hearing loss; early identification is important to prevent significant delays in developmental progress and school performance

i. Nurses should act as advocates for clients with hearing impairment and their families; nurses can provide support and appropriate referrals to the child and family dealing with this disability

6. Child and family education

a. Teach parents means of communicating with their children

b. Encourage parents to enroll their child in early intervention to promote speech development

7. Evaluation: the child develops communication skills; hearing evaluations do not deteriorate

II. Disorders of the Eye

A. *Conjunctivitis*

1. Description: inflammation of the conjunctiva, also known as "pink eye"

2. Etiology and pathophysiology

a. The conjunctiva is a clear membrane lining the inside of the eyelids and sclera; it is normally pink and clear, smooth and moist

b. Bacteria, viruses, allergens, trauma, or other irritants can cause the conjunctiva to become reddened (erythematous) and edematous

c. A yellow, white, or green purulent exudate may be present in the affected eye; there is excessive tearing of the affected eye

d. Bacterial conjunctivitis is contagious

3. Assessment

a. Conjunctiva reddened and edematous

b. Yellow, white, or green purulent exudate

c. Crusting present on eyelids and lashes

4. Priority nursing diagnoses

a. Pain

b. Knowledge deficit: safe administration of eye drops and ointments

NCLEX!

5. Planning and implementation

a. Nursing care focuses on measures to prevent the spread of infection

b. Although the eye may feel itchy, children should avoid rubbing their eyes; careful attention to handwashing and avoiding shared items is important

c. The eye should be cleansed with warm water and any crusting or exudate removed before instilling eye drops or eye ointment

6. Medication therapy: antibiotic drops or ointment will be ordered if infection is bacterial

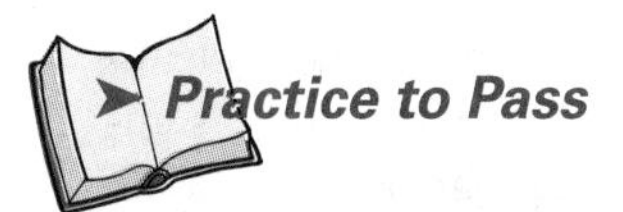

Parents of a 2-year-old child just diagnosed with bacterial conjunctivitis with antibiotic ophthalmic ointment prescribed ask the nurse when the child can return to daycare. What is the nurse's correct response?

7. Child and family education
   a. Caregivers should be taught to instill antibiotic drops or ointment into the conjunctival sac
   b. Instructions are given on prevention measures to limit the spread of infection to the other eye or other people
7. Evaluation: parents demonstrate safe and effective administration of eye drops/ointment; infection does not spread to other family members

B. *Amblyopia*

1. Description
   a. Also known as "lazy eye"
   b. Reduction of central vision in an eye that is normal
2. Etiology and pathophysiology
   a. Results from untreated strabismus, and causes decreased vision in one or both eyes
   b. Visual loss is caused by suppression of the signals by the brain
3. Assessment
   a. The condition is diagnosed with assessment and vision testing by an optometrist or ophthalmologist
   b. Nursing assessments depend upon age of child

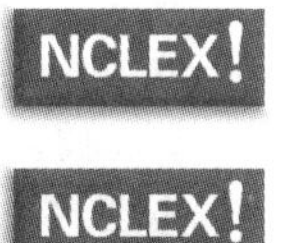

   c. Manifestations of visual impairment for infants include lack of tracking objects or lights with eyes, and poor or no eye contact
   d. Signs of visual impairment in toddlers and older children are excessive tearing, rubbing and squinting of the eyes, frequent blinking, and holding objects close to the eyes to see them or to read
4. Priority nursing diagnoses
   a. Sensory/perceptual alterations (visual)
   b. Body image disturbance
5. Planning and implementation

NCLEX!

   a. Medical treatment options include corrective lenses in eyeglasses, occluding the unaffected eye with a patch (occlusion therapy), eye muscle exercises
   b. Treatment is discontinued when vision has improved; however, 20/20 visual acuity is rarely attained
   c. Treatment of amblyopia is most successful when accomplished by age 7 to 8 years of age

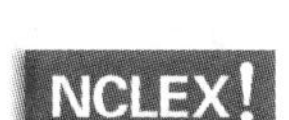

   d. Untreated amblyopia can lead to permanent visual impairment
   e. Nursing care involves educating the parents and child about the necessity of completing treatment

6. Child and family education
   a. Teach the parents means of patching the unaffected eye while maintaining skin integrity
   b. Child and parents need explanation of therapy and long term benefits
7. Evaluation: child completes treatment as prescribed

C. ***Strabismus***

1. Description: misalignment of the eyes
   a. Most common type is esotropia (crossed eyes)
   b. The eyes appear misaligned to the examiner
2. Etiology and pathophysiology
   a. Caused by the lack of coordination of the eye muscles
   b. Positive family history occurs in about 50 percent of the cases
3. Assessment: Screening tests include the cover-uncover test and the corneal light reflex (Hirschberg test)
   a. **Cover-uncover test:** ask the client to fix his or her gaze straight ahead, focusing on a distant object; cover one eye with an opaque card; as the eye is covered, observe the uncovered eye for movement; remove the card while observing the eye just uncovered for movement; this is a screening test for deviation in eye alignment and eye muscle weakness; eye muscle weakness is seen as movement of the "lazy eye" when it attempts to refocus during the cover test
   b. **Corneal light reflex (Hirschberg test):** this test is done to assess parallel symmetry of the eyes; the examiner shines a penlight directly onto the corneas of both eyes, holding the penlight about 12 inches away from the client's nasal bridge while the client focuses on a distant object; the examiner should see the light reflected at the same spot in both eyes; an asymmetric light reflex indicates a deviation in the alignment of the client's eyes (see Figure 3-2)
4. Priority nursing diagnoses
   a. Sensory/perceptual alterations (visual)
   b. Body image disturbance

Figure 3-2

Corneal light reflex results in strabismus.

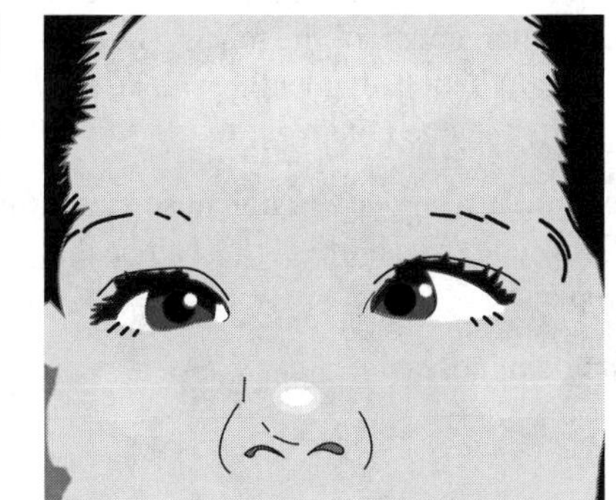

c. Risk for injury related to visual impairment

d. Risk for altered growth and development related to visual impairment

e. Risk for ineffective family coping related to caring for child with visual impairment

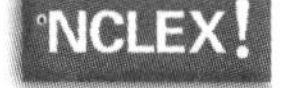

5. Planning and implementation: treatment of strabismus includes occlusion therapy ("good eye" is patched forcing the client to focus with weaker eye, thus strengthening the eye muscles), corrective lenses in eyeglasses, eye drops to cause blurred vision in "good eye," eye muscle exercises

6. Surgical treatment

a. Strabismus can be corrected surgically if conservative treatment has failed to correct the condition; surgery on the rectus muscles of the eyes can achieve normal eye alignment

b. Congenital strabismus should be corrected before 24 months of age to prevent amblyopia (decreased vision of one or both eyes)

Practice to Pass

The nurse is assessing a 14-month-old client brought to the clinic by the mother who states, "I'm concerned about her crossed eyes." What assessments can the nurse perform to screen the child for strabismus?

7. Child and family education: explanation of eye patching is given to the parents; preoperative teaching includes the benefits and risks of surgery, as well as maintaining NPO status prior to surgery

8. Evaluation: parents maintain eye patching as ordered; client and parents are prepared for surgical procedure

III. Disorders of the Throat

A. *Pharyngitis*

1. Description: an infection of the pharynx, often involving tonsils

2. Etiology and pathophysiology

a. A common disorder in children aged 4 to 7 years of age

b. Pharyngitis is rare in infancy

c. Approximately 80 percent of pharyngitis is of viral etiology, and relief of symptoms is indicated

d. Bacterial pharyngitis is most often caused by *group A beta-hemolytic streptcoccus* and requires antibiotic therapy

3. Assessment

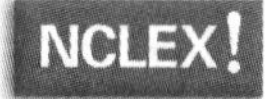

a. Symptoms include sore throat, difficulty swallowing, drooling caused by sore throat, and inability to swallow saliva secretions; inflammation of pharynx and enlargement of the tonsils (with or without exudate), fever, vomiting, cough, lymphadenopathy, and headache; hoarseness or a change in voice quality may be noted

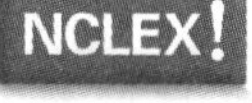

b. A throat culture is necessary to diagnose viral or bacterial etiology of pharyngitis; streptococcal infections can be diagnosed within minutes using a rapid strep test

4. Priority nursing diagnoses

a. Pain

b. Fluid volume deficit

c. Risk for hyperthermia

d. Risk for injury (seizures secondary to high temperature)

5. Planning and implementation

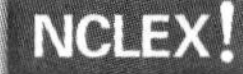

a. In viral pharyngitis, relief of symptoms is indicated; offer diet that is easy to swallow (soft or liquids) and soothing to the sore throat (no citrus juices or other foods that could cause burning or increased irritation)

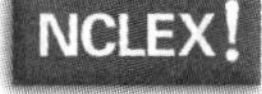

b. Saltwater gargles, throat lozenges, or anesthetic sprays can be used to promote pain relief

6. Medication therapy

a. Administer analgesics (acetaminophen) as ordered

b. Administer antibiotics as ordered for bacterial infections

7. Child and family education

a. Stress to parents the importance of completing the full course of antibiotic therapy to eradicate the infectious organisms

b. Untreated or inadequately treated streptococcal infections can result in acute rheumatic fever, glomerulonephritis, or other serious sequelae

8. Evaluation: client recovers from pharyngitis without sequelae; client completes antibiotic therapy

B. ***Tonsillitis***

1. Description: inflammation of the tonsils located in the posterior pharynx

2. Etiology and pathophysiology

a. Inflammation occurs as a result of viral or bacterial infection

b. Causative organism in bacterial infection can be *group A beta-hemolytic streptococcus,* which is particularly virulent

3. Assessment

a. Diagnosis of bacterial or viral etiology is made by throat culture

b. Streptococcal infection can be diagnosed within minutes using a rapid strep test

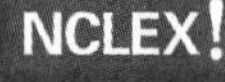

c. Symptoms

1) Enlarged, reddened tonsils, with or without exudate

2) Sore throat, difficulty swallowing because of severe sore throat

3) Drooling, caused by the inability to swallow saliva secretions

4) Lymphadenopathy

5) Mouth breathing

4. Priority nursing diagnoses

a. Pain

b. Fluid volume deficit

c. Risk for hyperthermia

d. Risk for injury (seizures secondary to hyperthermia)

5. Planning and implementation

   a. Management for viral tonsillitis is symptom relief, i.e., promoting comfort, pain relief with acetaminophen (Tylenol); management is similar to that of viral pharyngitis

   b. Management for bacterial tonsillitis is antibiotic therapy as well as symptom relief

NCLEX!

   c. Nursing management: offer diet that is easy to swallow (soft or liquids) and soothing to the sore throat (no citrus juices or other foods that could cause burning or increased irritation)

   d. Use of saltwater gargles, throat lozenges, or anesthetic sprays can promote pain relief

NCLEX!

6. Medication therapy: analgesics (acetaminophen) for comfort and hyperthermia; administer antibiotics as ordered for bacterial infections

7. Child and family education: stress to parents the importance of completing the full course of antibiotic therapy to eradicate the infectious organisms; explain how to manage the symptoms

Practice to Pass

The nurse is evaluating a child who was seen in the clinic 6 days ago for streptococcal pharyngitis. The child complains of a sore throat today, and reports that the oral antibiotic medication prescribed was finished "a few days ago." How should the nurse proceed with assessment?

8. Evaluation: client recovers from tonsillitis without sequelae; client completes antibiotic therapy as ordered

C. Tonsillectomy

1. Description: surgical removal of the tonsils to prevent recurrent tonsillitis

2. Etiology and pathophysiology

   a. Tonsillectomy may be indicated for recurrent tonsillitis, peritonsillar abcess, or respiratory compromise from airway obstruction

   b. Tonsillectomy is one of the most common surgical procedures performed on children

   c. Tonsillectomy is commonly performed in a day-surgery setting, ambulatory surgical setting, or may require an overnight stay in the hospital

3. Assessment: children should be free from symptoms of tonsillitis for at least 1 week prior to the surgery

4. Priority nursing diagnoses

   a. Preoperative

      1) Knowledge deficit (surgical procedure)

      2) Anxiety (parents)

   b. Postoperative

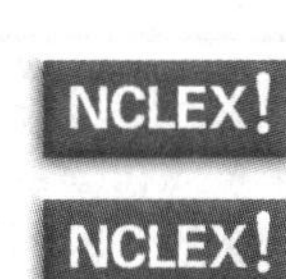

      1) Risk for aspiration

      2) Ineffective airway clearance

      3) Fluid volume deficit

      4) Pain

5. Planning and implemenation

a. Preoperative nursing management: includes client and family preoperative teaching, baseline lab data, including bleeding and clotting times

NCLEX!

b. Postoperative nursing management

1) Provide pain control with analgesic medications and ice collar

2) One of the most common complications is excessive bleeding or hemorrhaging from the operative site; observe the child for frequent or continual swallowing, vomiting bright red blood, and changes in vital signs

3) Offer clear, chilled fluids when awake and alert; red-colored fluids should be avoided because emesis of these fluids could be mistaken for blood

4) Teach the child and parents that a sore throat is to be expected for approximately 1 week postoperatively

6. Child and family education

a. Discharge teaching includes teaching about analgesic medications to be given at home

b. Instruct parents to assess the child for signs of complications such as hemorrhage from the operative site

c. Instruct parents to ensure adequate fluid intake that is necessary to prevent dehydration, advance the child's diet as tolerated to include soft, nonirritating foods, and avoid strenuous activity for about 1 week

d. The child may return to school in 10 days, when the operative site is adequately healed

7. Evaluation: the parents describe signs and symptoms of bleeding; the parents state fluids and foods appropriate for the postoperative child

IV. Disorders of the Nose: Epistaxis

A. Description: also known as nosebleed

B. Etiology and pathophysiology

1. Very common in children, especially boys

2. Superficial veins in the nares are a common source of bleeding

3. Bleeding can occur from irritation, drying of the mucosa from low humidity, or from picking the nose

C. Assessment

NCLEX!

1. The child brought to the Emergency Department or clinic with uncontrolled epistaxis should have vital signs assessed while simultaneous efforts to control the bleeding are being performed

2. If the child has experienced significant blood loss, the hemoglobin and hematocrit may be measured

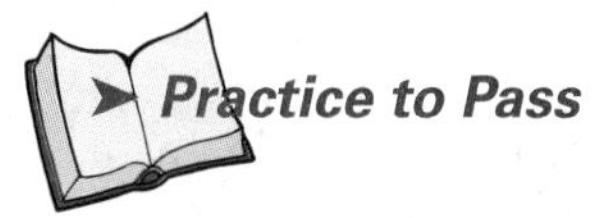

Following an Emergency Department visit for epistaxis, the parent of an 11-year-old child with a history of recurrent epistaxis states, "I wish we could prevent these nosebleeds." What teaching regarding home care can the nurse provide?

D. Priority nursing diagnoses

1. Risk for altered tissue perfusion
2. Risk for impaired airway clearance

E. Planning and implementation

1. Teach the parents and child to humidify the air (especially during winter months and nighttime hours) and have the child sleep with head elevated to prevent recurrence
2. Following an episode of nosebleed, the child is prone to rebleeding; the child should not bend forward, drink hot liquids, exercise excessively, or take hot baths or showers for 3 to 4 days following an episode of nosebleed

F. Medical management

1. If bleeding cannot be controlled by applying pressure, topical vasoconstrictive agents may be used, such as Neo-Synephrine, epinephrine, or thrombin
2. Cautery may be required with silver nitrate or electrocautery
3. If the bleeding cannot be stopped, the nose may be packed with absorbent packing material by the healthcare provider to stop the bleeding

G. Child and family education

1. Teach parents how to stop a nosebleed at home by applying steady pressure to both nostrils just below the nasal bone for 10 to 15 minutes

NCLEX!

2. Instruct parents to have child sit upright and slightly forward to be best able to apply pressure to nostrils and prevent excessive swallowing of blood
3. Instruct parents to seek health care if the bleeding cannot be stopped
4. Teach child to avoid picking at nose or forcefully blowing the nose; teach to release sneezes through the mouth

H. Evaluation: parents describe appropriate means of controlling bleeding; parents identify ways they can reduce the liklihood of recurrence; parents describe symptoms that necessitate physician intervention

Case Study

A 7-year-old child has experienced recurrent tonsillitis for the past year. He is scheduled for a tonsillectomy later in the day. The nurse is assessing the child to obtain a database and is providing preoperative teaching and a tour of the recovery room and day surgery area to the child and parents.

1. What health history data is important to elicit from the family?
2. What laboratory tests can the nurse anticipate that will need to be completed prior to surgery?
3. What content should the nurse emphasize in preoperative teaching directed toward the parents?
4. What content should the nurse emphasize in preoperative teaching that is directed toward the child undergoing surgery?
5. What physical assessments of the child are indicated?

For suggested responses, see pages 407–408.

Posttest

1 A client is to receive eye drops that are ordered to be given "OS." The nurse would administer the eye drops:

(1) To the left eye.
(2) To the right eye.
(3) In both eyes.
(4) In alternating eyes.

2 The nurse is caring for a 6-year-old child who just returned to the day-surgery recovery area from surgery following a tonsillectomy, adenoidectomy, and bilateral myringotomy with insertion of tympanostomy tubes. Which assessment data would indicate that the child is experiencing active, uncontrolled bleeding at the operative site?

(1) Tachycardia, hypertension, hemoptysis
(2) Bradycardia, hypotension, increased swallowing
(3) Tachycardia, hypotension, decreased swallowing
(4) Tachycardia, hypotension, increased swallowing

3 The nurse is planning postoperative care for a pediatric client following tonsillectomy. Nursing considerations include which of the following?

(1) A child's behavioral response to pain is affected by age and developmental level.
(2) Recovery from a painful procedure occurs at a faster rate in children as compared to adults.
(3) Opioid analgesic use in children is dangerous because of increased risk of addiction and respiratory depression.
(4) The immaturity of the nervous system in young children provides them with an increased pain threshold.

4 The nurse is beginning an otoscopic examination of the ear of a 2-year-old child. The child cries, kicks, and pulls away from the nurse. How should the nurse proceed?

(1) Explain to the child why the ear must be examined.
(2) Postpone the examination until the next clinic visit in one year.
(3) State, "I thought you were going to be grown up for me today."
(4) Get assistance to restrain the child to proceed with the exam.

5 During a day-surgery hospitalization experience for tonsillectomy, a 3-year-old child will most likely be fearful of:

(1) Intrusive procedures.
(2) Perceived abandonment.
(3) Premature death.
(4) Unfamiliar caregivers.

6 The nurse is performing an assessment of a 14-month-old toddler admitted to the day-surgery unit for bilateral myringotomy and placement of tympanostomy tubes. How should the nurse obtain the child's temperature?

(1) The nurse should use a tympanic thermometer with disposable speculum.
(2) The nurse should use an oral thermometer with disposable plastic sheath.
(3) The nurse should use a rectal thermometer with disposable plastic sheath.
(4) The nurse should use a temperature strip placed on the child's forehead.

7 Which of the following care measures is indicated in teaching home care of a child with bilateral bacterial conjunctivitis?

(1) Use of warm, moist, disposable compresses to remove crusting
(2) Use of oral antihistamine medication to relieve eye itching
(3) Use of ophthalmic corticosteroids to decrease inflammatory response
(4) Use of topical anesthetics applied to relieve discomfort

8 The parent of an infant diagnosed with viral nasopharyngitis should be taught to notify the health care provider:

(1) Of increased fussiness.
(2) If the infant develops a cough.
(3) Of temperature above 98.6°F.
(4) If the infant develops signs of ear infection.

9 Decongestant nasal drops are prescribed for an infant with nasopharyngitis. Instructions for administering the drops should include which one of the following?

(1) Do not use the drops or dropper for any other family member.
(2) Save any remaining medication for the next time the child is congested.
(3) Administer the drops frequently until the nasal congestion subsides.
(4) Insert the dropper tip as far into the infant's nose as is possible.

10 The nurse teaches the family of a toddler with streptococcal pharyngitis the importance of finishing the full course of oral antibiotic therapy. The nurse explains that a potential complication of untreated streptococcal infection is:

(1) Otitis media.
(2) Diabetes insipidus.
(3) Nephrotic syndrome.
(4) Acute rheumatic fever.

See pages 73–74 for Answers and Rationales.

Answers and Rationales

Pretest

1 **Answer: 1** ***Rationale:*** Amoxicillin is given only by the oral route.
Cognitive Level: Application
Nursing Process: Planning; ***Test Plan:*** PHYS

2 **Answer: 3** ***Rationale:*** Candida infections are a common side effect of antibiotic therapy because of alteration of the normal bacterial flora by the antibiotic agent.
Cognitive Level: Application
Nursing Process: Analysis; ***Test Plan:*** PHYS

3 **Answer: 2** ***Rationale:*** The nurse must emphasize the importance of completing the full course of antibiotic therapy, even though symptoms may have resolved before the antibiotic is finished.
Cognitive Level: Analysis
Nursing Process: Analysis; ***Test Plan:*** PHYS

4 **Answer: 2** ***Rationale:*** The nurse must observe the post-tonsillectomy client for signs of excessive bleeding or hemorrhage from the operative site. In the posterior pharynx, the bleeding can be concealed by the child swallowing the blood. Applying heat to the neck, warm liquids, or giving a straw would be contraindicated, as this could cause bleeding.
Cognitive Level: Application
Nursing Process: Implementation; ***Test Plan:*** PHYS

5 **Answer: 3** ***Rationale:*** The common cold is a viral infection. It is self-limiting, with symptoms lasting about 4 to 10 days. Antibiotics are not indicated for a viral infection. The other options are incorrect.
Cognitive Level: Analysis
Nursing Process: Planning; ***Test Plan:*** PHYS

6 **Answer: 3** ***Rationale:*** Turning up the volume loudly is a behavioral indicator suggesting hearing impairment. The other options are incorrect.
Cognitive Level: Application
Nursing Process: Assessment; ***Test Plan:*** PHYS

7 **Answer: 2** ***Rationale:*** Development of parent–infant attachment is important in promoting developmental progress. Parents are encouraged to talk, sing, and interact with their baby to learn about their infant's response, and to provide appropriate stimulation at 1 month of age. The other options are incorrect.
Cognitive Level: Analysis
Nursing Process: Planning; ***Test Plan:*** PHYS

8 **Answer: 4** ***Rationale:*** Purulent exudate and crusting are characteristic of conjunctivitis. Conjunctivitis associated with foreign body can cause severe eye pain. The other options are incorrect.
Cognitive Level: Application
Nursing Process: Analysis; ***Test Plan:*** PHYS

9 **Answer: 4** ***Rationale:*** The infected area should be cleansed with a disposable tissue after a single use. Handwashing is important to prevent the spread of infection. Items that come in contact with the infected eye are considered contaminated.
Cognitive Level: Analysis
Nursing Process: Evaluation; ***Test Plan:*** PHYS

10 **Answer: 3** ***Rationale:*** Saline nose drops will loosen secretions and crusting. The bulb syringe is necessary because infants cannot blow their own noses. The other options are incorrect.
Cognitive Level: Analysis
Nursing Process: Implementation; ***Test Plan:*** PHYS

Posttest

1 **Answer: 1** ***Rationale:*** OS is the abbreviation for left eye. OD is the abbreviation for right eye. OU is the abbreviation for both eyes.
Cognitive Level: Application
Nursing Process: Implementation; ***Test Plan:*** PHYS

2 **Answer: 4** ***Rationale:*** The nurse observes increased swallowing. Tachycardia and hypotension are late signs of significant blood loss. The other options are incorrect.
Cognitive Level: Analysis
Nursing Process: Assessment; ***Test Plan:*** PHYS

3 **Answer: 1** ***Rationale:*** Option 1 is the only true statement. Infants are less able to communicate their feelings than an older child and usually demonstrate restlessness and crying behaviors. Adolescents are able to describe their pain sensations.
Cognitive Level: Application
Nursing Process: Planning; ***Test Plan:*** PHYS

4 **Answer: 4** ***Rationale:*** Uncooperative pediatric clients may need to be restrained long enough to accomplish the assessment or procedure that is necessary. Other options are incorrect.
Cognitive Level: Analysis
Nursing Process: Implementation; ***Test Plan:*** PHYS

5 **Answer: 1** ***Rationale:*** One of the greatest fears of preschoolers is fear of mutilation. Other options are not developmentally appropriate responses for a preschooler.
Cognitive Level: Application
Nursing Process: Planning; ***Test Plan:*** PSYC

6 **Answer: 1** ***Rationale:*** The tympanic method is preferred. It is quick, accurate, and convenient. Oral temperature can be obtained on a cooperative child aged 3 and older. A rectal temperature is obtained as a last resort, when other methods are not possible.
Cognitive Level: Analysis
Nursing Process: Assessment; ***Test Plan:*** PHYS

7 **Answer: 1** ***Rationale:*** Crusting of dried exudate is common with bacterial conjunctivitis. Other options

are not indicated in the management of bacterial conjunctivitis.
Cognitive Level: Application
Nursing Process: Implementation; ***Test Plan:*** PHYS

8 **Answer: 4** ***Rationale:*** Options 1 to 3 are expected symptoms of viral pharyngitis in infants. Symptoms of ear infection should be reported to the health care provider.
Cognitive Level: Analysis
Nursing Process: Implementation; ***Test Plan:*** PHYS

9 **Answer: 1** ***Rationale:*** Eliminating contact or sharing of items with the infected person can reduce the potential spread of infection to other family members. The other options are incorrect.
Cognitive Level: Analysis
Nursing Process: Implementation; ***Test Plan:*** PHYS

10 **Answer: 4** ***Rationale:*** Rheumatic fever can follow an infection of certain strains of group A beta-hemolytic streptococci. Other options are incorrect.
Cognitive Level: Application
Nursing Process: Planning; ***Test Plan:*** PHYS

References

Ball, J. & Bindler, R. (1999). *Pediatric nursing: Caring for children* (2nd ed.). Stamford, CT: Appleton & Lange, pp. 119, 242–245, 271, 496, 714–746, 926.

Bindler, R. & Ball, J. (1999). *Quick reference to pediatric clinical skills*. Stamford, CT: Appleton & Lange, pp. 23–26.

Jarvis, C. (2000). *Physical examination and health assessment* (3rd ed.). Philadelphia: Saunders, pp. 297–414.

Taketomo, C. K., Hodding, J. H., & Kraus, D. M. (2000). *Pediatric dosage handbook* (7th ed.). Hudson, OH: Lexi-comp, Inc., p. 73.

Wong, D. L., Hockenberry-Eaton, M., Wilson, D., Winkelstein, M., Ahmann, E., & DiVito-Thomas, P. (1999). *Whaley and Wong's nursing care of infants and children* (6th ed.). St. Louis: Mosby, pp. 1259, 1418–1529.

CHAPTER 4

Respiratory Health Problems

Jennifer Jeames Coleman, MSN, RN

CHAPTER OUTLINE

OBJECTIVES

- Identify data essential to the assessment of alterations in health of the respiratory system in a child.
- Discuss the clinical manifestations and pathophysiology of alterations in health of the respiratory system of a child.
- Discuss therapeutic management of a child with alterations in health of the respiratory system.
- Describe nursing management of a child with alterations in health of the respiratory system.

[Media Link]

Use the CD-ROM enclosed with this text, or log onto the address given to access the free, interactive Companion Website created for this series. The CD-ROM and Companion Website accompanying this book offer additional practice opportunities and information—NCLEX Review, Case Studies, Glossary, In Depth with NCLEX, and more.

www.prenhall.com/hogan

Review at a Glance

alveoli *small, saclike dilatations of the terminal bronchioles where oxygen–carbon dioxide gas exchange takes place*

atelectasis *incomplete expansion or collapse of the lung caused by obstruction of the airway from secretions or a foreign body*

barrel chest *anteroposterior diameter of chest is increased to give chest a rounded appearance; caused by air trapping and hyperinflation of the alveoli*

bronchopulmonary dysplasia (BPD) *chronic obstructive pulmonary disease occurring in infants after prolonged exposure to mechanical ventilation and oxygen therapy*

digital clubbing *Increased rounding of the nails of the fingers and toes with a loss of the normal angle at the base of the nail; an indication of hypoxia*

dyspnea *difficult breathing*

epiglottis *structure that covers the larynx during swallowing to prevent food from entering the trachea*

foreign body aspiration *inhalation, intentional or otherwise, of an object into the respiratory tract*

hypercapnia *excessive carbon dioxide in the blood*

hypoxemia *deficiency of oxygen in the blood*

laryngotracheobronchitis *a viral infection that causes inflammation, edema, and narrowing of the larynx, trachea and bronchi*

peak expiratory flow rate *the maximum amount of air that can be forcibly exhaled*

surfactant *phospholipid produced by the alveoli that reduces surface tension of fluids and aids in lung expansion*

sweat test *measures sweat sodium and chloride concentrations; sample is collected from child's forearm on absorbent material; a level greater than 60 mEq/L is diagnostic for cystic fibrosis*

tachypnea *rapid respirations*

trigger *the initiator of an asthmatic episode*

Pretest

1 The mother of an infant who has had recurrent respiratory infections asks the nurse why infants are at increased risk for complications from respiratory infections. The best response by the nurse explains that in infants, the:

(1) Airway structures are larger, allowing for larger numbers of organisms.
(2) Respiratory rate is slower than in adults.
(3) Parents are unable to accurately assess respiratory problems.
(4) Airways are narrower and more easily obstructed.

2 The mother of a neonate hospitalized with an upper respiratory tract infection asks why her baby won't take her bottle. The nurse's best answer would be:

(1) "She's probably not hungry."
(2) "It's okay because we're giving her intravenous fluids, therefore she is not hungry."
(3) "Newborns breathe through their noses. Congestion may be interfering with her breathing and eating at the same time."
(4) "She might need a different type of formula. We'll call the physician to get a new order."

3 A 4-year-old female child presents to the emergency department with a sore throat, difficulty swallowing and a suspected diagnosis of acute epiglottitis. Which of the following should not be included in her initial assessment?

(1) Throat culture
(2) Vital signs
(3) Past medical history
(4) Auscultation of chest

4 The nurse is providing homecare instructions to the parents of a child with cystic fibrosis. Which statement by the parents indicates that they do not understand the treatment regimen?

(1) "We will perform chest physiotherapy and postural drainage four times a day."
(2) "We will keep her away from the church nursery if any of the children are coughing and have fever or runny noses."
(3) "If her bowel movements are normal and her appetite is good, she does not need her pancreatic enzymes."
(4) "The relay races and swimming at our Sunday school picnic next week will be good exercise for her."

5 A 2-year-old child is being discharged after bronchoscopy for removal of a coin from his esophagus. The most important topic of discharge teaching would be the importance of:

(1) Reassuring the child that he is fine.
(2) Proper nutrition for the next few days.
(3) Restricting his access to small toys or objects.
(4) Administering acetaminophen for his sore throat.

6 A 15-year-old child with a history of cystic fibrosis is admitted to the pediatric unit with assessment findings of crackles, increased cough, and greenish sputum. A 2-week hospitalization is anticipated. Which nursing intervention holds the highest priority?

(1) Referral to Child Life Services for school lesson plans
(2) Arranging for liberal visitation from peers
(3) Taking a diet history
(4) Gaining intravenous access

7 A 7-year-old child is brought to the Emergency Department for an acute asthma attack. He is wheezing, tachypneic, diaphoretic, and looks frightened. The nurse should prepare to administer:

(1) IV methylprednisolone.
(2) Racemic epinephrine.
(3) Oral prednisone.
(4) Cromolyn sodium.

8 An appropriate nursing diagnosis for the family of a toddler being treated for acute laryngotracheobronchitis is:

(1) Anticipatory grieving.
(2) Altered growth and development related to acute onset of illness.
(3) Impaired social interaction related to confinement in hospital.
(4) Fear/anxiety related to dyspnea and noisy breathing.

9 A child with bacterial pneumonia is crying and says it hurts when he coughs. The nurse would teach the child to:

(1) Hug his teddy bear when he coughs.
(2) Ask for pain medicine before he coughs.
(3) Take a sip of water before coughing.
(4) Try very hard not to cough.

10 An infant with chronic bronchopulmonary dysplasia (BPD) and a tracheostomy is being discharged on home oxygen therapy. Which statement by the mother indicates that further teaching is needed before discharge?

(1) "I will call my pediatrician if she gets a fever or has more secretions than usual from her tracheostomy."
(2) "I have a cute bib to loosely cover her tracheostomy when she eats and when we go outside in the wind."
(3) "We are so glad the baby will get to go with us on our camping trip to Yellowstone National Park. We have been waiting for her to get well so we can go."
(4) "We have already notified Alabama Power Company that our baby is coming home today."

See pages 99–100 for Answers and Rationales.

I. Overview of the Anatomy and Physiology of the Respiratory System

A. Structures

1. Upper airways: nose, pharynx, and larynx provide the pathway for air to enter the body and ultimately the lungs; the **epiglottis** covers the larynx, which is located between the pharynx and trachea, and keeps food from entering the lower respiratory tract; these upper structures also warm, humidify, and filter inspired air
2. Lower airways: trachea, bronchi, bronchioles, and **alveoli** conduct air and produce surfactant; alveoli are small, saclike extensions of the terminal

bronchioles where gas exchange takes place and blood is reoxygenated; hair-like projections called cilia provide mucus to the upper airway to aid in trapping of debris and foreign particles; **surfactant** is a phospholipid that aids in lung elasticity and alveoli expansion

B. Physiology

1. Prenatal development

   a. Development of the respiratory system should be complete prior to birth in order to establish breathing and oxygen–carbon dioxide exchange at birth; premature infants lack sufficient surfactant and have many underdeveloped and uninflatable alveoli, which compromise gas exchange

   b. Oxygenation is the responsibility of the placenta in utero; fetal pulmonary blood flow is minimal, there is little lung movement, and the collapsed lungs are filled with fluid excreted through the alveoli; pulmonary vascular resistance is increased and most blood is shunted away from the lungs by the foramen ovale and ductus arteriosus

2. Postnatal changes

   a. The birth process and delivery stimulate breathing and inflation of the lungs; a decreased oxygen level in the blood (**hypoxemia**), an increased carbon dioxide level (**hypercapnia**), and acidosis stimulate the respiratory center in the medulla of the brainstem and cause initiation of breathing

   b. Compression of the chest through the birth canal squeezes fetal lung fluid from the lungs, and the abrupt coolness of the outside environment sends impulses to the respiratory center in the medulla

   c. Surfactant reduces the surface tension of the fluid lining the alveoli to facilitate entry of air into the lungs; inspiration causes the diaphragm to contract, lengthen, and decrease intrapulmonic pressure; gases then move from an area of higher concentration to an area of lesser concentration; oxygen and carbon dioxide exchange that occurs in the alveoli and blood provides the body tissues with oxygen needed for survival

C. Pediatric differences

1. Size

   a. There is a shorter distance between structures in young children

   b. The lumen of the young child's respiratory tract is smaller and, thus, more easily obstructed; the diameter of the trachea is approximately the size of the child's little finger

   c. There are fewer alveoli at birth; numbers, size, and shape continue to increase until puberty

   d. Eustachian tubes are shorter and more horizontal, facilitating transfer of pathogens into the middle ear; lymphoid and tonsillar tissue is normally enlarged and may obstruct the passage of air

2. Function

   a. Neonates are nose-breathers; therefore, any obstruction in nasal passages interferes with breathing and eating

b. Narrower airways increase airway resistance and the child's risk for obstruction by edema, mucus, or foreign objects

c. Infant's airway walls have less cartilage, and are more flexible and more prone to collapse; intercostal muscles are immature; the chest wall is less stable, and retractions are more common

d. Newborns have less respiratory mucus to function as a cleaning agent

e. Increased respiratory and metabolic rates increase the need for oxygen

II. Diagnostic Tests of the Respiratory System

NCLEX!

A. Chest x-ray: visualization of size and shape of airways, lungs, heart, diaphragm, and rib cage; posterior, anterior, lateral, and oblique views may be taken; no preparation or discomfort occurs other than wearing lead apron if repeated x-rays are taken; female adolescents should be protected with a lead apron if there is any possibility of pregnancy

B. Computed tomography (CT scan): visualization of tumors or lesions; contrast medium may be used, necessitating that the child not eat or drink for 3 to 4 hours prior to the procedure; this procedure requires immobilization and possibly sedation

C. Bronchoscopy: a bronchoscope is utilized to visualize the trachea and bronchi directly; lesions can be located and sized; secretions and foreign bodies can be cleared from the airway

1. Preprocedure care

a. Obtain informed consent: procedure is done under local or general anesthesia; assess client and family's understanding and anxiety level

NCLEX!

b. Child should be NPO to guard against aspiration when gag reflex is suppressed

c. Administer prescribed sedative or narcotic as premedication; observe for bradycardia and hypotension

2. Postprocedure care

a. Assess for return of swallow and gag reflexes; keep NPO until reflexes return position flat and side-lying if not fully alert

b. Observe for signs of airway obstruction: dyspnea, cyanosis, stridor

c. Expect blood-streaked sputum for several hours; report any frank blood (may indicate hemorrhage)

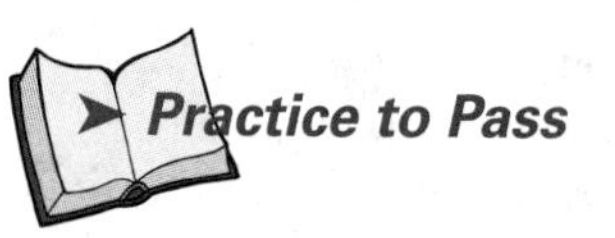

A 12-month-old child returns to the pediatric unit after a bronchoscopy. His mother is concerned that he has not eaten today and starts to prepare a bottle of formula. How will you respond to her?

D. Pulmonary function tests measure the child's respiratory ability, response to treatment, and degree of lung disease; a child as young as 5 or 6 years is usually able to follow commands and cooperate; **peak expiratory flow rate** (PEFR), the maximum amount of air that can be exhaled after a normal inspiration, is a very useful test of function; a spirometer is used and the child is allowed to become familiar with the equipment; instructions include practice in breathing normally through the mouth and blowing into the spirometer

E. Sputum culture

1. Isolates pathogens and identifies sensitivities for antibiotic selection if needed

2. Best collected in early morning as secretions accumulate during sleep and thus contain the most organisms

3. Young children are unable to produce sputum; nasal or gastric washing with sterile saline is performed to obtain a sample; maintain standard precautions and wear protective eyewear and masks if splashing is a possibility

F. Arterial blood gases

1. Determine the level of oxygen and carbon dioxide circulating in an arterial blood sample

2. Provide information about acid–base balance

NCLEX!

3. Collect in a heparinized syringe; place on ice and transport to lab immediately; apply pressure to the puncture site for at least 5 minutes and monitor for hematoma formation and peripheral circulation

G. Pulse oximetry measures oxygen saturation and the need for oxygen therapy; it is noninvasive and measures the amount of infrared light waves absorbed as they travel through perfused areas of the body

III. Congenital Respiratory Health Problems

A. Cystic fibrosis (CF)

1. Description

a. Multisystem disorder of exocrine glands, leading to increased production of thick mucus in bronchioles, small intestines, and pancreatic and bile ducts

b. Increased viscosity of secretions obstructs small passageways of these organs and interferes with normal pulmonary and digestive functioning

1) Lung problems are the most serious threat to life; thick, sticky secretions pool in the bronchioles, cause **atelectasis** (collapse of the lungs) and serve as a medium for bacterial growth

2) Pancreatic ducts become clogged with the thick secretions and prevent pancreatic enzymes from reaching the duodenum, impairing digestion and absorption.

3) Small intestines, in the absence of pancreatic enzymes, are unable to absorb fats and protein; thus, growth and puberty are retarded

2. Etiology and pathophysiology

a. Inherited as an autosomal recessive trait; the gene on chromosome 7 responsible for functioning of the cystic fibrosis transmembrane regulator (CFTR) is defective; absence of CTFR as a chloride channel interferes with sodium-chloride transport, prohibiting movement of water across the cell membranes

b. Usually diagnosed in infancy and early childhood; affects white children primarily; rarely seen in blacks and children of Asian descent; males and females are affected equally

c. Life expectancy has increased to median age of 30 years, but the disease is terminal; death is usually the result of resistant pulmonary organisms and fibrosis and destruction of lung tissues

3. Assessment

a. Diagnostic

1) **Sweat test** (pilocarpine iontophoreses) analyzes sodium and chloride content in sweat; a chloride concentration greater than 60 meq/L is diagnostic of cystic fibrosis; parents often report that infants taste salty when kissed

2) 72-hour fecal fat

3) Chest x-ray

4) Prior to delivery, prenatal DNA analysis of amniotic fluid shows intestinal alkaline phosphatase is reduced in a fetus with cystic fibrosis

b. Nursing

1) History usually reveals frequent bouts of respiratory infections

2) Observe for any respiratory impairment, i.e., cough, presence and color of sputum, **dyspnea** (difficulty breathing), color of nailbeds and mucous membranes, pulse oximetry; auscultate breath sounds for equality, crackles, wheezes, or any increased effort during breathing; observe for clubbing of fingers and toes; **digital clubbing,** an indication of hypoxia, produces nails with increased rounding and a loss of the normal angle at the base of the nail

3) Assess nutritional status by obtaining height and weight and plot on growth charts; skin turgor and mucous membranes reveal hydration status; record diet history and activity tolerance; signs of malabsorption include bulky, frothy, foul-smelling stools called steatorrhea, and unusually protruberant abdomen and thin extremities; often the first sign of CF is meconium ileus, where the intestine is blocked with thick, tenacous secretions in the newborn period and the neonate is unable to pass the first meconium stool

4. Priority nursing diagnoses

a. Ineffective airway clearance

b. Impaired gas exchange

c. Risk for infection

d. Alteration in nutrition

e. Activity intolerance

f. Fear/anxiety

g. Knowledge deficit

h. Risk for ineffective family coping

5. Planning and implementation

a. Respiratory: monitor for retractions, dyspnea, cyanosis, color of sputum, quality of cough; ensure pulmonary toilet is performed, auscultate breath sounds before and after treatments; encourage coughing and deep breathing exercises and physical activity as tolerated; administer prescribed antibiotics and bronchodilator

b. Digestive: provide high-calorie (150 percent above normal recommendations), high-protein diet and snacks; infants are given a predigested formula such as pregestimil or nutramigen; administer pancreatic enzymes with all meals and snacks; individualize to achieve stools as near normal as possible; administer fat-soluble vitamins; determine food preferences to encourage acceptance of diet; weigh daily; avoid pulmonary treatments immediately after meals to decrease risk of vomiting

6. Medications: antibiotics for treatment of pulmonary infection and purulent secretions, pancreatic enzymes for fat absorption, vitamin supplementation, mucolytics to decrease viscosity of sputum, bronchodilators to improve lung function; see Table 4-1 for overview of commonly ordered respiratory care medications

Table 4-1

Medications Commonly Used to Treat Respiratory Problems

Medication	Use	Action	Nursing Considerations
Bronchodilators Albuterol (Proventil) Epinephrine (Adrenalin) Metaproterenol (Alupent) Terbutaline (Brethaire)	May be used for acute and daily therapy; routes of admnistration include oral, inhaled, and parenteral	Relax smooth muscles in the airways	Tachycardia, restlessness and increased activity may be side effects; reduction in dose usually lessens the undesired effects; inhaled drugs have more rapid onset; to prevent exercise-induced asthma episode, give drug at least 15 minutes before sustained activity
Anti-inflammatory corticosteroids Prednisone (Deltasone and others) Methylprednisolone (Medrol) Beclomethasone (Vanceril)	Used to reduce the inflammatory response during or to prevent an asthmatic attack; oral, inhaled, intravenous preparations are available	Reduce inflammation and mucosal edema in airways	Lowest possible dose of steroids to avoid side effects of growth retardation, fluid retention, increased appetite, mood changes; inhaled steroids have fewer side effects than oral administration; rinse mouth after inhalation to prevent oral candidiasis; take oral drug with food or milk to minimize stomach upset; give at least 15 minutes before prolonged exercise to prevent exercise-induced asthma episode
Nonsteroidal anti-inflammatory drugs (NSAIDs) Cromolyn sodium (Intal) Nedrocromil sodium (Tilade)	Used as prophylaxis or treatment of asthma; oral, nasal, and inhaled preparations are available (Cromalyn); inhaled preparation only (Nedrocromil)	Used prophylactically and for prevention of exercise-induced asthma episode	Should be taken regularly for proper effect

Table 4-1 *(continued)*

Medication	Use	Action	Nursing Considerations
Diuretic Furosemide (Lasix)	Diuretic; oral, intravenous preparations are available	Removes excess fluid from lungs	Monitor for electrolyte changes; maintain strict intake and output; advise clients to take drug in morning to avoid sleep disturbances from increased urination
Mucolytics Dornase alfa (Pulmozyme) Acetylcysteine (Mucomyst)	Used in cystic fibrosis as inhalation drug	Loosen and thin pulmonary secretions to facilitate removal by coughing	Teach proper use of inhaler
Antibiotics Penicillins Cephalosporins Aminoglycosides	Used for bacterial infections in pneumonia, epiglottis after cultures to determine sensitivities; available in oral or parenteral forms	Kill bacteria to cure infection	Obtain specimens for cultures and sensitivities; ascertain client allergies and drug reactions; administer drugs as scheduled; course of drug therapy may be prolonged, teach family to complete the entire antibiotic dose for the time prescribed; family should observe for signs of superinfection, such as thrush or monilial diaper dermatitis
Antiviral Ribavirin (Virazole)	Used against respiratory syncytial virus (RSV) and influenzae virus; administered via small particle aerosol generator	Inhibits viral replication and reduces severity of RSV	Drug is given by oxygen tent for 12 to 18 hours over 3 to 7 days; ensure proper operation of small particle aerosol generator; pregnant health care workers should not care for child; drug is teratogenic to fetus; caregiver side effects include headache, burning eyes, and crystallization of soft contact lenses
Pancreatic enzymes Pancrelipase (Pancrease, Cotazym, Ultrase)	Used in cystic fibrosis to aid in digestion and absorption of nutrients; supplied in capsule form that can be opened and the powder sprinkled on a small amount of food	Pancreatic enzyme replacement	Enzymes must be consumed before or with every meal or snack; capsules can be swallowed whole; if taken apart do not add powder to hot foods or enzyme activity will be compromised; enzyme dosage is adjusted based on number and consistency of stools and whether or not adequate weight gain is maintained

7. Child and family education

NCLEX!

a. Avoid exposure to respiratory infections; report immediately any fever, increase in cough, or change in sputum

b. Chest percussion and postural drainage must be performed three to four times daily; noncompliance will result in increased hospitalizations and infections; see Box 4-1 for instructions on chest physiotherapy and postural drainage

c. High-calorie, high-protein diet is essential; give pancreatic enzymes with all meals and snacks; may need extra salt in hot weather

d. Physical activity and exercise loosen secretions and promote lung expansion

e. Provide information on community resources, such as Cystic Fibrosis Foundation, American Lung Association; provide social service consults, home-health referrals with visiting nurses and respiratory therapists

f. Genetic counseling

g. Provide written information on medications, breathing exercises, chest physiotherapy, and postural drainage

h. Suggest clergy, mental health services, respite care, and families of other children with CF to assist with psychologic and emotional coping with chronic, progressive illness

8. Evaluation: Family demonstrates and verbalizes intent to adhere to homecare regimen of pulmonary treatments, medications, diet, and exercises; child gains weight consistently, participates in self-care and age-appropriate activities; child demonstrates ability to clear secretions from airway by productive cough, oxygen saturation greater than 94 percent and decreased respiratory distress

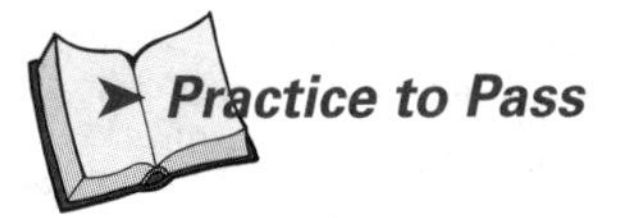

A 6-year-old child has cystic fibrosis and is hospitalized for an acute respiratory infection. The playroom has scheduled a puppet show and the child's mother asks you if he can get his antibiotics later so he won't miss the show. What facts will you consider as you decide how to respond?

IV. Acquired Respiratory Health Problems

A. *Bronchopulmonary dysplasia (BPD)*

1. Description

a. Chronic obstructive pulmonary disease occurring in infants after prolonged oxygen therapy and mechanical ventilation

Box 4-1

Chest Physiotherapy (CPT)

- Child is dressed in a lightweight shirt.
- Percussion is performed with a cupped hand striking the chest over a portion of the lung; if done properly, a popping sound will be heard.
- Postural drainage facilitates removal of secretions that are loosened during percussion; for drainage, various head-down positions drain all lung segments.
- Positioning for bronchial drainage can be achieved by child standing on his head, hanging upside down on monkey bars, and other playground activities that are fun for the child.
- Avoid performing CPT immediately after eating.

b. Premature infants with BPD have usually survived respiratory distress syndrome; term infants generally have serious respiratory problems, also requiring ventilatory assistance

2. Etiology and pathophysiology

a. High oxygen concentrations and mechanical ventilation damage bronchial epithelium and alveoli; thickened alveolar walls, scarring, and fibrosis lead to atelectasis, poor airway clearance of mucus and poor gas exchange; chronic low oxygenation results in decreased lung compliance and altered function

b. Lung immaturity is a major contributor to occurrence of BPD, and improved survival rates of premature infants have increased the incidence of BPD; as little as three days of positive pressure ventilation can increase an infant's risk of developing BPD

c. There may be a genetic predisposition; males have increased morbidity

3. Assessments

a. Diagnosed by chest x-ray, which reveals lung changes and air trapping with or without hyperinflation

b. Blood gases reveal hypercapnia and respiratory acidosis

c. Respiratory observations include **tachypnea** (rapid respirations), tachycardia, increased work of breathing, retractions, wheezing, and **barrel chest** (rounding of the chest caused by trapped air) (Figure 4-1)

d. Pallor, activity intolerance and poor feeding result from chronic hypoxia

4. Priority nursing diagnoses

a. Impaired gas exchange

b. Ineffective airway clearance

Figure 4-1

Barrel chest.
Source: Ball, J. & Bindler, R. (1999). *Pediatric nursing: Caring for children* (2nd ed.). Stamford, CT: Appleton & Lange, p. 439.

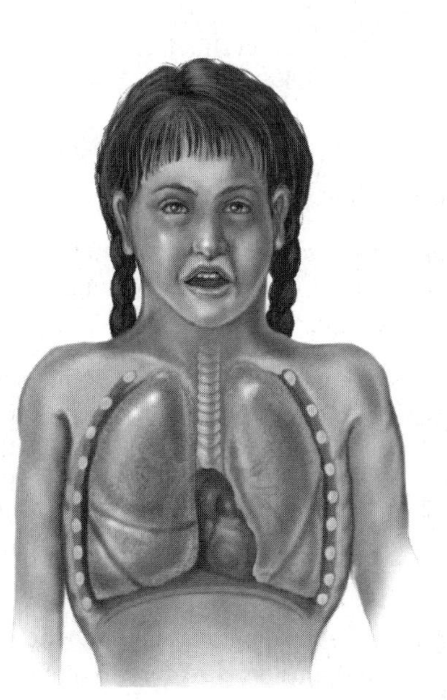

c. Altered nutrition

d. Altered growth and development

e. Risk for infection

f. Anxiety/fear

5. Planning and implementation

a. Infants with BPD are cared for in intensive care units and require an artificial airway; avoid pressure or trauma to the endotracheal tube and infant's airway

b. Suctioning, turning, and weighing is done carefully to ensure oxygen saturations are maintained

c. Monitor respiratory status continuously; infants' condition can worsen in a short period of time

d. Monitor for fluid overload; infants are at increased risk for pulmonary edema; weigh daily; maintain strict intake and output

e. Strict handwashing; avoid exposure to respiratory infections

f. Cluster nursing care to minimize oxygen requirements and caloric expenditure

g. Plan quiet stimulation and activities to foster normal infant development and parental bonding given the extended, and often repeated, hospitalizations of infants with BPD

6. Medications (see Table 4-1)

a. Bronchodilators open airways and increase lung compliance

b. Corticosteroids reduce edema and inflammation in the airways

c. Diuretics remove excess fluid from the lungs and help prevent pulmonary edema

d. Antibiotics may be given prophylactically

7. Child and family education

a. Infants are discharged with multiple needs; assess family's understanding and ability to follow treatment regimen

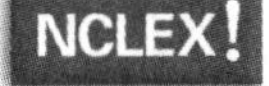

b. Teach parents cardiopulmonary resuscitation (CPR), use of home monitoring equipment and oxygen therapy; infants are usually discharged with a tracheostomy when oxygen concentration requirements are low

c. Review infection control practices, i.e., handwashing, avoidance of family members with respiratory infections; teach warning signs of illness

d. Teach safety precautions regarding oxygen therapy and tracheostomy care; see Box 4-2 for instructions on home tracheostomy care; contact utility companies, emergency services, and the telephone companies before discharge of a technology-dependent child

e. Review basic care—feeding, bathing, playing, holding—with parents; allow parents the opportunity to care for child in the hospital before dis-

Box 4-2

Tracheostomy Home Care and Oxygen Therapy

Discharge instructions for a child with a tracheostomy should include the following:

- Keep small toys, talcum powder, plastic bibs and bedding, and any small particles away from child to decrease risk for aspiration or occlusion of trachea.
- Be sure child wears cloth bib loosely over tracheostomy when eating to prevent food particles from entering tube.
- Be careful when bathing to keep water from entering trachea; showers are not recommended.
- Cover tracheostomy loosely when outside in strong wind and cold to prevent tracheal spasms.
- Observe skin around tracheostomy daily for redness, breakdown, or any signs of infection.
- Change tracheostomy ties weekly; be sure to use nonfraying material; always have assistance to change ties.
- Clean area around tracheostomy daily with half-strength saline and hydrogen peroxide and cotton applicators.
- Suction tracheostomy tube when needed to remove secretions from the child's airway; use sterile gloves and limit suctioning to 5 seconds. Insert suction catheter only to the length of the tracheostomy tube and apply intermittent suction while withdrawing the catheter.
- Be sure child is allowed to rest between suctioning if catheter is passed more than once.
- Notify physician if tracheal secretions are increased or become purulent, or if child develops a fever.
- Keep written instructions available at all times.
- Keep emergency bag with extra suction catheters and tracheostomy tubes available.
- Notify utility companies and emergency medical services that child in the home requires emergency equipment.
- Do not allow smoking in the home of child with oxygen therapy.
- Keep oxygen tanks away from any heat source; keep a fire extinguisher nearby.

charge; after basic care is mastered, the medical treatment plan is developed with assistance of parents

f. Make referrals to community agencies for supplies, medications, nutrition, parental support, and stimulation programs to foster growth and development

8. Evaluation: family demonstrates ability to care for child and seek medical attention when needed; infant maintains blood gases within normal range; infant demonstrates ability to clear airway by respiratory rate and rhythm within normal limits; infant demonstrates consistent growth and performs age-appropriate developmental tasks

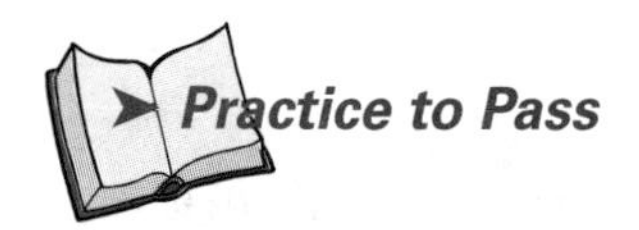

What are the risk factors contributing to the development of bronchopulmonary dysplasia (BPD)?

B. Asthma

1. Description

a. Chronic inflammatory disorder in which airways narrow and are hyperreactive to stimuli that do not affect nonasthmatic individuals

b. Exposure to an irritant causes bronchial muscles to go into spasm, leading to increased respiratory effort; increased airway resistance, air trapping, and exhaustion results

2. Etiology and pathophysiology

a. Exposure to an irritant causes constriction of bronchial smooth muscle, edema, increased secretion of thick mucus, and airway narrowing; expiration through the narrowed lumen is impaired, resulting in air trapping and hyperinflation of the alveoli

NCLEX!

b. The initiator of an asthmatic episode, called a **trigger,** can be any number of stimuli, including inhalants, airborne pollens, stress, weather changes, exercise, viral or bacterial agents, food additives, etc

c. It is unclear exactly how heredity factors into the occurrence of asthma, but there is a familial tendency; although the incidence of asthma has risen, the severity of attacks may lessen as child grows and airway increases in size

3. Assessments

a. Diagnostic

1) Chest x-ray reveals hyperinflation of the airways

2) Pulmonary function tests reveal reduced peak expiratory flow rate (PEFR)

b. Wheezing and dry cough indicate an asthma episode; prolonged expiration, restlessness, fatigue, and tachypnea are observed as the child struggles to breathe despite hyperinflated, poorly ventilated alveoli

c. Chronic use of accessory muscles for respiration leads to a barrel chest in children with frequent exacerbations

4. Priority nursing diagnoses

a. Ineffective airway clearance

b. Activity intolerance/fatigue

c. Altered family processes

d. Risk for suffocation

e. Knowledge deficit

5. Planning and implementation

a. Assess for cyanosis or marked respiratory distress; administer humidified oxygen if needed; monitor pulse oximetry

b. Maintain IV access to ensure sufficient intake of fluids to replace insensible losses from hyperventilation and for medication administration; avoid cold liquids to decrease risk of bronchospasm

NCLEX!

c. Monitor airway response to treatment; sudden cessation of wheezing and decreased breath sounds with increased respirations may indicate worsening of child's condition

d. Position in high-Fowler's and cluster nursing care to conserve child's energy

6. Medications for asthma include bronchodilators and anti-inflammatory agents administered orally, parenterally, or by inhalation (see Table 4-1)

7. Child and family education

a. Explain that the goal is to prevent acute asthma episodes and to ensure optimal physical and psychologic health

b. Teach family to identify and avoid potential triggers

c. Assess family's coping skills and ability and willingness to care for child and adhere to therapy

d. Review parents' understanding of asthma and how to recognize signs and symptoms of an impending attack

e. Teach parents to monitor child's condition with peak expiratory flow rates

f. Arrange for additional support and continuous education through special camps, clinics, schools, and community agencies such as the American Lung Association

NCLEX!

8. Evaluation: the family verbalizes accurate knowledge of asthma and plans to adhere to therapy; the child engages in age-appropriate activities; the child maintains clear airway with normal respiratory effort; the child maintains adequate ventilatory capacity as evidenced by PEFR at personal best

V. Infectious Respiratory Health Problems

A. Acute *laryngotracheobronchitis* (LTB)

1. Description

a. Viral infection that causes inflammation, edema, and narrowing of the larynx, trachea, and bronchi; usually LTB is preceded by a recent upper respiratory infection

b. LTB is most common in infants and toddlers and affects boys more often than girls; it is the most common of the croup syndromes

2. Etiology and pathophysiology

a. LTB is usually caused by parainfluenzae virus, influenzae A and B, respiratory syncytial virus (RSV) and mycoplasma pneumoniae

b. Inflammation and narrowing of the airways cause inspiratory stridor and suprasternal retractions as the child struggles to inhale air; increased production of thick secretions and edema further obstruct the airway and cause hypoxia, and carbon dioxide to accumulate; respiratory acidosis and failure is the outcome

3. Assessments

a. Onset is gradual after upper respiratory infection

NCLEX!

b. Child awakens with low-grade fever, barking cough, and acute stridor; noisy breathing and the use of accessory muscles increase

c. Child is agitated, restless, has a frightened appearance, sore throat, and rhinorrhea

d. Pulse oximetry is used to detect hypoxemia; anteroposterior (AP) and lateral upper airway x-rays are ordered

4. Priority nursing diagnoses
   a. Ineffective breathing pattern
   b. Fear/anxiety
   c. Knowledge deficit
   d. Risk for fluid volume deficit
5. Planning and implementation
   a. Monitor child's respiratory effort continuously to ensure a patent airway; observe for diminished breath sounds, circumoral cyanosis, cessation of noisy breathing, and drooling
   b. Quiet respiratory effort is a sign of physical exhaustion and impending respiratory failure (NCLEX!)
   c. Provide humidity and supplemental oxygen; intravenous fluids prevent dehydration and help liquefy secretions
   d. Assist child to assume upright position or any position of comfort; promote a calm, quiet environment; keep parents nearby to decrease child's stress and to lessen crying
   e. Keep emergency intubation equipment available at the bedside; the nurse is also immediately available (NCLEX!)
   f. Assess parental and child's anxiety level; provide emotional support
6. Medications (see Table 4-1)
   a. Bronchodilators decrease mucosal constriction and laryngeal edema; nebulized racemic epinephrine has a rapid onset with improvement of symptoms, although relapse may occur within 2 hours
   b. Corticosteroids decrease inflammation and edema
7. Child and family education
   a. Assess parental anxiety and ability to adhere to medical recommendations
   b. Symptoms are usually worse at night and may recur for several nights; instruct parents that child can be cared for at home if able to take fluids by mouth and has no stridor at rest
   c. Cool mist humidifier and the presence of parents can be the initial treatment of the crisis; comforting measures include cuddling, rocking, singing and any calming measures until breathing becomes easier
   d. Instruct parents to seek medical attention immediately if breathing becomes labored, child seems exhausted or very agitated, or if symptoms do not improve after cool air humidity treatment
   e. Teach parents that LTB is a viral illness; avoid contact with large groups of people and practice infection control measures
8. Evaluation: parents demonstrate understanding of home care and the need for medical attention; the child breathes without difficulty; breath sounds are clear; heart and respiratory rates are within normal for age

B. Epiglottis

1. Description

a. Inflammation and swelling of the epiglottis, primarily affecting children between the ages of 2 and 8

b. The site of obstruction is supraglottic and is life-threatening because edema in this area can obstruct the airway and occlude the trachea within minutes

2. Etiology and pathophysiology

a. Bacteria, usually *Haemophilus influenzae,* cause the epiglottis to become cherry red, swollen, and so edematous that it obstructs the airway; secretions pool in the pharynx and larynx; the child has a sore throat and is unable to swallow; complete airway obstruction can occur within 2 to 6 hours

b. Onset is sudden, in a previously healthy child; the Hib vaccine has contributed to a decreased incidence of epiglottitis, although the causative organisms may also be streptococcus and staphylococcus

3. Assessments

a. Child awakens with sudden onset of high fever (102.2°F), extremely sore throat, and pain on swallowing

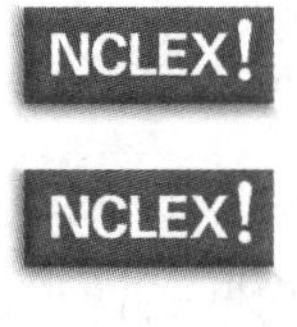

b. Child is very anxious, restless, looks ill, and insists on sitting upright leaning on arms, with chin thrust out and mouth open (tripod position)

c. Dysphonia (muffled voice), dysphagia (difficulty swallowing), drooling of saliva, and distressed respiratory effort are the classic signs of epiglottitis

d. Edematous, cherry-red epiglottis is the most reliable diagnostic sign

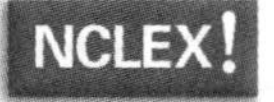

e. Examination of the throat is contraindicated, however, unless emergency intubation equipment and trained personnel are available; physical manipulation of the hypersensitive and irritated airway muscles may result in spasm and complete obstruction

f. Lateral neck x-ray confirms an enlarged epiglottis; x-rays are portable and completed in the examination room with the child on the parent's lap to minimize stress and maximize child's comfort and calm behavior

g. Complete blood count and blood cultures are taken once the child is intubated and stabilized

4. Priority nursing diagnoses

a. Fear

b. High risk for suffocation

c. Ineffective breathing pattern

d. Ineffective airway clearance

5. Planning and implementation

a. Assess continuously for respiratory distress and decrease in respiratory effort; report changes in status

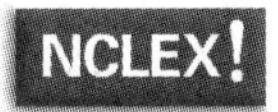

b. Never leave child unattended; support child in position of comfort; encourage parents to hug and cuddle their child

c. Keep endotracheal and tracheotomy tubes and suction equipment at bedside; assist with emergency ventilation if needed before child is taken to operating room for airway insertion

d. Child is usually intubated for 24 hours; restraints may be necessary to prevent dislodgment of the tube, as swelling of the epiglottis may prohibit reintubation

e. Provide support for child and family and alleviate anxiety; explain all procedures clearly and calmly

f. All invasive procedures, including starting an intravenous infusion, arterial blood gases, and blood cultures are performed in the operating room

g. Keep child NPO; intravenous fluids provide hydration; administer antipyretics and antibiotics as prescribed

h. After extubation, monitor the child closely in the intensive care unit to ensure immediate assessment if respiratory effort is compromised

6. Medications

a. Antibiotics treat the bacterial infection and are usually given for 7 to 10 days; child is discharged in about 3 days on oral antibiotics

b. Antipyretics treat fever and manage the pain of sore throat

c. Corticosteroids may be given for 24 hours before extubation to decrease edema

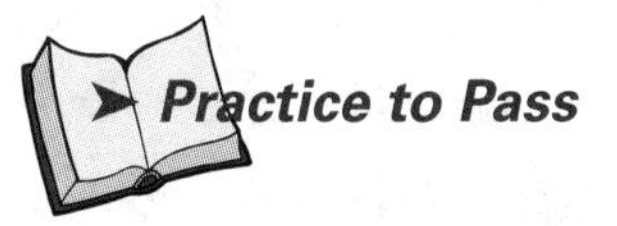

You are the nurse in the Emergency Department. The mother of a 2-year-old with epiglottitis tells you that she has to call her husband to come to the hospital. She saw a telephone down the hall and informs you that she will be right back. What are your concerns? How will you respond?

7. Child and family education

a. Provide emotional support and explain all procedures calmly; encourage parents to cuddle and comfort child

b. Prepare child and parents for airway insertion in operating room

c. Teach parents importance of completing antibiotic regimen after discharge; explain medications, how to administer, and any side effects to be expected

d. Discuss importance of Hib vaccine and reassure parents that recurrence of epiglottitis is uncommon

8. Evaluation: parents demonstrate understanding of home care and completion of antibiotics; the child breathes without difficulty and maintains pink mucous membranes and nail beds; the child demonstrates relaxed posture and sleeps quietly

C. Pneumonia

1. Description

a. Inflammation of the lungs that occurs most often in infants and young children; bronchioles and alveolar spaces are affected

b. Pneumonia may be a primary condition or can occur secondary to another illness

2. Etiology and pathophysiology

a. Viruses from the upper respiratory tract are the usual cause; the virus invades the alveoli and bronchial mucosa, causing sloughing and debris; respiratory syncytial virus (RSV) is the common organism and causes severe illness in the immunocompromised infant

b. Bacterial pneumonia occurs when organisms circulating in the bloodstream travel to the lungs, increase in number, and damage pulmonary cells; alveoli are filled with fluid and exudate and may involve one segment or the entire lung; a history of a viral infection usually precedes bacterial pneumonia

c. Mycoplasma pneumoniae infection is most common in older children in fall and winter, and occurs in crowded living conditions

3. Assessments

a. Viral pneumonia

1) Child usually presents with mild fever, nonproductive cough, and rhinitis

2) Disease is self-limiting and lasts 5 to 7 days; high-risk infants with RSV invasion may demonstrate wheezing, tachypnea, and increased respiratory distress

b. Bacterial pneumonia

1) Children with bacterial pneumonia usually present with high fever, productive cough, and ill appearance

2) There may be retractions, grunting respirations, chills, and chest pain; respiratory distress is significant and accompanied by restlessness and anxiety

c. Chest x-ray reveals density of lung tissue, patchy infiltrates, and increased fluid; pulse oximetry and blood gas measurements determine oxygen saturation; complete blood count and blood cultures determine if causative agent is viral or bacterial

4. Nursing diagnoses

a. Ineffective airway clearance

b. Ineffective breathing pattern

c. Risk for fluid volume deficit

d. Anxiety

e. Activity intolerance/pain

5. Planning and implementation

a. Monitor breath sounds, respiratory rate, use of accessory muscles, color, oxygen saturation levels, and level of activity and restlessness every 2 hours

b. Encourage child to assume position of comfort, usually upright; assist child to cough, deep breathe, and change position often; teach splinting to ease discomfort with coughing; lying on the affected side may also splint chest and decrease discomfort

c. Ensure chest physiotherapy is performed as ordered; administer oxygen if needed; encourage child to use the incentive spirometer

d. Administer antipyretics and analgesics for temperature control and pain relief

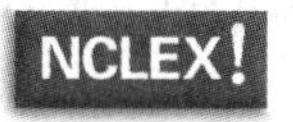

e. Administer oral and/or IV fluids as ordered to ensure hydration; keep strict intake and output records; weigh daily; assess for signs of dehydration

f. Provide cool mist to aid in temperature reduction; change linens and bedclothes often to prevent chilling from dampness

g. Assist infants and young children with clearing secretions by bulb syringe and/or deep suction as needed

h. Provide emotional support to parents

i. Cluster nursing care to allow for periods of undisturbed rest and a quiet environment

6. Medications

a. Antibiotics treat bacterial infection after culture and sensitivity reports indicate the causative organism

b. Acetaminophen and ibuprofen reduce fever and promote comfort

7. Child and family education

a. Explain all treatments and procedures to child and family; encourage parents to stay and participate in child's care

b. Assess ability of parents to care for child at home

c. Teach parents to take child's temperature; discuss importance of oral fluids and inform parents of recommended amounts appropriate to child's age

d. Child may go home on oral antibiotics; explain actions, dosage, times, and importance of continuing until entire prescription is completed; discuss any expected side effects

NCLEX!

e. Discuss infection control and prevention measures; explain importance of avoiding ill contacts and adhering to immunization schedule

f. Child will need additional rest periods after discharge

g. Lungs may not be completely healed when symptoms disappear; follow-up chest x-ray may be needed to determine status of lung tissue

8. Evaluation: parents verbalize knowledge and ability to adhere to treatment regimen with regard to medications, oral fluids, assistance with clearing of secretions; the child is afebrile, and respiratory rate and oxygen saturation levels are within normal limits for age; the child participates in activities of daily living and consumes adequate hydration

D. Bronchiolitis

1. Description

a. Inflammation of the bronchioles with edema and excess accumulation of mucus; air trapping and atelectasis result from increased airway resistance because of the small obstructed bronchioles

b. A major cause of hospitalization of high-risk infants

2. Etiology and pathophysiology

   a. Respiratory syncytial virus (RSV) is the primary causative organism; virus is spread by contact with contaminated objects; RSV is not airborne but can live for several hours on nonporous surfaces

   b. RSV bronchiolitis is most prevalent during the first 2 years of life, with most occurrences in spring and winter; bronchiolitis usually begins with a mild upper respiratory infection; as disease progresses, gas exchange is compromised, hypoxemia results, and metabolic acidosis develops

3. Assessments

   a. Clinical manifestations include worsening of an upper respiratory tract infection with tachypnea, retractions, low-grade fever, anorexia, thick nasal secretions, and increasingly labored breathing; older infants may have a frequent, dry cough

   b. Auscultation of the lungs reveal wheezing or crackles

   c. Nasopharyngeal washing to obtain respiratory secretions identifies the virus causing the condition; chest x-ray may be normal or indicate hyperinflation or nonspecific inflammation

4. Priority nursing diagnoses

   a. Ineffective airway clearance related to increased airway secretions

   b. Parental anxiety related to child's respiratory distress

   c. Fluid volume deficit related to decreased intake

5. Planning and implementation

   a. Complete a respiratory assessment hourly; provide humidified oxygen to ease respiratory effort; pulse oximetry to assess oxygen levels

   b. Clear nasal passages with bulb syringe; elevate head of bed

   c. Cluster nursing care to allow for rest; assess anxiety level of parents and provide support; maintain a calm environment

   d. Intravenous fluids may be needed if oral intake is compromised; monitor strict intake and output; weigh daily to assess fluid loss

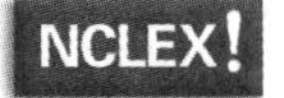

   e. Maintain strict handwashing and contact precautions; caregivers should not care for other high-risk children

6. Medications

   a. Ribavirin, a respiratory antiviral agent, is useful for premature and other high-risk infants (see Table 4-1)

   b. Bronchodilators and steroids are sometimes used

7. Child and family education

   a. Explain disease process and provide support to lessen anxiety

   b. Encourage parents to assist in care of their infant; explain all procedures and treatments

c. Parents should be taught to use bulb syringe as needed to keep nasal passages clear

d. Teach the parents to provide frequent oral fluids; notify physician if child demonstrates symptoms of dehydration, including crying without tears, sunken eyes, lethargy, or "acts sick"

e. Instruct the parents to notify physician if child refuses to eat or breathing becomes worse

f. Instruct the parents to use humidifier in child's bedroom

g. Teach the parents to avoid smoking in child's vicinity

h. Teach the parents to practice strict handwashing; keep child away from individuals with upper respiratory infections; RSV can reoccur

8. Evaluation: child demonstrates clear breath sounds and regular respirations; the child consumes adequate oral fluids and has moist mucous membranes; the parents verbalize understanding of disease and participate in child's care

VI. Accidents and Injuries Causing Respiratory Health Problems

A. Foreign body aspiration

1. Description

a. Inhalation of an object into the respiratory tract, intentional or otherwise

b. Peak age for foreign body aspiration is children less than 3 years of age; it is a leading cause of death in children under 1 year

2. Etiology and pathophysiology

a. Foreign bodies usually lodge in the right main bronchus because it is shorter and wider than the left; obstruction may be partial or complete and causes atelectasis, air trapping, and hyperinflation distal to the site of obstruction

b. The type and shape of the object, as well as the small diameter of an infant's airway, determines the severity of the problem; round objects such as hot dogs, round candy, nuts, and grapes do not break apart and are more likely to occlude the airway; latex balloons are particularly hazardous; objects with irregular shapes may irritate the airway and partially obstruct airflow

c. Failure to remove a foreign object is usually fatal; a delay in removal may cause aspiration pneumonia

3. Assessments

a. Sudden coughing and gagging is the first sign and objects in the upper airway may be expelled

b. Partial obstruction may cause symptoms of respiratory infection for days or even weeks; child may have hoarseness, croupy cough, wheezing, and dyspnea

NCLEX!

c. If obstruction is complete, child will demonstrate stridor, cyanosis, difficulty swallowing and speaking

d. A child who cannot speak, is cyanotic, and collapses requires immediate attention for complete airway obstruction

e. Fluoroscopy and chest x-ray reveal foreign body in respiratory tract

4. Priority nursing diagnoses

a. Ineffective airway clearance

b. Ineffective breathing pattern

c. Fear/anxiety

d. Knowledge deficit related to child safety

5. Planning and implementation

a. Respiratory assessment to determine severity of problem and degree of obstruction; continuous monitoring to provide assistance if obstruction worsens

b. If total airway obstruction occurs, perform back blows and chest thrusts for infants, and Heimlich maneuver in children older than 1 year

NCLEX!

c. Keep NPO; foreign body is usually removed in surgery

d. Position for comfort and to optimize airway; provide emotional support to parents and child and alleviate anxiety

Practice to Pass

The father of a 3-year-old child is feeding him peanut butter on a spoon at snack time. What information would be appropriate for this dad?

e. After removal of object, assess for additional obstruction that may be caused by laryngeal edema and tissue swelling

6. Medications

a. Antibiotics may be administered if secondary infection is suspected

b. They may also be used if purulent secretions are present in the airway, with or without signs of pneumonia

7. Child and family education

a. Teach parents about the hazards of aspiration and the importance of childproofing the home.

b. Review age-appropriate foods and discuss the most frequently aspirated objects: coins, hot dogs, balloons, nuts, popcorn, grapes, round candy, peanut butter

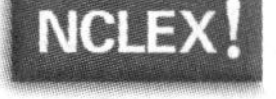

c. Discuss toy safety and avoidance of toys with small, removable parts; caution against allowing the child to run and play with objects in his/her mouth

d. Teach parents CPR and techniques of chest thrusts, back blows, and abdominal thrusts.

8. Evaluation: child maintains a patent airway and has normal breath sounds; the parents verbalize an understanding of needed child safety precautions

Case Study

A 7-year-old child is being discharged after initial diagnosis and treatment of acute asthma. You are the pediatric asthma educator completing the final education session with his parents.

1. What instructions regarding the peak expiratory flow meter will you discuss?
2. How will you respond when the child's parents tell you they plan to restrict him from physical education at school in order to prevent another attack?
3. What information will assist the child's parents in avoiding an exacerbation by recognizing subtle signs of an asthma episode?
4. What is the purpose of a spacer with the metered dose inhaler?
5. What is the overall goal of asthma education discharge teaching?

For suggested responses, see page 408.

Posttest

1 **The mother of an infant diagnosed with bronchiolitis asks the nurse what causes this disease. The nurse's response would be based on the knowledge that the majority of infections that cause bronchiolitis are a result of:**

(1) Ribavirin.
(2) Mycoplasma pneumoniae.
(3) Respiratory syncytial virus (RSV).
(4) Hemophilus influenzae.

2 **A child is brought to the Emergency Department with suspected epiglottitis. Which nursing intervention would be considered unsafe?**

4

(1) Allowing the child to remain in the position of choice
(2) Placing intubation equipment at the bedside
(3) Encouraging parents to comfort the child
(4) Examining the throat

3 **An 18-month-old child is seen in the Emergency Department with respiratory distress and is admitted with a diagnosis of pneumonia. Following the initial workup, the baby is still short of breath but is rubbing his eyes as if he is sleepy. The mother wants to lay the baby down for his nap. The infant refuses to lie down. The nurse would suggest:**

(1) Rocking the baby until he is asleep and then lay him down.
(2) The mother hold him in her arms while he sleeps.
(3) The mother allow the baby to sleep in an upright position.
(4) A sleeping pill to help the baby rest.

4 **Which statement by an 8-year-old child with asthma indicates that she understands the use of a peak expiratory flow meter?**

(1) "My peak flow meter can tell me if an asthma episode might be coming, even though I might still be feeling okay."
(2) "When I do my peak flow, it works best if I do three breaths without pausing in between breaths."
(3) "I always start with the meter reading about halfway up. That way I don't waste any breath."
(4) "If I use my peak flow meter every day, I will not have an asthma attack."

5 **A child with cystic fibrosis is hospitalized for a respiratory infection. Which documentation in the chart would indicate the need for counseling regarding nutrition and gastrointestinal complications?**

(1) Frothy, foul-smelling stools
(2) Weight unchanged from yesterday
(3) Consumed 80 percent of breakfast
(4) Eats three snacks every day

6 **An adolescent was diagnosed with cystic fibrosis as an infant. At this time, the adolescent will need additional teaching related to:**

(1) Obtaining a sweat chloride test.
(2) The effect of pancreatic enzymes on the sex hormones.
(3) Weight reduction diet.
(4) Reproductive ability.

7 **The parents of a child with cystic fibrosis inform the nurse that they will be unable to perform postural drainage at home because their bed does not recline like the hospital bed. The nurse's response is based on an understanding that:**

(1) Postural drainage is essential to mobilize secretions in the airways so they can be coughed out.
(2) Postural drainage is not necessary as long as the child takes his pulmozyme to decrease the viscosity of the mucus.
(3) Postural drainage does not influence the pulmonary status of a child with cystic fibrosis.
(4) The parents can be referred to the Cystic Fibrosis Foundation for a flexible bed.

8 **An 11-month-old child is being discharged home for the first time after being diagnosed with bronchopulmonary dysplasia (BPD). She will require home oxygen therapy. Which statement by the mother indicates that discharge teaching is incomplete?**

(1) "We will not allow any smoking at our home."
(2) "We have several fire extinguishers, and we know how to use them."
(3) "Her brother will blow out the birthday candles at her party."
(4) "We will return to the hospital if she seems irritable and won't play."

9 **The nurse is teaching home tracheostomy care to the parents of a toddler. What information is essential to include?**

(1) The importance of changing the tracheostomy every day
(2) How to recognize signs of infection and obstruction
(3) How to remove the tracheostomy so the child can talk
(4) Teaching the child to keep large objects away from the tube

10 **A child with a respiratory infection is scheduled to have a sweat test. The mother asks the purpose of this diagnostic test. The nurse's response would be based on the knowledge that the test:**

(1) Determines if the child is dehydrated.
(2) Asesses if the sweat glands are functioning.
(3) Identifies the infectious organism.
(4) Establishes a diagnosis of cystic fibrosis.

See pages 100–101 for Answers and Rationales.

Answers and Rationales

Pretest

1 **Answer: 4** ***Rationale:*** Infants and young children have narrower airways and shorter distance between structures; accessory muscles generally used for breathing are immature. The respiratory rate of infants is faster than adults, and parents can be taught to assess the child for respiratory problems.
Cognitive Level: Analysis
Nursing Process: Implementation; ***Test Plan:*** PHYS

2 **Answer: 3** ***Rationale:*** Newborns are unable to coordinate breathing and sucking simultaneously. They are nose-breathers, and anything that interferes with nasal patency impairs feeding as well.
Cognitive Level: Analysis
Nursing Process: Implementation; ***Test Plan:*** PHYS

3 **Answer: 1** ***Rationale:*** In epiglottitis, any manipulation of the throat can cause stimulation of the gag reflex. The inflamed, edematous epiglottis could then completely obstruct the airway. All other assessments should be made.
Cognitive Level: Application
Nursing Process: Assessment; ***Test Plan:*** SECE

4 **Answer: 3** ***Rationale:*** Children with cystic fibrosis require pancreatic enzymes with every meal and snack to counter malabsorption and nutritional problems. Normal bowel movements indicate that enzyme dosage is appropriate. It is important to avoid other children with infections, but physical activity is encouraged within the child's capability. Chest percussion is a normal part of health maintenance for this child.
Cognitive Level: Analysis
Nursing Process: Evaluation; ***Test Plan:*** HPM

5 **Answer: 3** ***Rationale:*** Developmentally, small children practice increased hand-to-mouth activity and explore objects with their mouths. Any small toy or food can be ingested and potentially obstruct the airway. All of the other choices are correct, but option 3 is most important.
Cognitive Level: Application
Nursing Process: Implementation; ***Test Plan:*** HPM

6 **Answer: 4** ***Rationale:*** Pulmonary pathogens are particularly detrimental to children with cystic fibrosis. Colonization of the lungs with resistant organisms often leads to poor survival rates. Aggressive intravenous administration of high-dose antibiotics is always a priority.
Cognitive Level: Analysis
Nursing Process: Planning; ***Test Plan:*** PHYS

7 **Answer: 2** ***Rationale:*** Epinephrine is a beta adrenergic drug given via inhalation for emergency relief of acute bronchospasm; action is immediate and the drug may be repeated in 3 to 5 minutes. Methylprednisolone and prednisone are both corticosteroids to reduce the inflammatory process but would not give immediate relief. Cromolyn sodium is a preventive medication.
Cognitive Level: Application
Nursing Process: Planning; ***Test Plan:*** PHYS

8 **Answer: 4** ***Rationale:*** The sudden onset of severe respiratory distress is frightening and very stressful for the family and child. There is no prolonged hospital confinement.
Cognitive Level: Analysis
Nursing Process: Planning; ***Test Plan:*** PSYC

9 **Answer: 1** ***Rationale:*** Splinting the affected side with a pillow or stuffed animal lessens the discomfort experienced with bacterial pneumonia.
Cognitive Level: Application
Nursing Process: Implementation; ***Test Plan:*** PHYS

10 **Answer: 3** ***Rationale:*** Home oxygen therapy and tracheostomy care require access to emergency equipment typically not available on a camping trip. Additionally, camp fires are hazardous. All other choices indicate correct information.
Cognitive Level: Analysis
Nursing Process: Evaluation; ***Test Plan:*** SECE

Posttest

1 **Answer: 3** ***Rationale:*** At least one-half of all cases of bronchiolitis are attributed to RSV. The other responses are incorrect.
Cognitive Level: Application
Nursing Process: Implementation; ***Test Plan:*** PHYS

2 **Answer: 4** ***Rationale:*** Any manipulation of the tongue or throat may stimulate the gag reflex and cause complete obstruction. Emergency intubation equipment should be readily available before any examination of the throat is attempted.
Cognitive Level: Application
Nursing Process: Implementation; ***Test Plan:*** SECE

3 **Answer: 3** ***Rationale:*** The child's respiratory distress makes lying down difficult. The child will breath more easily in a semi- to high-Fowler's position.
Cognitive Level: Analysis
Nursing Process: Implementation; ***Test Plan:*** PHYS

4 **Answer: 1** ***Rationale:*** Peak expiratory flow readings over time indicate the child's respiratory ability when she is well. Readings of 50 percent below "personal best" indicate an asthma episode is imminent. It does not prevent an attack.
Cognitive Level: Analysis
Nursing Process: Evaluation; ***Test Plan:*** HPM

5 **Answer: 1** ***Rationale:*** Frothy, foul-smelling stools reflect malabsorption and indicate that pancreatic enzymes are not being consumed or dosages may need adjustment. Maintenance of weight and consuming meals and snacks are positive nutrition goals for children with cystic fibrosis.
Cognitive Level: Application
Nursing Process: Assessment; ***Test Plan:*** PHYS

6 **Answer: 4** ***Rationale:*** The developmental task of adolescence is to set future goals, including marriage and family. Men are usually sterile, and women may have decreased fertility as thick cervical mucus interferes with mobility of sperm. The difference between sterility and impotence should also be addressed.
Cognitive Level: Application
Nursing Process: Planning; ***Test Plan:*** HPM

7 **Answer: 1** ***Rationale:*** The removal of thick, pulmonary secretions is critical to the maintenance of adequate lung function and prevention of infection. Daily chest physiotherapy, including postural drainage, is required and must be consistently performed. Playground activities such as monkey bars, trapeze bar, somersaults, and headstands can accomplish the purposes of postural drainage.
Cognitive Level: Analysis
Nursing Process: Analysis; ***Test Plan:*** HPM

8 **Answer: 3** ***Rationale:*** There should be no open flames when oxygen is in use; oxygen enhances combustion and is a fire hazard.
Cognitive Level: Analysis
Nursing Process: Evaluation; ***Test Plan:*** HPM

9 **Answer: 2** ***Rationale:*** Accumulating mucopurulent secretions may provide a medium for bacterial growth or can obstruct the lumen of the tube. Suctioning is another risk for introduction of bacteria. Early recognition of signs of infection is important.
Cognitive Level: Application
Nursing Process: Implementation; ***Test Plan:*** HPM

10 **Answer: 4** ***Rationale:*** Children with cystic fibrosis have elevated chloride concentrations of sweat because of the dysfunction of the exocrine glands.
Cognitive Level: Analysis
Nursing Process: Implementation; ***Test Plan:*** PHYS

References

Ball, J. & Bindler, R. (1999). *Pediatric nursing: Caring for children* (2nd ed.). Stamford, CT: Appleton & Lange, pp. 406–461.

Betz, C. L. & Sowden, L. A. (2000). *Mosby's pediatric nursing reference* (4th ed.). St. Louis: Mosby, pp. 29–33, 41–50, 101–111, 143–152.

Bindler, R. & Ball, J. (1999). *Quick reference to pediatric clinical skills.* Stamford, CT: Appleton & Lange, pp. 101–108.

Bouder, V. R., Dickey, S. B., & Greenbeg, C. S. (1998). *Children and their families: The continuum of care.* Philadelphia: Saunders, pp. 863–896, 914–972.

Christensen, B. L. & Kockrow, E. O. (1999). *Foundations of nursing* (3rd ed.). St. Louis: Mosby, p. 365.

deWit, S. C. (1998). *Essentials of medical-surgical nursing* (4th ed.). Philadelphia: Saunders, pp. 413–437.

deWit, S. C. (2001). *Fundamental concepts and skills for nursing.* Philadelphia: Saunders, pp. 669–670.

Dickinson-Herbst, D. (2001). Cystic fibrosis and lung transplantation: Ethical concerns. *Pediatric Nursing 27*(1): 87–89.

Dorland's illustrated medical dictionary (29th ed.). Philadelphia: Saunders, pp. 206, 707.

Fowler, C. (2001). Preventing and managing exercise induced asthma. *The Nurse Practitioner 26*(3): 25, 29–35.

Karch, A. (2001). *Lippincott's nursing drug guide.* Philadelphia: Lippincott Williams & Wilkins, pp. 448–451.

Kozier, B., Erb, G., & Justesen, S. L. (2000). *Procedures supplement for fundamentals of nursing* (6th ed.). Upper Saddle River, NJ: Prentice Hall, pp. 145–150.

Ladewig, P. W., Lorda, M. L., & Olds, S. B. (1998). *Maternal-newborn nursing care: The nurse, the family, and the community* (4th ed.). Menlo Park, CA: Addison-Wesley, pp. 628–629, 677–679.

McKinney, E., Ashwill, J., Mussay, S., James, S., Gorrie, T., & Droske, S. (2000). *Maternal-child nursing.* Philadelphia: Saunders, pp. 1235–1243.

Monahan, F. D. & Neighbors, M. (1998). *Medical-surgical nursing: Foundations for clinical practice* (2nd ed.). Philadelphia: Saunders, pp. 537–556, 566–567, 659–668.

Pillitteri, A. (1999). *Child health nursing: Care of the child and family.* Philadelphia: Lippincott, pp. 548–597.

Smith, S. F. & Duell, D. J. (1996). *Clinical nursing skills: Basic and advanced skills* (4th ed.). Stamford, CT: Appleton & Lange.

Steinbach, S. F. (2000). Four controversies in pediatric asthma care. *Contemporary Pediatrics 17*(10): 151–171.

Taylor, C., Lillis, C., & Lemone, P. (2001). *Fundamentals of nursing: The art and science of nursing care* (4th ed.). Philadelphia: Lippincott Williams & Wilkins, pp. 512–574, 1228–1245.

Vittone, S. (2001). Lung transplantation for cystic fibrosis: Additional considerations. *Pediatric Nursing 27*(1): 90–92.

Wong, D. L. & Hockenberry-Eaton, M. (2001). *Wong's essentials of pediatric nursing* (6th ed.). St. Louis: Mosby, pp. 433–434, 823–877.

CHAPTER 5

Cardiac Health Problems

Marilyn L. Weitzel, MSN, RN,
Doctoral Candidate

CHAPTER OUTLINE

OBJECTIVES

- Identify data essential to assessing alterations in health of the cardiac system in a child.
- Discuss the clinical manifestations and pathophysiology of alterations in health of the cardiac system of a child.
- Discuss therapeutic management of a child with alterations in health of the cardiac system.
- Describe nursing management of a child with alterations in health of the cardiac system.

[Media Link]

Use the CD-ROM enclosed with this text, or log onto the address given to access the free, interactive Companion Website created for this series. The CD-ROM and Companion Website accompanying this book offer additional practice opportunities and information—NCLEX Review, Case Studies, Glossary, In Depth with NCLEX, and more.

www.prenhall.com/hogan

REVIEW AT A GLANCE

acyanotic heart defect *a heart condition that does not cause deoxygenation, or low oxygen levels. The skin and mucous membrane color is usually normal pink*

cardiac catheterization *a test that examines the heart by placing a catheter into a vein or artery and advancing it to the heart in order to sample the oxygen levels and pressure measurements in the heart chambers*

cyanotic heart defect *a heart condition that causes the blood to contain less oxygen than required. The skin and mucous membrane color is usually pale to blue*

echocardiogram *a graphic record of walls, valves, and vessels of the heart produced by ultrasound*

Jones Criteria *guidelines for diagnosis of initial attack of rheumatic fever developed by Jones in 1992*

left to right shunt *movement of blood from the left side of the heart to the right side through an abnormal opening*

lymphadenopathy *a condition that causes swollen glands and can be caused by infection or cancer*

murmur *a heart sound resembling running water through a tight space; usually indicates a malfunctioning valve or an abnormal opening in the cardiac septum*

polycythemia *a condition of more red blood cells than normal; often indicates hypoxemia and the body's compensatory response*

prostaglandin E1 *a hormone that reopens the ductus arteriosus; it is used in cases where the blood is not oxygenating properly and the patent ductus arteriosus allows for mixing of saturated and unsaturated blood*

right to left shunt *movement of blood from the right side of the heart to the left side of the heart through an abnormal opening in the septum; this results in deoxygenated blood because the systemic blood bypasses the lungs and is ejected into the aorta*

vasculitis *inflammation of the tunica intima (inner lining) of the arteries and veins*

Pretest

1 An infant is admitted with an acyanotic heart defect. Which assessment finding should be discussed with the physician?

(1) Heart murmur
(2) Dyspnea
(3) Weight gain
(4) Eupnea

2 For an infant client with a cyanotic heart defect, which symptoms would indicate risk for congestive heart failure?

(1) Respiratory crackles and frothy secretions
(2) Decreased cyanosis
(3) Increased blood pressure
(4) Oxygen saturation increase

3 A child is admitted with a diagnosis of "rule out rheumatic fever." Which assessment finding supports this diagnosis?

(1) Elevated antistreptolysin-O (ASO)
(2) Elevated hematocrit
(3) Decreased hemoglobin
(4) Decreased salicylate level

4 A child is admitted with possible coarctation of the aorta. Which of the following orders should be questioned?

(1) Regular diet
(2) BP of upper and lower extremities q 4 hours
(3) Intake and output
(4) Vital signs on admission, then Q.D.

5 A child with tetralogy of Fallot becomes acutely ill with an increase in cyanosis, tachycardia, and tachypnea. Which nursing action would be most effective to relieve cardiac load?

(1) Place child in Trendelenburg position.
(2) Place child in knee-chest position.
(3) Have oxygen equipment available.
(4) Maintain suction equipment available.

6 A child with a cyanotic heart defect is being discharged home to await surgical repair. In the discharge teaching, the nurse instructs the parents:

(1) To prevent the child from crying at all.
(2) To observe the child for signs of increased intracranial pressure.
(3) In cardio-pulmonary resuscitation.
(4) To identify growth and development milestones.

7 **A client with rheumatic fever is admitted to the nursing unit. The nurse's most important intervention is to:**

(1) Prevent spread of rheumatic fever.
(2) Provide comfort from arthralgia.
(3) Evaluate for nervous system complications.
(4) Teach parents about cardiopulmonary resuscitation (CPR).

8 **A child with Kawasaki's disease is admitted to the pediatric unit. Since promotion of comfort is an appropriate nursing goal, the nurse:**

(1) Administers aspirin and immunoglobulins as ordered.
(2) Administers Tylenol and immunoglobulins as ordered.
(3) Keeps child NPO for the first 24 hours.
(4) Encourages a vigorous exercise program.

9 **A pediatric client is discharged after an acute phase of rheumatic fever. The priority discharge instruction given by the nurse is that the child:**

(1) Is to resume regular activities.
(2) Needs to take antibiotics as ordered.
(3) Needs to maintain complete bedrest.
(4) Will experience central nervous system (CNS) complications.

10 **A pediatric client with a cyanotic heart defect experiences a cyanotic episode. Symptoms consistent with this cyanotic episode would include:**

(1) Skin is ruddy or mottled prior to cyanosis.
(2) Decreased rate of respirations.
(3) Decreased heart rate.
(4) Lethargy.

See page 122 for Answers and Rationales.

I. Overview of the Anatomy and Physiology of the Cardiac System

A. Heart has four chambers: right and left atria (upper chambers), and right and left ventricles (lower chambers)

B. Heart has four valves: pulmonic (right ventricle to pulmonary artery), aortic (left ventricle to aorta), tricuspid (right atrium to right ventricle) and mitral (left atrium to left ventricle)

C. Fetal circulation

1. Ductus venosus

a. Umbilical vein carries oxygenated blood from the placenta to the infant

b. Blood bypasses liver through the ductus venosus

c. When umbilical cord is clamped and cut, blood flow ceases and ductus venosus closes

d. Blood flows into liver

2. Foramen ovale

a. Systemic blood enters right atrium

b. Oxygenated blood flows from right to left atria through the foramen ovale

c. Blood bypasses the lungs which are nonfunctional

d. Blood flows from left atria to left ventricle and out to aorta

e. Foramen ovale closes after birth with the change in pressure in cardiac chambers

3. Ductus arteriosus

a. A fistula between aorta and pulmonary artery allows for mixing of blood

b. Blood flowing through pulmonary artery may enter aorta through a patent ductus arteriosus

c. Ductus arteriosus closes after birth with first few breaths

D. Oxygenation

1. Oxygen is bound to hemoglobin on red blood cells

2. Hematocrit and hemoglobin facilitate oxygenation

3. Desaturated blood contains more than 5 g of unoxygenated hemoglobin per 100 mL of blood

E. Cardiac function

1. Heart rate is sensitive to oxygen level

2. Cardiac output is dependent on heart rate until child is 5 years old

3. Child has an increased risk of heart failure

a. Immature heart is sensitive to volume or pressure overload

b. Muscle fibers are less developed

F. Diagnostic tests for cardiac system

1. Radiography (x-ray)

a. Reveals size and contour of heart

b. Visualizes characteristics of pulmonary vascular markings

c. Nursing: no special care

2. Echocardiography (ultrasound)

a. Identifies heart structure

b. Identifies pattern of movement, hemodynamics

c. Nursing: no special care

3. Electrocardiogram (ECG)

a. Records quality of major electrical activity of the heart

b. Identifies arrhythmias

c. Nursing: no special care

4. Holter monitor: 24 hour monitoring of the ECG

5. Stress ECG: ECG done after exercise

6. Cardiac catheterization

a. Description: examines the heart by placing a catheter into an artery or vein and advancing it to the heart

b. Measurements

1) Oxygen levels in each chamber

2) Pressure in each chamber

c. Identifies anatomic alterations

d. Pre-procedure care

1) Age-appropriate teaching including information of what child will feel, see, and hear

2) Family support

3) NPO after midnight

4) Oral sedation is given

5) Obtain baseline vital signs, hemoglobin, hematocrit, and pedal pulses

e. Post-procedure care

1) Monitor for bleeding: hematoma, hemorrhage, thrombus

a) Maintain direct pressure to insertion site for 15 minutes and a pressure dressing for 6 hours

b) Obtain vital signs, neurovascular signs q 15 minutes for the first hour, then q 30 minutes for 1 hour or longer until stable

c) Maintain bedrest for 6 hours

2) Monitor for arrhythmias

3) Monitor for infection

4) Assess insertion site

5) Assess for diuresis related to dye

f. Discharge teaching

1) Teach signs of complications to family (bleeding, infection, thrombosis)

2) Encourage quiet play only for first 24 hours to avoid disturbing insertion site

3) Encourage increased fluid intake to maintain hydration to offset diuretic effect of contrast dye

G. Surgical procedures

1. Palliative: surgery designed to improve the overall condition of the child; does not correct the disorder; many palliative surgeries may create additional defects that allow for better exchange of blood between the chambers

2. Correction: surgery designed to resolve the cardiac problem

II. Congenital Cardiac Health Problems

A. Acyanotic heart defects: heart conditions that do not cause deoxygenation or low oxygen levels; the skin and mucous membrane color is usually normal pink

1. Atrial septal defect (see Figure 5-1)

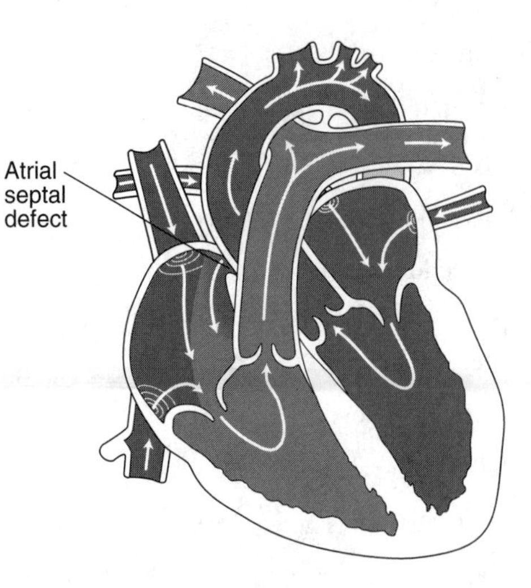

Figure 5-1

Atrial septal defect.
Source: Ball, J. & Bindler, R. (1999). *Pediatric nursing: Caring for children* (2nd ed.). Stamford, CT: Appleton & Lange, p. 480.

a. Description

1) Defect between the atria
2) Septal wall defect allowing blood to flow from left atrium to right atrium, called a **left to right shunt**

b. Etiology and pathophysiology

1) Opening between the atria
2) Foramen ovale fails to close
3) Sometimes much of septum is absent
4) Increased pulmonary blood flow

NCLEX!

c. Assessment

1) Often asymptomatic if small defect
2) Dyspnea
3) Fatigue, poor growth
4) Soft systolic **murmur** (abnormal heart sound) in pulmonic area, splitting S_2
5) **Echocardiogram:** a diagnostic test that utilizes ultrasound; shows right ventricular overload and shunt size
6) Congestive heart failure
7) Cardiac catheterization: visualization of defect

d. Priority nursing diagnoses

1) Anxiety
2) Ineffective family coping: disabling
3) Risk for impaired growth and development
4) Risk for infection

5) Altered nutrition: Less than body requirements

6) Impaired gas exchange

e. Planning and intervention

1) Surgical closure or patch of defect

2) Transcatheter device closure during cardiac catheterization

NCLEX!

3) Nursing management of child with acyanotic heart disease (see Table 5-1)

f. Child and family education

1) Explain to parents the purpose of the tests and procedures

2) Teach parents ways to support nutrition, reduce stress on heart, promote rest, and support growth and development during preoperative period

3) Teach parents signs of congestive heart failure and infection

4) Prepare parents and child for surgery by visiting the intensive care unit, explaining equipment and sounds

5) Prepare older child for postoperative experience, including coughing and deep breathing and need for movement

6) Teach the need for antibiotic prophylaxis to prevent subacute bacterial endocarditis

g. Evaluation: child's growth and development progresses regularly; child's gas exchange is maximized; workload of the heart is minimized

Table 5-1

Nursing Care of the Child with an Acyanotic Heart Defect

Nursing Diagnosis	Nursing Care
Anxiety; Ineffective family coping: disabling	1. Assess coping mechanisms of family. 2. Provide family with information about condition. 3. Refer family to American Heart Association.
Risk for impaired growth and development	1. Treat the child as normally as possible. Teach parents that children are more comfortable when they know what to expect. 2. Promote mental development activities as appropriate for age and condition.
Risk for infection	1. Limit exposure to individuals with infections. 2. Promote good pulmonary hygiene—change position, use percussion and postural drainage. 3. Prophylactic antibiotics when undergoing surgical or dental treatments to prevent subacute bacterial endocarditis.
Altered nutrition: Less than body requirements	1. Offer small frequent feedings. 2. Use soft nipple for infant to ease the stress of sucking. 3. Organize nursing care to allow for rest.
Impaired gas exchange	1. Promote good pulmonary hygiene. 2. Monitor intake and output. Limit fluids as ordered. 3 Administer diuretics as ordered. 4. Change position every two hours.

2. Ventricular septal defect (VSD)

a. Description (see Figure 5-2)

1) Defect between the ventricles

2) Septal wall incomplete allowing blood to flow from left ventricle to right ventricle (left to right shunt)

b. Etiology and pathophysiology

1) Increased pulmonary blood flow

2) Left to right shunting of blood flow is caused by the higher pressure in the left ventricle

3) The shunting of blood causes an increased load on the right ventricle

NCLEX!

c. Assessment

1) Tachypnea, dyspnea

2) Poor growth, reduced fluid intake

3) Palpable thrill

4) Systolic murmur at left lower sternal border

5) ECG and radiology detect larger septal defects

6) Signs of congestive heart failure

d. Priority nursing diagnoses (see Table 5-1)

e. Planning and intervention

1) Occasionally spontaneous closure occurs

2) Surgical patching if failure to thrive occurs

3) Prophylactic antibiotics treatment to prevent endocarditis

4) Preoperative nursing care involves promoting growth and development and promoting oxygenation (see Table 5-1)

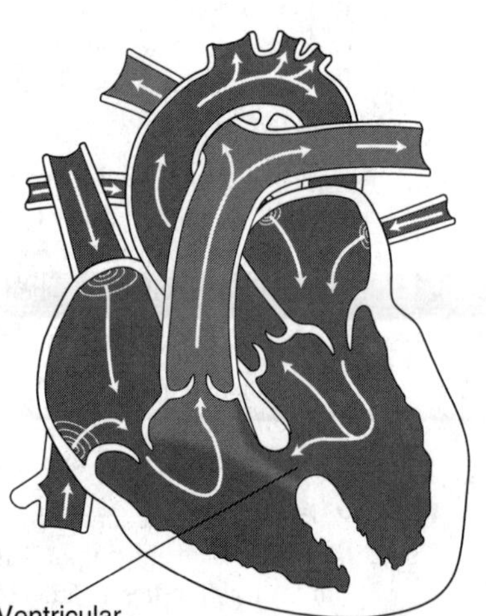

Figure 5-2

Ventricular septal defect. *Source:* Ball, J. & Bindler, R. (1999). *Pediatric nursing: Caring for children* (2nd ed.). Stamford, CT: Appleton & Lange, p. 481.

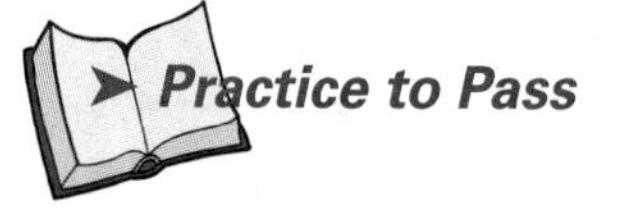

A child is being discharged after a surgical repair of a ventricular septal defect. What does the nurse include in the discharge teaching plan?

5) Postoperative nursing care continues with the activities of pre-op care, while providing analgesics as necessary to provide comfort and using sterile dressings on the incision

f. Child and family education

1) Explain to parents the purpose of the tests and procedures
2) Teach parents ways to support nutrition, reduce stress on heart, promote rest, support growth and development during preoperative period
3) Teach parents signs of congestive heart failure and infection
4) Prepare parents and child for surgery by visiting the intensive care unit, explaining equipment and sounds
5) Prepare older child for postoperative experience including coughing and deep breathing and need for movement

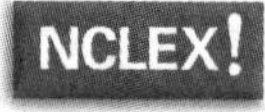

6) Teach the need for antibiotic prophylaxis to prevent subacute bacterial endocarditis

g. Evaluation: child's growth and development progresses regularly; child's gas exchange is maximized; work load of the heart is minimized

3. Coarctation of aorta

a. Description (see Figure 5-3)

1) Narrowing of the descending aorta
2) Restricts blood flow leaving the heart

b. Etiology and pathophysiology

1) Narrowing or constriction of descending aorta
2) Often near ductus arteriosus
3) Progressive disorder that leads to congestive heart failure

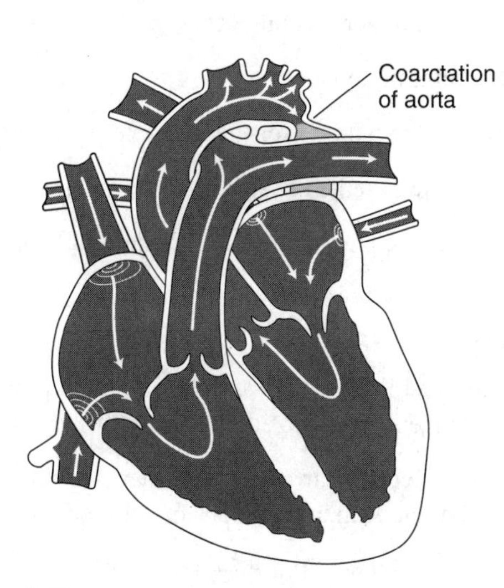

Figure 5-3

Coarctation of aorta. *Source:* Ball, J. & Bindler, R. (1999). *Pediatric nursing: Caring for children* (2nd ed.). Stamford, CT: Appleton & Lange, p. 483.

NCLEX!

c. Assessment

1) May be asymptomatic
2) Blood pressure difference of 20 mm between upper and lower extremities
3) Brachial and radial pulses full, femoral pulses weak
4) Headache, vertigo, and epistaxis
5) Exercise intolerance
6) Left ventricular hypertrophy
7) Dyspnea
8) Cerebrovascular accident (CVA) secondary to hypertension in upper circulation

d. Priority nursing diagnoses

1) Altered tissue perfusion (renal)
2) Risk for injury
3) Activity intolerance
4) Knowledge deficit
5) Others as previously listed in Table 5-1

NCLEX!

e. Therapeutic management

1) Balloon cardiac catheterization
2) Surgical resection and patch of coarctation
3) Prophylaxis for endocarditis when undergoing surgical or dental procedures
4) Prior to correction, monitor BP in upper and lower extremities
5) Rebound hypertension occurs in the immediate postoperative period

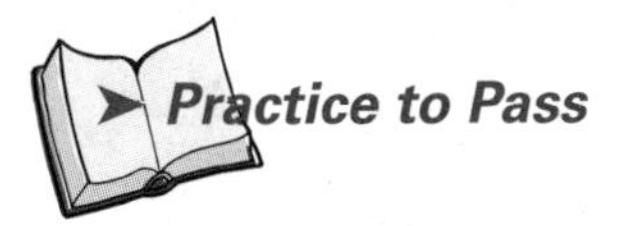

A pediatric client is being discharged to home following a cardiac catheterization. What are three priority points in the nurse's discharge teaching to the family?

f. Child and family education

1) Prepare the parents for the tests and procedures the child will undergo
2) Teach the parents the signs and symptoms of worsening condition
3) Educate the parents on administration of cardiac and vasoactive drugs
4) The child will need prophylactic antibiotics for all surgical and dental procedures

g. Evaluation: child's growth and development progresses regularly; child's gas exchange is maximized; workload of the heart is minimized

B. Cyanotic heart defects: heart conditions that cause the blood to contain less oxygen than required; the skin and mucous membrane color is usually pale to blue

1. Tetralogy of Fallot (see Figure 5-4)

a. Description

Figure 5-4

Tetrology of Fallot.
Source: Ball, J. & Bindler, R. (1999). *Pediatric nursing: Caring for children* (2nd ed.). Stamford, CT: Appleton & Lange, p. 490.

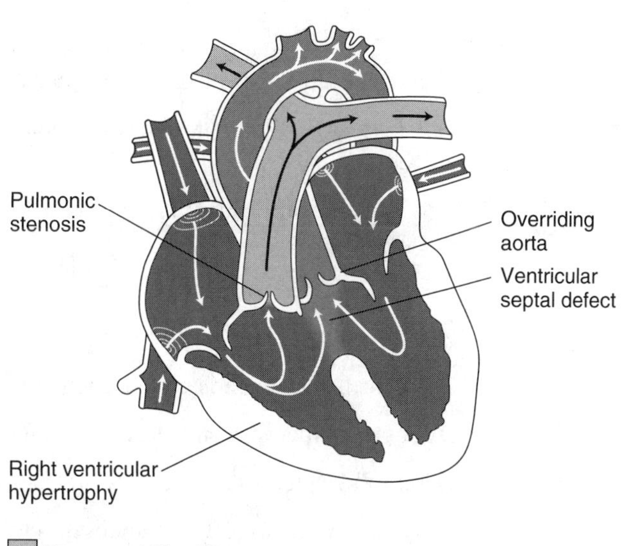

1) Four defects that combine to allow blood flow to bypass the lungs and enter the left side of the heart, called a **right to left shunt**
2) Unoxygenated blood enters the body circulation accounting for the cyanosis

b. Etiology and pathophysiology

1) Four defects: pulmonic stenosis, right ventricular hypertrophy, ventricular septal defect, and overriding aorta
2) Atrial septal defect occurs at times
3) Deficient oxygen in the tissues leads to acidosis
4) Hypercyanosis (TET) spells occur, which are transient periods when there is an increase in the right to left shunting of blood

NCLEX!

c. Assessment

1) TET spells characterized by hypoxia, pallor, and tachypnea; precipitated by crying, defecation, and feeding; older children will assume a squatting position to decrease blood return from the lower extremities; treatment involves placing the child in knee-chest position, administering morphine or propranolol and oxygen
2) Clubbing of digits
3) **Polycythemia** (excess number of red blood cells), metabolic acidosis
4) Poor growth, exercise intolerance
5) Systolic murmur in pulmonic area
6) Right ventricular hypertrophy
7) Cardiac catheterization visualizes anomalous structures

d. Priority nursing diagnoses (see Table 5-2)

e. Therapeutic management

1) **Prostaglandin E1:** to maintain open ductus arteriosus

2) Palliative surgery to improve oxygenation includes shunting procedures

3) Corrective surgery includes patching the VSD and relieving the pulmonary stenosis

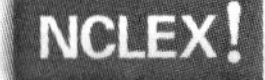

4) See Table 5-2 for associated nursing care

f. Child and family education

1) Teach the parents to promote nutrition in light of weak suck

2) Discuss activities to promote oxygenation

3) Describe symptoms of respiratory infections

4) Describe treatments and procedures the child will undergo

Table 5-2

Nursing Care of the Child with Cyanotic Heart Disease

Nursing Diagnosis	Nursing Care
Altered cardiopulmonary tissue perfusion	1. Monitor hemoglobin and hematocrit levels. 2. Keep the child calm. Do not allow long periods of crying. 3. When hypercyanosis occurs, assist the child to squatting or knee-chest position. 4. Administer oxygen and morphine as ordered during these spells.
High risk for infection	1. Limit exposure to individuals with infections. 2. Promote good pulmonary toilet—change position, percussion, and postural drainage. 3. Prophylactic antibiotics when undergoing surgical or dental treatments to prevent subacute bacterial endocarditis.
Altered nutrition	1. Offer small frequent feedings. 2. Use soft nipple for infant to ease the stress of sucking. 3. Organize nursing care to allow for rest.
Risk for impaired gas exchange	1. Limit activity. 2. Maintain clear airways. 3. Monitor electrolytes.
Risk for decreased cardiac output	1. Assess vital signs. 2. Monitor for signs of congestive heart failure. 3. Note peripheral edema. 4. Weigh child q day. 5. Maintain strict intake and output measurement. 6. Administer diuretics as ordered. 7. Administer oxygen as ordered. 8. Palpate liver every 4 to 12 hours (indicates right-sided failure). 9. Administer digoxin as ordered: a. Assess for apical pulse—monitor for bradycardia or arrhythmias. b. Be consistent in measurement of medication and time of administration. c. Do not repeat dose if child vomits.
Risk for injury	1. Monitor hemoglobin and hematocrit. 2. Observe for signs of thrombus formation.

g. Evaluation

1) Parents and child describe treatments and procedures
2) Child gains weight steadily
3) Child's mental development progresses
4) Child remains free of symptoms of respiratory infections

2. Transposition of the great vessels

a. Description (see Figure 5-5)

1) Aorta arises from right ventricle, and pulmonary artery arises from left ventricle
2) Other anomalies exist that increase mixing of blood between the two separate circulations; these anomalies promote oxygenation
3) Right to left shunting of blood occurs

b. Etiology and pathophysiology

1) Pulmonary artery originates from left ventricle; blood travels from the left ventricle to the pulmonary artery, then to the lungs, and then back into the left atrium
2) Aorta originates from right ventricle; blood leaves the right ventricle by the aorta, travels to the body cells and returns to the right atrium by way of the vena cava
3) There are two closed circulation pathways
4) Survival depends on foramen ovale remaining open to mix oxygenated and deoxygenated blood

NCLEX!

c. Assessment

1) Progressive cyanosis → hypoxia → acidosis
2) Sign and symptoms of congestive heart failure
3) Tachypnea

Figure 5-5

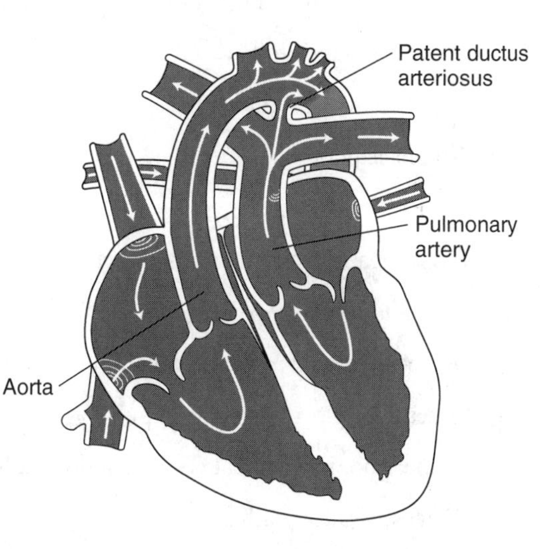

Transposition of great vessels. *Source:* Ball, J. & Bindler, R. (1999). *Pediatric nursing: Caring for children* (2nd ed.). Stamford, CT: Appleton & Lange, p. 491.

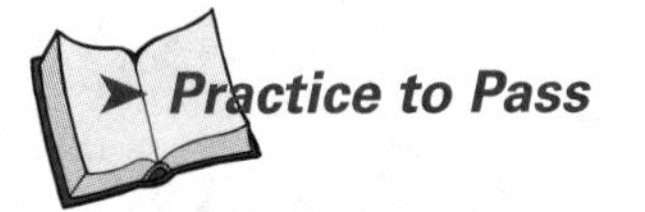

A child has been given a diagnosis of transposition of the great vessels. How would you explain the disorder to the family? What is the most important point that the family needs to understand and implement prior to surgery?

4) Poor feeding

5) Failure to grow

6) Echocardiogram identifies misplacement of arteries

d. Priority nursing diagnoses (see Table 5-2)

e. Therapeutic management

1) Prostaglandin E1 to maintain open ductus arteriosus

2) Palliative surgical interventions

3) Corrective surgery

4) Prophylactic antibiotic therapy to prevent endocarditis

5) Nursing activities to promote nutrition and reduce respiratory congestion (see Table 5-2)

f. Child and family education

1) Home care requirements related to nutrition, rest, and oxygenation

2) Preparation for procedures and treatments

3) Safe administration of cardiac drugs and diuretics

g. Evaluation: parents and child describe treatments and surgical procedures; child's growth and development progresses steadily; child maintains adequate gas exchange; parents administer medications effectively and safely

3. Hypoplastic left heart syndrome

a. Description

1) Abnormally small left ventricle noted at birth

2) Inability of the heart to supply the oxygen needs of the body

b. Etiology and pathophysiology

1) Absent or stenotic mitral and aortic valves

2) Abnormally small left ventricle and aortic arch

3) Major resistance to aortic flow

4) Hypertrophy of right ventricle

5) Prognosis poor

NCLEX!

c. Assessment

1) Tachypnea, chest retractions, dyspnea

2) Cyanosis

3) Decreased pulses, poor peripheral perfusion

4) Increased right ventricular impulse

5) Echocardiogram indicates small and weak left ventricle

6) Congestive heart failure

d. Priority nursing diagnosis

1) Anticipatory grieving

2) Anxiety

3) Ineffective individual (or family) coping

4) Others as previously outlined in Table 5-2

NCLEX!

e. Planning and interventions

1) Prostaglandin E1 given to prevent closure of patent ductus arteriosus

2) Palliative surgery

3) Transplant may be performed

4) Survival rate low

f. Evaluation: parents describe treatments and procedures their child is undergoing; parents accept diagnosis and display appropriate grieving behaviors

III. Acquired Cardiac Health Problems

A. Rheumatic fever

1. Description

a. Systemic inflammatory disease that involves the heart and joints; CNS and connective tissue involvement may also occur

b. Occurs secondary to an infection by group A beta-hemolytic streptococcus

2. Etiology and pathophysiology

a. Follows 2 to 6 weeks after a group A beta-hemolytic streptococcal infection

b. It may be an autoimmune reaction against beta-hemolytic streptococcus; strep organisms cannot be cultured out of the lesions of rheumatic fever

c. Acute phase lasts 2 to 3 weeks and is characterized by inflammation of connective tissue in the heart, joints, and skin

d. Proliferative phase affects primarily the heart with Aschoff bodies developing on the heart valves; cardiac valve leaflets scar and lead to valvular stenosis and regurgitation

e. Episode of rheumatic fever lasts up to 3 months and is self-limiting

f. Long-term consequence is rheumatic heart disease, which is often manifested in valvular damage

g. Difficult to diagnose as mimics other diseases; diagnosis is usually based on **Jones Criteria,** which describe frequent symptoms of rheumatic fever; symptoms are listed according to the likelihood of rheumatic fever infection as major manifestations and minor manifestations; diagnosis is based on the presence of two major or one major and two minor criteria

NCLEX!

3. Assessment using Jones Criteria (1992)

a. Major criteria include

1) Multiple joints may be involved in the inflammatory process; joints affected are most frequently the large joints—knees, elbows, and wrists

2) Carditis is most severe symptom of rheumatic fever; symptoms of carditis include a new murmur, pericardial friction rub, changes on the ECG; tachycardia may be noted by the nurse in the form of a sleeping pulse greater than 100

3) Chorea is the CNS symptom of rheumatic fever and involves the involuntary movement of limbs; emotional lability and slurred speech may occur; this symptom tends to have a latent period of 2 months or more from the strep infection

4) Erythema marginatum is a erythematous, macular rash which occurs primarily on the trunk and proximal limbs; this symptom is frequently associated with carditis

5) Subcutaneous nodules are nontender nodules that develop on the skin over the flexor surfaces of joints and the vertebrae

b. Minor criteria

1) Fever: spiking temperature

2) Arthralgia

3) Elevated erythrocyte sedimentation rate (ESR), C-reactive protein, and decreased red blood cell (RBC) count

4) Prolonged P-R and/or Q-T interval on ECG

c. Supporting evidence (of recent streptococcal infection)

1) History of streptococcal infection

2) History of scarlet fever

3) Positive throat culture for streptococcus

4) Elevated anti-streptolysin-O (ASO) titer

4. Priority nursing diagnoses

a. High risk for injury—carditis

b. Pain

c. High risk for diversional activity deficit

5. Planning and interventions

a. Bedrest until ESR returns to normal

b. Use aspirin and prednisone as ordered anti-inflammatory agents to reduce the inflammation; aspirin will also promote comfort from the painful joints

c. Monitor the client for cardiac function

d. Give penicillin as ordered in either an oral daily dose or monthly long-acting injection after recovery from rheumatic heart disease to reduce the risk of recurrence of the strep infection; erythromycin given if allergic to penicillin

e. Design nursing activities to promote rest and to encourage diversional activities which do not stress the heart; maintain bedrest with bathroom privileges

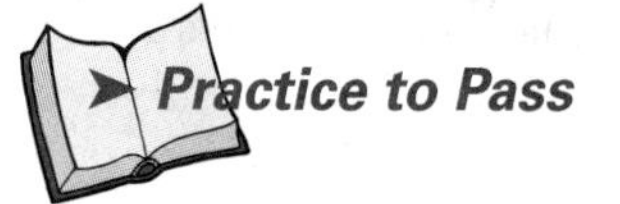

The mother of a pediatric client diagnosed with rheumatic fever asks why the client cannot resume activities normal for age. How does the nurse discuss the potential complications?

6. Child and family education
   a. Client and parents need to understand the pathology of the disease as well as the rationale for the bedrest
   b. Diversional activities are discussed that allow for mental stimulation without physical activity
   c. Assist parents in planning for home care of the child
7. Evaluation: the child remains free of cardiac complications; the parents and child describe safe and effective administration of the prophylactic antibiotic

B. Kawasaki's disease

1. Description
   a. A multisystem disorder involving **vasculitis** (inflammation of the tunica intima or inner lining of the arteries and veins)
   b. Also called mucocutaneous lymph node syndrome
2. Etiology and pathophysiology
   a. Unknown cause but generally affects young children; most frequently affected are boys under 2 years of age
   b. Three phases of disease
      1) Acute phase characterized by fever, conjunctival hyperemia, swollen hands and feet, rash, and enlarged cervical lymph nodes
      2) Subacute phase is characterized by cracking lips, desquamation of skin on tips of fingers and toes, cardiac disease, and thrombocytosis
      3) Convalescent phase has lingering signs of inflammation
   c. Significantly increased platelet count
   d. Possible cardiac pathology including arrhythmias, congestive heart failure, and myocardial infarction

NCLEX!

3. Assessment
   a. Phase one (days 1 to 10): fever lasting longer than 5 days that is unresponsive to antipyretics, conjunctivitis, crusted and fissured lips, swelling of hands and feet, erythema, **lymphadenopathy** (a condition that causes swollen glands and can be caused by infection or cancer)
   b. Phase two (days 10 to 25): fever diminishes, irritability, anorexia, desquamation of hands and feet, arthritis and arthralgia, cardiovascular manifestations
   c. Phase three (days 26 to 40): drop in ESR, and diminishing signs of illness
4. Priority nursing diagnoses
   a. High risk for injury
   b. Hyperthermia
   c. High risk for altered home health maintenance
5. Planning and intervention
   a. Administer aspirin 80 to 100 mg/kg/day as ordered while temperature is elevated

b. Administer gamma globulin (IVIG) as ordered to reduce risk of coronary artery lesions and aneurysms

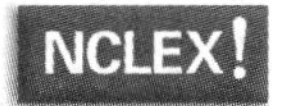

c. Nursing management

1) Promote comfort
2) Small frequent feedings
3) Passive range of motion to extremities
4) Cool baths
5) Gentle oral care
6) Encourage fluids
7) Monitor for complications
    a) Aneurysms
    b) Side effects of aspirin therapy: bleeding, GI upset
    c) Side effects of IVIG therapy: elevated blood pressure, facial flushing, tightness in chest
8) Monitor temperature
9) Monitor eyes for conjunctivitis

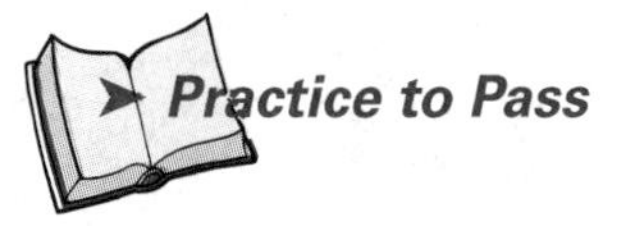

The parent of a preschool child reports that the child's hands are peeling, eyes are red, and the child has joint pain. What should the school nurse suggest to the parents, and what is the immediate concern?

6. Child and family education

a. Safe administration of aspirin therapy

b. Teach parents to keep the skin clean and avoid soaps and lotions

c. Offer liquids high in calories, low in acids

d. Low-cholesterol diet

e. Call physician if child refuses to walk

f. Monitor temperature in A.M. and P.M. prior to giving aspirin

7. Evaluation: the client recovers without serious sequelae; the parents describe temperature control means

Case Study

A 1-week-old client is scheduled for palliative surgery for transposition of the great vessels. You are the nurse who is supporting the parents through this illness.

❶ What questions will you ask the parents prior to surgery?

❷ What assessments do you make preoperatively?

❸ What are the priority postoperative nursing interventions?

❹ What discharge instructions will you give the parents?

❺ The parents ask what emergency situations may arise and how they should respond. What do you say?

For suggested responses, see page 408.

Posttest

1 A toddler has been diagnosed with an acyanotic cardiac defect. Which assessment data would most likely indicate congestive heart failure?

(1) Heart murmur
(2) Cardiac volume overload
(3) Anuria
(4) Excitability

2 An infant who has a congenital heart defect comes into the clinic with complaints of irritability, pallor, and increased cyanosis that began quickly over the last 30 minutes. As the nurse assesses the infant, the parent asks why the child's color is bluish. The best response by the nurse is, "Skin color is:

(1) Related to the time of day."
(2) Related to brain function."
(3) Related to hemoglobin level and oxygen saturation."
(4) Unrelated to your child's condition."

3 A client is admitted with a diagnosis of "rule out rheumatic fever." Based on Jones Criteria, the nurse assesses for:

(1) Polyarthritis and dental caries.
(2) Fever, headache, and low red blood cell count.
(3) Chorea, muscle weakness, and decreased erythrocyte sedimentation rate.
(4) Erythema, polyarthritis, and elevated antistreptolysin-O (ASO) titer.

4 A toddler with Kawasaki's disease is ordered to receive aspirin therapy. Typical administration of aspirin for Kawasaki's disease would include which of the following principles?

(1) High doses of aspirin should be given while fever is high.
(2) Length of aspirin therapy is related to child's response.
(3) Aspirin dose increases after fever is gone.
(4) Aspirin dosage is unrelated to platelet count.

5 A newborn with possible hypoplastic left heart disease is to be admitted to the nursing unit. Which drug should be available for use?

(1) Digitoxin (Crystodigin)
(2) Prostaglandin E1 (Prostin VR)
(3) Morphine
(4) Testosterone (Andro)

6 A 2-year-old child is being discharged home and will have palliative surgery for tetralogy of Fallot at a later date. The mother wants to know about how much physical activity she can allow for the child. The nurse's best answer is:

(1) "Allow the child to regulate her activity."
(2) "Keep her on complete bedrest."
(3) "Limit her activities to a few hours."
(4) "Keep the child from crying."

7 After a pediatric client has a cardiac catheterization, which intervention would have the highest priority in the immediate postoperative period?

(1) Encourage intake of small amounts of fluid.
(2) Teach the parents signs of congestive heart failure.
(3) Monitor the site for signs of infection.
(4) Apply direct pressure to entry site for 15 minutes.

8 A child is being seen in the ambulatory clinic for a sore throat diagnosed as caused by group A beta-hemolytic streptococcus. The nurse provides care with the understanding that the risk of developing rheumatic fever is greatest:

(1) Two weeks later.
(2) Prior to administering an antibiotic.
(3) Once the child has begun antibiotic therapy.
(4) With the onset of the strep infection.

9 Which evaluation would indicate a toxic dose of digoxin?

(1) Tachycardia and dysrhythmia
(2) Headache and diarrhea
(3) Bradycardia and nausea and vomiting
(4) Tinnitus and nuchal rigidity

10 **The nurse is developing a discharge teaching plan for the family of a child with Kawasaki's disease. Which of the following is the first priority?**

(1) Teaching parents to administer aspirin and watch for side effects
(2) Recommending the child avoid contact sports
(3) Monitoring the child's temperature and notifying the doctor if it is over 98.6°F
(4) Establishing home schooling for 6 months

See page 123 for Answers and Rationales.

Answers and Rationales

Pretest

1 **Answer: 2** ***Rationale:*** Children with acyanotic heart defects may have a murmur without other symptoms. Dyspnea and tachycardia are early signs of pulmonary edema, which may lead to congestive heart failure.
Cognitive Level: Analysis
Nursing Process: Assessment; ***Test Plan:*** PHYS

2 **Answer: 1** ***Rationale:*** Pulmonary overload occurs prior to congestive heart failure. Crackles and frothy secretions are signs of moist respirations, a symptom of pulmonary overload.
Cognitive Level: Analysis
Nursing Process: Assessment; ***Test Plan:*** PHYS

3 **Answer: 1** ***Rationale:*** ASO titers indicate history of streptococcal infection, which is a precursor to rheumatic fever. The other symptoms are not related to this diagnosis.
Cognitive Level: Analysis
Nursing Process: Assessment; ***Test Plan:*** PHYS

4 **Answer: 4** ***Rationale:*** Blood pressure will be elevated in upper extremities and reduced in lower extremities with presence of coarctation of aorta. The constriction of the aorta may be progressive. Vital sign assessments provide data related to this progression and should be more frequent than once a day.
Cognitive Level: Analysis
Nursing Process: Analysis; ***Test Plan:*** PHYS

5 **Answer: 2** ***Rationale:*** The knee-chest position decreases venous return to the heart and thereby increases systemic vascular resistance, which leads to decreased cardiac output.
Cognitive Level: Application
Nursing Process: Implementation; ***Test Plan:*** PHYS

6 **Answer: 3** ***Rationale:*** Parents need to be prepared for emergencies. Crying for short periods is effective as deep breathing exercises. Increased intracranial pressure is not associated with cardiac failure. Monitoring growth and development would not be the primary concern.
Cognitive Level: Application
Nursing Process: Implementation; ***Test Plan:*** SECE

7 **Answer: 2** ***Rationale:*** Among the symptoms of rheumatic fever is migratory polyarthritis. The child will complain of aching joints. At the time of diagnosis, the child is not infectious. CPR is not a priority at this time because the child is hospitalized.
Cognitive Level: Application
Nursing Process: Implementation; ***Test Plan:*** PHYS

8 **Answer: 1** ***Rationale:*** Aspirin is ordered as an antipyretic and anti-clotting agent, while immunoglobulins decrease fever and inflammation. Reducing symptoms of the disease will increase client comfort. The child's lips are cracked, and soft foods and liquids are comforting. The child will be lethargic and passive range of motion exercises are utilized to facilitate joint movement.
Cognitive Level: Application
Nursing Process: Implementation; ***Test Plan:*** PHYS

9 **Answer: 2** ***Rationale:*** The child needs to take prescribed antibiotics indefinitely to prevent future infection and possible endocarditis from streptococcal infection. Complete bedrest is not required in the recovery period, but the child is maintained with limited activities. Complications of rheumatic fever are cardiac, not CNS.
Cognitive Level: Application
Nursing Process: Evaluation; ***Test Plan:*** HPM

10 **Answer: 1** ***Rationale:*** When pulmonary circulation is impaired, hemoglobin may not be reoxygenated which leads to the cyanotic appearance. The respirations and heart rate increase during a cyanotic episode and the child experiences agitation or irritability.
Cognitive Level: Analysis
Nursing Process: Assessment; ***Test Plan:*** HPM

Posttest

1 **Answer: 2** ***Rationale:*** Congestive heart failure may occur when the amount of blood passing from left to right side of the heart overloads the pulmonary system.
Cognitive Level: Application
Nursing Process: Assessment; ***Test Plan:*** PHYS

2 **Answer: 3** ***Rationale:*** The hemoglobin molecule carries oxygen. The oxyhemoglobin gives the skin the pink color. In the absence of oxyhemoglobin, the skin color darkens.
Cognitive Level: Application
Nursing Process: Implementation; ***Test Plan:*** PSYC

3 **Answer: 4** ***Rationale:*** Jones Criteria is a protocol to assist in identifying rheumatic fever. It consists of major symptoms, minor symptoms, and supporting evidence. Erythema, polyarthritis, and elevated ASO titer are among the major and minor symptoms and supporting evidence.
Cognitive Level: Analysis
Nursing Process: Assessment; ***Test Plan:*** PHYS

4 **Answer: 2** ***Rationale:*** Aspirin therapy is ordered 80 to 100 mg/kg/day until fever drops. Then aspirin is continued at 10 mg/kg/day until platelet count drops. Aspirin is used as an antipyretic and anti-agglutination drug.
Cognitive Level: Application
Nursing Process: Analysis; ***Test Plan:*** PHYS

5 **Answer: 2** ***Rationale:*** Prostaglandin E1 prevents closure of ductus arteriosus and thereby allows for mixing of oxygenated and unoxygenated blood until palliative surgery can be done.
Cognitive Level: Application
Nursing Process: Planning; ***Test Plan:*** PHYS

6 **Answer: 1** ***Rationale:*** Although a child requiring surgery for tetralogy of Fallot may have a need for additional services, such as supplemental oxygen at home, the child should be able to play and move about in the environment to meet both physiological and developmental needs.
Cognitive Level: Application
Nursing Process: Implementation; ***Test Plan:*** PHYS

7 **Answer: 4** ***Rationale:*** Direct pressure on wound site helps to form clot and reduce bleeding. Hemorrhage can be life-threatening in the immediate postoperative period.
Cognitive Level: Application
Nursing Process: Implementation; ***Test Plan:*** PHYS

8 **Answer: 1** ***Rationale:*** Rheumatic fever often follows 2 weeks after a streptococcal infection regardless of treatment.
Cognitive Level: Analysis
Nursing Process: Implementation; ***Test Plan:*** HPM

9 **Answer: 3** ***Rationale:*** Signs of digoxin toxicity include bradycardia, arrhythmia, nausea, vomiting, anorexia, dizziness, headache, weakness and fatigue.
Cognitive Level: Application
Nursing Process: Evaluation; ***Test Plan:*** PHYS

10 **Answer: 1** ***Rationale:*** Aspirin is an anti-inflammatory and antipyretic. The child may experience bleeding and G.I. upset as side effects.
Cognitive Level: Application
Nursing Process: Implementation; ***Test Plan:*** PHYS

References

Ashwill, H. J. & Droske, S. C. (1997). *Nursing care of children: Principles and practice.* Philadelphia: W. B. Saunders, pp. 651–665, 906–950.

Ball, J. & Bindler, R. (1999). *Pediatric nursing: Caring for children* (2nd ed.). Stamford, CT: Appleton & Lange, pp. 466–501.

Doenges, M. E. & Moorehouse, M. F. (1998). *Nurses' pocket guide: Diagnosis, interventions and rationales* (6th ed.). Philadelphia: F. A. Davis Company, pp. 545, 575, 589, 619.

Pillitteri, A. (1998). *Child health nursing: Care of the child and family.* Philadelphia: Lippincott, pp. 599–633.

CHAPTER 6

Neurologic Health Problems

Donna Miles Curry, RN, PhD

CHAPTER OUTLINE

OBJECTIVES

- Identify data essential to the assessment of alterations in health of the neurologic system in a child.
- Discuss the clinical manifestations and pathophysiology of alterations in the health of the neurologic system of a child.
- Discuss therapeutic management of a child with alterations in health of the neurologic system.
- Describe nursing management of a child with alterations in health of the neurologic system.

[Media Link]

Use the CD-ROM enclosed with this text, or log onto the address given to access the free, interactive Companion Website created for this series. The CD-ROM and Companion Website accompanying this book offer additional practice opportunities and information—NCLEX Review, Case Studies, Glossary, In Depth with NCLEX, and more.

www.prenhall.com/hogan

REVIEW AT A GLANCE

Brudzinski's sign *noted when the child's head is flexed while in the supine position, resulting in involuntary flexion of knees or hips; a positive Brudzinski's sign is a common sign in meningitis*

coma *level of unconsciousness in which client cannot be aroused even with painful stimuli*

Cushing's triad *a late sign of increased intracranial pressure characterized by increased systolic blood pressure, bradycardia, and irregular respirations*

epidural hematoma *bleeding between the dura and the cranium*

intracranial pressure (ICP) *the force exerted by brain tissue, cerebrospinal fluid, and blood within the cranial vault; normal ICP is 4 to 12 mm*

Kernig's sign *demonstrated when the leg of a client is raised with the knee flexed and any resistance or pain is felt; it is a common finding indicative of meningeal irritation in meningitis*

level of consciousness (LOC) *a measure of the degree of responsiveness of the mind to sensory stimuli; lower levels indicate decreased neurologic functioning; the levels can be categorized (in order of decreasing level of functioning) as confusion, delirium, obtunded, stupor, and coma*

meninges *fibrous membrane that covers brain and lines the vertebral canal; consists of three layers: the dura, arachnoid, and pia mater*

myelin *a sheath made of a fatty substance that covers the axon process of the neuron or nerve fibers and increases the speed and accuracy of nerve impulses; the myelination process is not complete at birth, but proceeds in a head to toe direction and accounts for the gradual development of fine and gross motor skills during early childhood*

neurogenic *refers to a lack of innervation to an organ*

nuchal rigidity *stiffness of the neck or resistance to neck flexion, often seen in infections of the central nervous system*

opisthotonus *client positions self hyperextending the head and neck; this is seen in meningitis and felt to relieve some of the discomfort from the meningeal irritation*

photophobia *sensitivity to light, seen in some clients with migraine headaches or viral infections such as measles and encephalitis*

subdural hematoma *bleeding between the dura and the cerebrum*

spasticity *tenseness of muscles, uncoordinated, stiff movements; can be seen as scissoring or crossing of the legs; exaggerated reflex reactions*

tonic-clonic *term frequently used to describe characteristics of certain seizures; tonic indicates continuous muscle contraction; clonic indicates alternating contraction and relaxation of muscles*

Pretest

1 **A child has been admitted with a history of a seizure 2 hours ago. The history reports fever, chills, and vomiting for the past 24 hours. In report, the nurse is told that the child has a positive Brudzinski's sign. The nurse knows that this is most likely caused by:**

(1) Increased intracranial pressure.
(2) Meningeal irritation.
(3) Encephalitis.
(4) Intraventricular hemorrhage.

2 **A nurse is assessing a new admission. The 6-month-old infant displays irritability, bulging fontanels, and setting-sun eyes. The nurse would suspect:**

(1) Increased intracranial pressure.
(2) Hypertension.
(3) Skull fracture.
(4) Myelomeningocele.

3 **An 8-year-old client with a ventriculoperitoneal shunt was admitted for shunt malfunction. He presents with symptoms of increased intracranial pressure. The mechanism of the development of his symptoms is most probably related to:**

(1) Increased flow of cerebrospinal fluid.
(2) Increased reabsorption of cerebrospinal fluid.
(3) Obstructed flow of cerebrospinal fluid.
(4) Decreased production of cerebrospinal fluid.

4 **A child with a myelomeningocele is started on a bowel management plan. The child's mother questions why this is being done. The nurse's response will be based on the understanding that:**

(1) Lack of innervation to the colon predisposes the child to diarrhea.
(2) Lack of innervation to the anal spinchter predisposes the child to being incontinent.
(3) Lack of mobility increases the gastric-colic reflex.
(4) Lack of mobility decreases the need for regular bowel movements.

5 A child has just been diagnosed with bacterial meningitis. The parent asks the nurse how long the child will be in isolation. The nurse's reply will be based on a protocol that isolation continues until:

(1) The organism is located.
(2) The antibiotics are initiated.
(3) The antibiotics have been administered for 24 hours.
(4) Ten days of antibiotic therapy have been completed.

6 The nurse observes a client with the neck and back arched and extremities severely extended. The mother asks why the child is doing that. The nurse explains that this posturing is called:

(1) Decerebrate.
(2) Decorticate.
(3) Jacksonian seizure.
(4) Opisthotonos.

7 A child is being treated for increased intracranial pressure (ICP). Which intervention would be contraindicated to order to decrease ICP?

(1) Keeping head of bed at a 30-degree angle
(2) Providing supplemental oxygen
(3) Turning head to one side
(4) Administering IV osmotic diuretics as ordered

8 A 10-year-old boy receives a blow to his head with a hard baseball and is admitted to the hospital for observation. If the child were to develop an epidural hematoma, the child would most like display symptoms:

(1) In the emergency room or soon after arriving on the unit.
(2) On the unit over the next few days.
(3) After discharge home.
(4) Over the next two months.

9 A 15-year-old client is seen in the emergency department following a head injury from football. During the first few hours after admission, he sleeps unless awakened, but he can be aroused easily and is oriented. In charting assessment findings, the nurse would describe this level of consciousness as:

(1) Semicomatose.
(2) Lethargy.
(3) Obtunded.
(4) Stuporous.

10 A young child has just been diagnosed with cerebral palsy. The nurse is teaching the parents how to meet the dietary needs of their child. The nurse would explain that children with cerebral palsy frequently have special dietary needs or feeding challenges because:

(1) The paralysis of their muscles decreases their caloric need.
(2) The spasticity of muscles increases their caloric need.
(3) All children with cerebral palsy require assistance with feedings.
(4) The child's inactivity increases the risk of obesity.

See pages 154–155 for Answers and Rationales.

I. Overview of the Anatomy and Physiology of the Nervous System: Several key points must be remembered when considering the nervous system of the infant and young child in contrast to the adolescent and adult

A. **The brain and spinal cord develop during the first trimester,** they are very susceptible to malformations caused by some insult such as infection, substance abuse, or maternal dietary deficiency

B. **The nervous system is not mature at birth,** but as the number of glial cells and dendrites increase, refinement continues until about 4 years of age

C. **Myelination is also incomplete; *myelin*** (a sheath made of a fatty substance that covers the axon process of the neuron or nerve fibers) is essential to increase the speed and accuracy of nerve impulses, providing the child with fine and gross motor skills and coordination

D. Development is in a cephalocaudal or "head to tail" direction

E. At birth and during early childhood, fontanels are not closed, and cranial bones have yet to ossify; this allows the head to expand to accommodate increased swelling or other causes of intracranial pressure

F. Young infants have a proportionately large, heavy head compared to adults, and they lack neck strength

G. An infant's brain is highly vascular, and the dura can strip away from the pericranium; the brain is more prone to hemorrhage when shaken or when another force is applied

H. Vertebrae are not completely ossified, placing young children at greater risk for cervical spine injury and compression fractures

II. Diagnostic Tests and Assessments of the Nervous System

A. Physical assessment

1. Level of consciousness (LOC)

a. This is a measure of the responsiveness of the brain to stimuli and has two components: alertness and cognitive power

b. Levels of decreasing consciousness include confusion, delirium, obtunded, stupor and **coma** (unarousable to painful stimuli)

c. Glasgow coma scale: an established instrument used to quantify the LOC

1) There are two versions based on the child's development level; one for the infant and young child (preverbal) and the older child and adult

2) Scores on the three subscales range from 1 to 4 for eye opening, 1 to 5 for verbal response, and 1 to 6 for motor response

3) The highest level of functioning would be scored 15, while the lowest level of functioning would score a 3 (see Table 6-1)

Table 6-1

Glasgow Coma Scale

Assessment	Response	Score*
Eyes open	Spontaneously	4
(Record C if eyes are closed by swelling)	To speech	3
	To pain	2
	No response	1
Best motor response	Obeys commands	6
(Record best upper arm response.)	Localized pain	5
	Flexion-withdrawal	4
	Abnormal flexion	3
	Abnormal extension	2
	No response	1
Best verbal response	Oriented	5
(Record T if an endotracheal or tracheostomy tube is in place)	Confused	4
	Inappropriate words	3
	Incomprehensible sounds	2
	No response	1
Total Score:		___

*A higher score indicates a higher level of functioning.

Source: LeMone, P. & Burke, K. M. (2000). *Medical surgical nursing: Critical thinking in client care* (2nd ed.). Upper Saddle River, NJ: Prentice-Hall, Inc., p. 1683.

2. **Intracranial pressure (ICP)**

    a. Is the pressure within the cranium or skull that surrounds the brain, normally 4 to 12 mm

    b. Pressure is caused by the volume of brain mass, cerebrospinal fluid (CSF), and blood

    c. An increase in any of these three must be compensated for by the others

    d. Fortunately for young children whose sutures have not closed, their cranium can expand to a point if there is increased pressure

3. Fontanels

    a. Membranes at the juncture of unclosed sutures

    b. Two prominent fontanels: the anterior and the posterior

4. Developmental milestones

    a. Specific criteria for comparing a child to other children of the same age on specific fine or gross motor, social, and cognitive skills

    b. Most criteria have been validated through cross-sectional and longitudinal studies

    c. Many of these criteria are incorporated into standardized developmental screening instruments such as the Denver II

5. Neurological exam: a specialized physical examination to determine neurologic function; it includes the following criteria:

    a. Description of behavior

    b. Vital signs: pulse, respiration, blood pressure, body temperature

    c. Eyes: pupil size and reactivity, movements, and blinking are assessed; in addition a funduscopic exam may be done to check for papilledema and preretinal hemorrhages

    d. Motor function: presence of spontaneous activity or response to pain; tremors, twitching or seizures may be observed

    e. Posturing

    1) When cortical control over motor function is lost, primitive posturing reflexes are apparent

    2) Decorticate posturing is seen with a severe dysfunction of the cerebral cortex; it includes adduction of the arms at the shoulders, arms flexed at the chest, wrists flexed, hands fisted, and lower extremities flexed

    3) Decerebrate posturing is seen with dysfunction at the level of the midbrain; it includes rigid extension and pronation of arms and legs (see Figure 6-1)

    f. Reflexes

    1) Specific reflexes are absent in deep coma such as corneal, pupillary, muscle-stretch, superficial, and plantar

Figure 6-1

A. Decorticate posturing,
B. Decerebrate posturing.

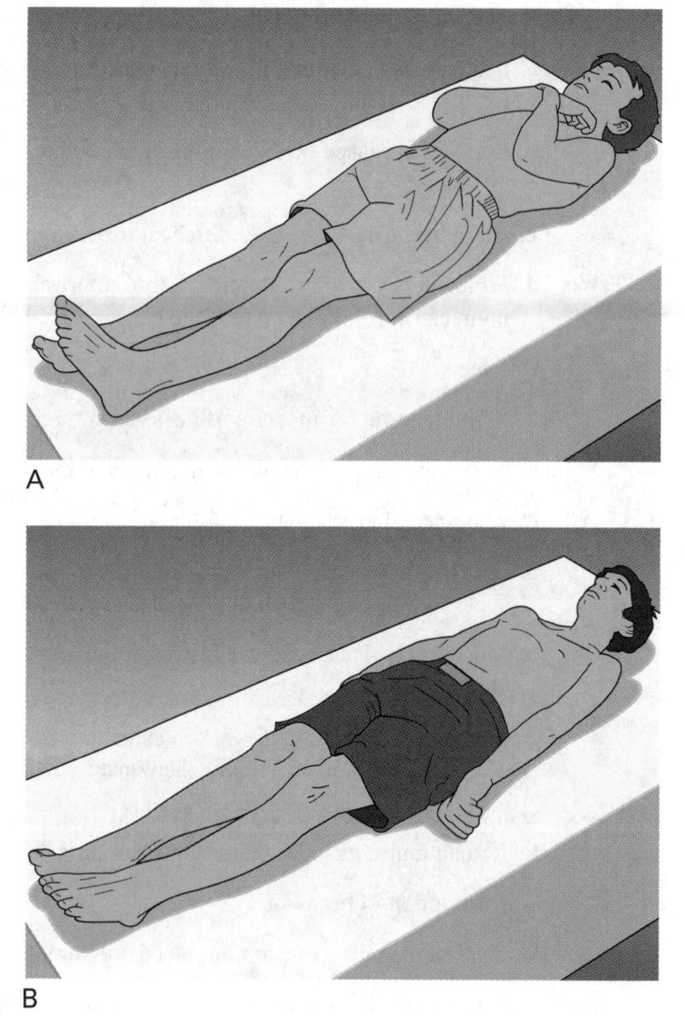

2) Specific neonatal reflexes such as the Moro, tonic neck, and withdrawal reflexes are evidence of normal neurological functioning, but the persistence of these and other neonatal or primitive reflexes after certain ages can indicate areas of dysfunction

6. Kernig's and Brudzinski's signs: specialized approaches that demonstrate meningeal irritation

   a. **Kernig's sign:** positive or present when the leg of a client is raised with the knee flexed and any resistance or pain is felt; this is a common finding indicative of meningeal irritation in meningitis

   b. **Brudzinski's sign:** positive or present when the child's head is flexed while in the supine position, resulting in involuntary flexion of knees or hips; this is a common sign in meningitis

B. Diagnostic tests

1. Lumbar puncture (LP): insertion of needle to obtain cerebrospinal fluid (CSF) to assess for blood, glucose, or proteins

2. Magnetic resonance imaging (MRI): a noninvasive procedure usually conducted in radiology department that permits visualization of neurologic structures using radio frequency emissions from elements

3. Computed tomography (CT): radiological procedure where pinpoint x-ray beams are directed on horizontal or vertical plane which, when entered on a computer, provide "slices" or pictures of cross sections of the brain at any axis

4. Electromyogram (EMG): a procedure that measures the electric potentials of individual muscles

5. Electroencephalogram (EEG): procedure using multiple electrodes placed on the head to record changes in electric potentials or impulses of the brain; it can be used to diagnose seizures and determine brain death

III. Congenital Neurologic Health Problems

A. Cerebral palsy

1. Description

   a. A nonprogressive motor disorder of the CNS resulting in alteration in movement and posture

   b. Classified as spastic, athetoid, ataxic, or mixed

   c. Topographic descriptions explain the part(s) of the body affected by cerebral palsy and include hemiplegia, diplegia, and quadriplegia

2. Etiology and pathophysiology

   a. The cause is trauma, hemorrhage, anoxia, or infection before, during, or after birth

   b. One-third of children with cerebral palsy also have some degree of mental retardation

3. Assessment

   a. Abnormal muscle tone and coordination: the child with spastic cerebral palsy presents with **spasticity** (hypertonicity of muscle groups); the child with athetoid cerebral palsy presents with wormlike movements of the extremities; the ataxic form of cerebral palsy involves disturbed coordination

   b. May display hypertonia or hypotonia and may have varying degrees of tonicity on different extremities

   c. May have scissoring of the legs

   d. Absence of expected reflexes or presence of reflexes that extend beyond the expected age are suggestive of cerebral palsy

   e. Failure to meet developmental norms may be the first suggestion of "something wrong"

   f. Physical symptoms include altered speech and difficulty with swallowing; visual and hearing defects may be present; the nurse may note scissoring of the lower extremities

   g. Seizures may accompany cerebral palsy and may be another indication of the brain injury

4. Priority nursing diagnoses
   a. Impaired physical mobility
   b. Self-care deficit
   c. Altered nutrition: less than body requirements
   d. High risk for injury related to neuromuscular, perceptual, or cognitive impairments
   e. Impaired verbal communication
   f. Fatigue
5. Planning and implementation

NCLEX!

   a. Many individuals with cerebral palsy require increased calorie intake because of spasticity or increased motor functioning
   b. If the motor involvement causes the child to have poor coordination or if the child has seizure activity, there is a need to provide safe environment such as protective headgear or a padded bed
   c. Communication can be a problem if there is oral involvement; the child may need to use a communication board or computer-assisted communication; the use of touch is an excellent means to communicate caring to a child with limited intelligence
   d. Self-care is a goal for all children; extensive collaboration with occupational therapists for strategies and devices to assist in this area may be necessary

NCLEX!

   e. Risk for aspiration is present if oral muscles are involved; use of adaptive feeding devices and positioning during feedings can decrease risk; for some clients with severe spasticity, a gastrostomy tube might be surgically placed for enteral feedings
   f. Collaborate with multidisciplinary team for speech, nutrition, occupation, and physical therapies; child and family must be the center of this team
   g. Regional early-intervention consortiums conduct community-based developmental screenings to find children who might be at risk or have developmental delays from disorders such as cerebral palsy; these children can then be referred for further assessment so that possible delays can be identified and appropriate early intervention initiated; the most widely used developmental screening test is the Denver II
   h. Provide adequate nutrition and rest
   i. Maintain a safe environment
6. Surgical procedures and medication therapy
   a. To control spasticity, traditional treatments have included surgery to release tendons to promote mobility, rehabilitation therapies, oral medications, and intramuscular injections of phenol and botulinum toxin
   b. New treatment is the use of a surgically implanted intrathecal pump, which administers a continuous infusion of baclofen; potential pump-related problems include infection and overdose; benefits include improved function, gait, and motor control and generally improved health

7. Child and family education

   a. Teach parents use of physical therapy strategies such as range-of-motion exercises to use at home

   b. Child will need to learn self-care skills such as how to feed and dress self and perform hygiene activities

   c. Teach parents special feeding techniques and use of adaptive devices such as special silverware and dishes; parents may need to be taught how to do gastrostomy tube feedings if indicated

8. Evaluation

   a. Child establishes optimal physical mobility and self-care skills

   b. Child demonstrates adequate nutrition, as evidenced by age-appropriate maintenance or increase in height and weight

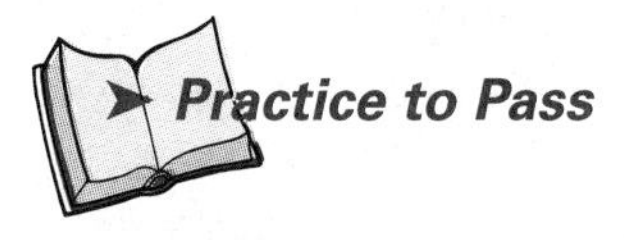

Describe the multidisplinary team that will be needed in the rehabilitation of the child with cerebral palsy.

   c. Child is free from injury

   d. All individuals interacting with the child are able to comprehend the child's communication

   e. Child demonstrates adequate energy level, as evidenced by ability to participate in daily routine

   f. Family copes with the management of the child's health problems

B. Neural tube defects

1. Description: neural tube defects (also known as spina bifida or myelodysplasia) develop during the first trimester of fetal development; the defect can occur at any place along the spinal canal (see Figure 6-2)

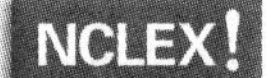

2. Etiology and pathophysiology

   a. Etiology is unknown but thought to be associated with folic acid deficiency in mother's diet; the degree of disability is determined by the location of

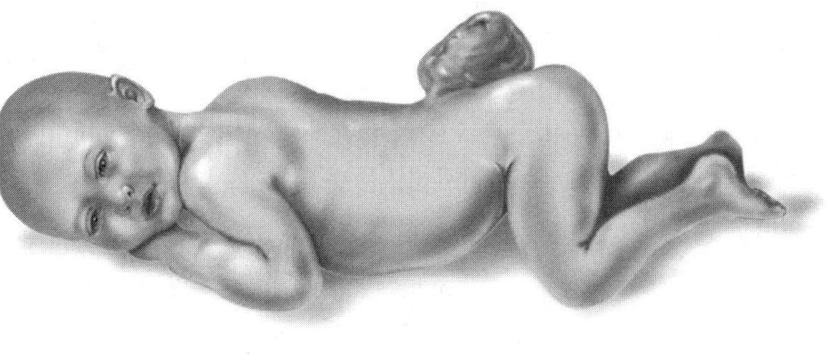

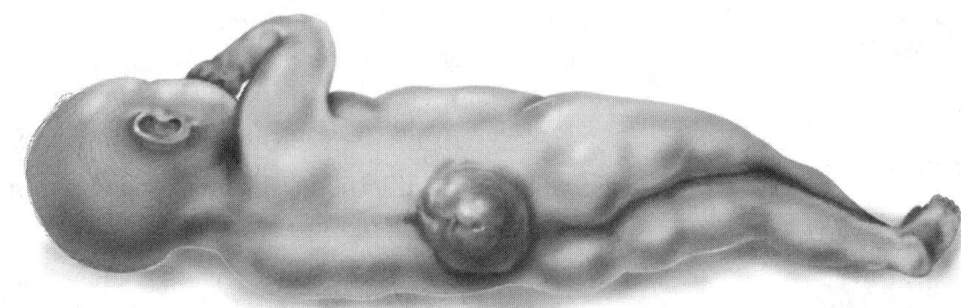

Figure 6-2

Infant with lumbarsacral myelomeningocele. *Source:* Ball, J. & Bindler, R. (1999). *Pediatric nursing: Caring for children* (2nd ed.). Stamford, CT: Appleton & Lange, p. 787.

the defect and amount of spinal nerves encased in the sac; the higher the defect, the greater the neurologic dysfunction

b. There are several types of spina bifida or neural tube defects

1) Spina bifida occulta: posterior vertebral arches fail to fuse, but there is not herniation of spinal cord or **meninges** (fibrous membrane that covers brain and lines vertebral canal); no loss of function

2) Meningocele: posterior vertebral arches fail to fuse, and there is a saclike protrusion at some point along the posterior vertebrae; sac does contain meninges and cerebral spinal fluid

3) Myelomeningocele: posterior vertebral arches fail to fuse; saclike herniation contains meninges, cerebrospinal fluid, as well as a portion of spinal cord or nerve roots; sometimes leakage of CSF occurs

4) Encephalocele: brain and meninges herniate through defect in the skull into a sac

3. Assessment

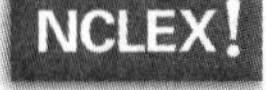

a. Prenatal diagnosis can be determined by elevated levels of alpha-fetoprotein (AFP) in fluid obtained by amniocentesis; defect can also be assessed on prenatal ultrasound

NCLEX!

b. During postnatal period, monitor for leakage of spinal fluid from sac as well as skin integrity of sac; assess for infection around sac as well as possible systemic or CNS infection

c. Assess degree of sensation at or below level of lesion; this can be evidenced by lack of movement or sensation in legs, and a **neurogenic** (lacking innervation) bladder or bowel

d. Measure head circumference since there is a high risk of hydrocephalus

4. Priority nursing diagnoses

a. High risk for infection

b. High risk for impaired skin integrity

c. Altered urinary elimination

d. Bowel incontinence/colonic constipation

e. Impaired physical immobility

5. Planning and implementation

a. Collaborative management: the defect/sac is surgically repaired during the first 48 hours postnatal

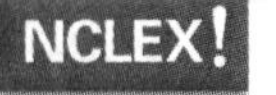

b. Preoperative care should be focused on maintaining skin integrity of sac and keeping it free of infection; positioning the infant on the side or abdomen can attain this; the sac is kept moist with sterile, saline-soaked dressings; avoid contamination of sac area by urine or feces

c. Individuals with myelodysplasia have an increased incidence of latex allergies; monitor for this

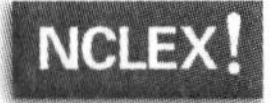

d. Neurogenic bladder: frequent, clean straight catheterization is preferred method of management; maintain home schedule as much as possible

NCLEX!

e. Neurogenic bowel: work with family to develop a bowel management plan using control of high-fiber diet, adequate fluid intake, and pattern for evacuation of bowels; in some cases, laxatives and enemas are used as prescribed by physician

f. Collaborate with physical therapy to develop modes of transport, such as using braces with crutches or wheelchair

g. Since areas with altered sensation are prone to skin breakdown, teach child and family to reposition frequently and inspect affected areas on a regular basis

6. Medication therapy: Low-dose antibiotics may be prescribed to prevent urinary tract infections (UTIs)

7. Child and family education

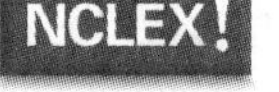

a. Teach family about possibility of child developing hydrocephalus and signs/symptoms of increased intracranial pressure and what to do if changes develop

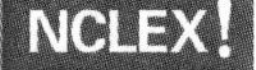

b. Since most children with neural tube defects except for those with spina bifida occulta have some neurogenic bladder, teaching about clean intermittent straight catheterization is important; work with family to develop bowel management program also

8. Evaluation

a. Child does not develop CNS or wound infection

b. Child does not develop pressure ulcers

c. Child demonstrates normal renal functioning and adequate urinary elimination by having infrequent UTIs

d. Child evacuates bowels on a routine basis

e. Child becomes physically mobile within limits of neuromuscular potential

C. Hydrocephalus

1. Description: a condition characterized by imbalance between cerebrospinal fluid (CSF) production and absorption resulting in enlarged ventricles and an increase in intracranial pressure; if untreated, this condition can cause permanent brain damage

2. Etiology and pathophysiology

a. Congenital causes include Arnold Chiari formation associated with myelomeningocele

b. Can be acquired from meningitis, trauma, or intraventricular hemorrhage in premature infants

c. Etiology is idiopathic in up to 50 percent of cases

3. Assessment

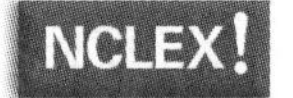

a. For infants, increased head circumference, split cranial sutures, high-pitched cry, bulging fontanel, irritability when awake and seizures (see Figure 6-3)

Figure 6-3

Development of hydrocephalus in young child. A. Normal ventricles. B. Enlarged ventricles and bulging fontanel.
Source: Ball, J. & Bindler, R. (1999). *Pediatric nursing: Caring for children* (2nd ed.). Stamford, CT: Appleton & Lange, p. 783.

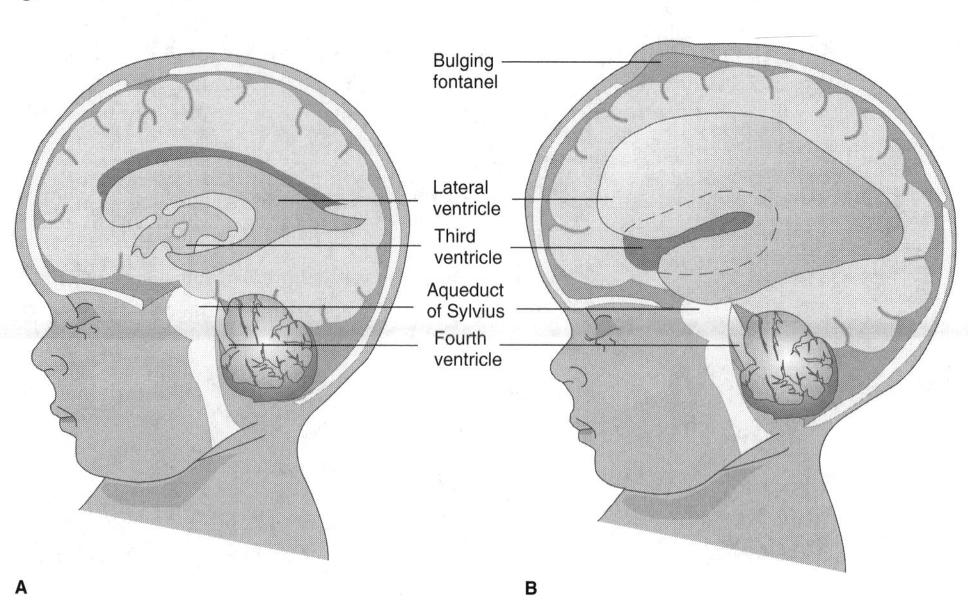

NCLEX!

b. Toddlers and older children may also present with setting-sun eyes, seizures, irritability, papilledema, decreased LOC, and change in vital signs (increased blood pressure and widening pulse pressure)

c. Older children may complain of headaches and have difficulty with balance or coordination

NCLEX!

d. All children can present with vomiting, lethargy, and Cheyne-Stokes respiratory pattern

e. Diagnosis confirmed using CT and MRI to reveal location of CSF obstruction

4. Priority nursing diagnoses

a. Altered tissue perfusion (cerebral)

b. High risk for infection

c. Risk for impaired skin integrity related to large size of head and inability to move

5. Planning and implementation

NCLEX!

a. Surgical insertion of a tube (the consistency of a piece of spaghetti) into the ventricles with the end in either the peritoneum or atrium; the most common version of this "shunt" is the ventriculoperitoneal; preoperatively the child is monitored for symptoms of increased ICP; postoperatively the child is placed flat and on the unoperative side; if held, it is important not to allow the head to be elevated

NCLEX!

b. Postoperatively, the child should also be monitored for symptoms of infection; notify the physician if symptoms are present: fever, change in LOC, excessive redness at incision site or along shunt tract, elevated WBC count with leukocytosis or left shift

6. Medication therapy: client may be on prophylactic antibiotics postoperatively

7. Child and family education

a. Teach the caregiver the symptoms of shunt infection and malfunction and what actions to take should symptoms develop

NCLEX!

b. Signs of shunt malfunction

1) Infant whose cranial suture lines have not fused; signs include increased head circumference, high-pitched cry, bulging fontanel, irritability when awake, and seizures

2) Toddlers and older children display vomiting, irritability, and headache; as condition persists, setting-sun eyes, seizures, papilledema, decreased LOC, and change in vital signs (increased BP and widening pulse pressure) occur

3) Older children have difficulty with balance or coordination

4) All children may have lethargy and Cheyne-Stokes repirations

c. Some children with hydrocephalus have brain damage that results in motor, language, perceptual, and intellectual disabilities; their parents may need referrals to early-intervention professionals to provide long-term rehabilitation services

NCLEX!

d. Children with hydrocephalus and myelomeningocele have an increased risk of latex allergies; parents should be taught to avoid nipples, pacifiers, and toys made of latex products

8. Evaluation

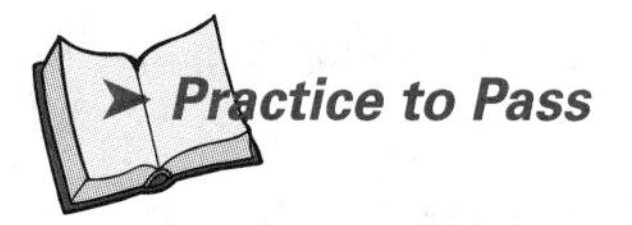

Practice to Pass

Identify the age-related differences in discharge instructions to a parent whose child has a ventriculoperitoneal shunt.

a. Child demonstrates cerebral perfusion as evidenced by age-appropriate response to the environment and vital signs within normal limits

b. Child does not demonstrate any signs or symptoms of infection

c. Caregivers verbalize the purpose of the shunt and how to detect infection or malfunction

IV. Acquired Neurologic Health Problems

A. Seizures

1. Description

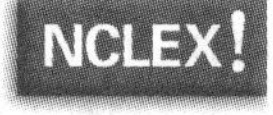

a. Seizures are alterations in the firing of neurons in the brain; this malfunction of the electrical systems or "wiring" is the result of cortical neuronal discharge; the result of this discharge depends on where in the brain the discharges begin and how they spread

b. Seizures can be divided into two categories: partial seizures, which begin locally in one hemisphere of the brain, and generalized seizures, which begin in both hemispheres of the brain

c. Seizures are the most common alteration in the nervous system seen in children; they are present with numerous different conditions involving the CNS

d. Epilepsy is a chronic disorder characterized by recurrent seizures

e. Determining the type of seizure is done based on history and EEG results

2. Etiology and pathophysiology

   a. Seizures have many causes; most seizures are "idiopathic," that is, the cause is unknown; somehow the seizure threshold has been altered to influence neuronal discharge

   b. Common etiologies of seizures during infancy include perinatal hypoxia, congenital diseases, infections, metabolic or degenerative diseases, drug withdrawal, and neoplasms; common etiologies of seizures during childhood include febrile infections, head injury, lead toxicity, drugs, genetic disorders, and neoplasms

3. Assessment

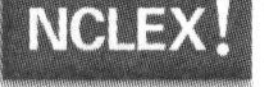

   a. During actual seizure activity, it is important to observe the order of events and duration of the seizure; for **tonic-clonic** seizures, be certain to time the length of seizure until jerking stops; tonic indicates continuous muscle contraction; clonic indicates alternating contraction and relaxation of muscles; for all other types of seizures, note the duration from start of seizure to time that consciousness is regained; describe any precipitating events or unusual behavior; note the parts of the body involved and if it begins in any particular body part

NCLEX!

   b. Observe the face for any color change, perspiration, and lack of expression; note if the mouth has any deviation to one side or the other, teeth clenched, tongue bitten, frothing at mouth, and/or flecks of blood or bleeding; if able to access the pupils, note any change in size, equality, reaction to light, and accommodation

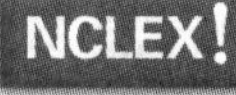

   c. Observe for presence or length of apnea; other general observations might be involuntary urination or defecation

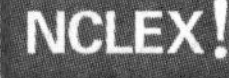

   d. Postictally, it is important to note the duration of the postictal period; level of consciousness; orientation to time, person, place; and any alterations in motor ability or speech

4. Priority nursing diagnoses

   a. Risk for injury related to type of seizure and possible loss of consciousness

   b. Risk for aspiration

   c. Altered family processes related to having child with chronic illness

5. Planning and implementation

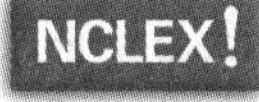

   a. Protect child during a seizure: place child on his or her side and monitor vital signs

   b. Administer anticonvulsant medications as ordered

   c. Assist parents in understanding and accepting the diagnosis

   d. Promote the development of a positive self-image for the child; talk with the child about his or her feelings; plan strategies to promote acceptance and decrease fear among peers

6. Medication therapy

   a. Since seizures are felt to be caused by a heightened sensitivity to neuronal firing, most medication therapy involves using drugs whose actions decrease this sensitivity; eighty-five percent of children with epilepsy have seizures that are well controlled by one antiepileptic medication; choice of medication by physician will vary depending on the type of seizures the child has

b. Phenobarbital is one the oldest medications used; one of the most commonly used currently is carbamazepine (Tegretol)

c. Unfortunately, 15 percent of children with epilepsy are difficult to manage, and their seizures are not easily controlled; these children can suffer from poor self-esteem, academic failure, and poor social relationships; for some of these children, if the focus of the epilepsy can be pinpointed, surgery may be an option to control the seizures

7. Child and family education

a. Families need to know what to do when the child has a seizure; safety measures should be taught and when to call the EMS; children with frequent seizures are advised to wear some form of medical alert identification

b. Combination of barbiturates with carbamazepine can potentiate drugs levels; parents need to be advised to not use any over-the-counter medications prior to consulting with their health care professional (for example, cold products containing antihistamine since the side effects are increased)

c. Parents and older children should be educated as to the type of seizure the child has, the medication currently taken and in the past, and should be able to give a record/history of seizure control or number of seizures experienced and their timing

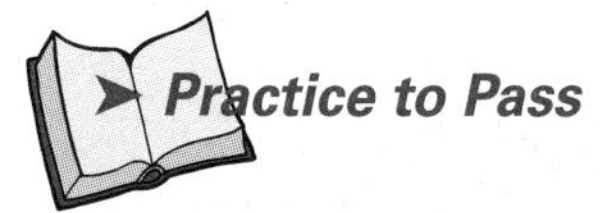

Parents of a child who has had his or her first seizure have gone through a fairly stressful and frightening experience. Keeping in mind that preparing for discharge can be equally stressful, what are key points the nurse should discuss with the parents in preparation for discharge?

8. Evaluation

a. The child is free from injury during seizures

b. The child experiences as few seizures as possible

c. The family and child cope with the management of the seizures

d. The child has a positive self-image

B. Craniosynostosis

1. Description: the premature closure of the cranial sutures in young children; there is some relationship between craniosynostosis and several inherited syndromes

2. Etiology and pathophysiology

a. Etiology is unknown; it can be diagnosed by clinical exam; diagnosis is confirmed through skull films, CT scan, and MRI

b. Premature closure of the skull may lead to increased ICP and resulting brain damage

3. Assessment: a bony ridge is palpated along a suture line; compensatory growth of the skull in directions parallel to the closed suture line creates skull deformities; the nurse should monitor fontanels all infants for the premature closure of the fontanels; measuring head circumference also provide data related to this diagosis

4. Priority nursing diagnoses
    a. Knowledge deficit
    b. High risk for injury
    c. Body image disturbance
    d. Ineffective family coping
5. Planning and implementation
    a. Medical treatment is surgical correction of the skeletal defect

NCLEX!

    b. All principles of good postoperative care should be followed: incision should be kept dry and intact; monitor for signs of increased ICP, changing LOC, and infection during the postoperative period
    c. Parents and child should be prepared for the child's postoperative appearance; in addition to the large, turban-like bandage, the child will have orbital edema and bruising; long-term results of the surgery should be discussed and "before and after" pictures may assist the family in mentally preparing for surgery

NCLEX!

    d. Fluid restrictions may be ordered in the postoperative period; the child may be maintained with the head of the bed elevated to a 30-degree angle
6. Child and family education
    a. Parent education should include reassurance that the surgery will improve the child's appearance and that most children postoperatively are healthy and have normal brain development
    b. Parents may need instructions about how to change the dressing at home
7. Evaluation
    a. Family verbalizes understanding of the perioperative experience
    b. Client does not demonstrate any brain injury or infection as evidenced by age-appropriate response to the environment, intact sensation/motion to extremities, age-appropriate speech patterns, normal urine output, absence of fever, and no other symptoms of infection

V. Infectious Neurologic Health Problems

A. Meningitis

1. Description: inflammation of the meninges; this is the most common infection of the CNS; two primary classifications include viral or aseptic and bacterial
2. Etiology and pathophysiology
    a. Viral etiology is a wide variety of viral agents or enteroviruses

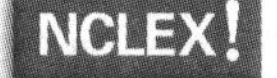

    b. Bacterial causative organisms include *haemophilus influenzae* (type B), *streptococcus pneumoniae* and *neisseria meningitides* (meningococcal)
3. Assessment

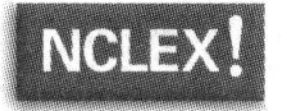

    a. Viral meningitis clinical manifestations in infants and toddlers are irritability, lethargy, vomiting, and change in appetite; for the older child, the infection is usually preceded by a nonspecific febrile illness; the child presents with headache, malaise, muscle aches, nausea/vomiting, **photophobia** (sensitivity to light) and nuchal/spinal rigidity

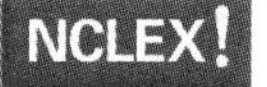

b. Bacterial meningitis clinical manifestations in infants and toddlers present with poor feeding/suck, vomiting, high-pitched cry, bulging fontanel, fever or hypothermia depending on the maturity of the infant's neurological system, and poor muscle tone; children and adolescents will present with abrupt onset, fever and chills, headache, and **nuchal rigidity** (stiffness of the neck); the child may also display vomiting, alterations in sensorium, photophobia, delirium, extreme irritability, aggressive or maniacal behavior, seizures and/or drowsiness; positive Kernig or Brudzinski's signs indicates meningeal irritation; **opisthotonus** posture (hyperextending the head and neck) is believed to relieve some of the discomfort from the meningeal irritation; petechial or purpuric rash will be seen if it is a meningococcal infection

c. Meningitis is diagnosed by laboratory findings; cerebral spinal fluid is obtained by lumbar puncture for analysis; findings can differentiate between viral and bacterial meningitis (see Table 6-2); cultures can determine the causative agent

4. Priority nursing diagnoses

a. Risk for ineffective breathing pattern

b. Pain

c. Risk for injury

d. Risk for ineffective thermoregulation

5. Planning and implementation

a. Monitor respiratory status and administer oxygen and maintain artificial airway

NCLEX!

b. Provide an environment that will minimize ICP elevation; this can include elevating head of bed 15 to 30 degrees, avoiding neck extension or flexion, and maintaining the head in a neutral position; keep environment quiet and subdued, and handle child in a gentle manner

NCLEX!

c. Monitor for cerebral edema; child may be at risk for syndrome of inappropriate antidiuretic hormone (SIADH); suspect this if the urine output decreases but the serum sodium also decreases; restrict oral fluids and monitor IV fluids to prevent fluid overload

d. Administer antipyretics as needed for temperature elevation

Table 6-2

Comparison of Cerebrospinal Fluid in Meningitis

	Normal	**Viral Meningitis**	**Bacterial Meningitis**
Pressure	5–15 mm Hg	Normal or slightly elevated	Elevated
Appearance	Clear	Clear	Cloudy
Leukocytes (mm^3)	0–5	Slightly elevated	Elevated
Protein (mg/dL)	10–30	Slightly elevated	Elevated
Sugar (mg/dL)	40–80	Normal or decreased	Decreased

e. Assess for evidence of pain with all routine assessments; administer pain medication as prescribed; however, narcotics should be avoided; this should promote rest and reduce risk of increased ICP; elevated ICP can be masked by narcotic analgesics

f. Children with bacterial meningitis will need to be isolated until at least 24 hours of antibiotic therapy have been completed

NCLEX!

g. Monitor the child for complications of meningitis (seizures, hearing loss, visual alterations); neurologic sequelae such as mental retardation, cerebral palsy, and hydrocephalus may occur; a complication of meningococcal meningitis is meningococcemia, an overwhelming septic infection that can lead to circulatory collapse and tissue necrosis

h. Viral meningitis is treated symptomatically; usually only infants are hospitalized for viral meningitis

NCLEX!

6. Medication therapy: bacterial meningitis is treated with intravenous antibiotics sensitive to the causative organism; treatment usually continues for 7 to 14 days; preventive care includes a vaccine that is currently available to protect all young children from haemophilus influenzae infection; individuals who have close contact with children diagnosed with meningococcal and *H. influenzae* meningitis may receive rifampin (Rifadin) prophylactically

7. Child and family education

NCLEX!

a. Provide information to the parents about the disease and its transmission; provide information about the need for isolation and antibiotic therapy; also explain the need for prophylactic treatment for those in contact with the child

b. Provide parents with information about the possible development of sequelae from the disease and possible side effects of medications

c. Share information about followup as well as rehabilitation services with the family

8. Evaluation

a. Child demonstrates vital signs within normal limits

b. Child's pain is controlled as evidenced by vital signs within normal limits and relaxed muscle tone

c. Child demonstrates adequate cerebral perfusion

d. Child recovers without sequelae

B. Encephalitis

1. Description

a. Encephalitis is an inflammation of the brain

b. Presenting symptoms will vary depending on the causative organism and location of the infection in the brain; classic symptoms include the child presenting with an acute febrile illness with neurologic signs

2. Etiology and pathophysiology

a. Etiology is usually a viral organism; herpes simplex type 1 is the most common cause during the neonatal period; enteroviruses are frequently identified as causative agents; nonviral agents include bacteria, parasites, fungi, and rickettsiae

b. The infectious process usually begins elsewhere in body

c. Prognosis depends on degree of CNS involvement; permanent neurologic sequelae may result

3. Assessment

a. In addition to fever, the child may have a severe headache, nausea, or vomiting, and signs of an upper respiratory infection

b. Neurologic symptoms include those of nuchal rigidity, photophobia, and positive Kernig's and Brudzinski's signs

c. The child may also be disoriented, confused with personality or behavior changes; other signs are speech disturbances, motor dysfunction, cranial nerve deficits, and focal or generalized seizures that alternate with periods of screaming, hallucinating and bizarre movement; the LOC can change from stupor to coma

5. Priority nursing diagnoses

a. Risk for injury related to seizures

b. Risk for ineffective breathing patterns

c. Pain

6. Planning and implementation

a. Monitor the child's vital signs, respiratory status, oxygenation, and urine output

b. Provide seizure precautions and have resuscitation materials close to bed; these children are best managed in intensive care settings during the acute phase

c. Measures must be taken to maintain skin integrity and other complications of immobility; theses include proper positioning, frequent turning, and chest physiotherapy

d. Work with parents in planning for discharge; since many of these children have neurologic sequelae, the family will need support giving physical and emotional care to the child at home; parents will play an active role in rehabilitation process; follow-up visits need to be coordinated; parents may need referral to home care, counseling, social services, and support groups in their community

7. Medication therapy: if suspected organism is bacterial, appropriate antibiotics will be ordered; acyclovir or other antiviral agents are administered for herpes virus infection

8. Child and family education

a. Parents and child will need information about causative agent and plan of treatment

b. Discharge plans need to be started early; because of neurologic sequelae, plans for rehabilitation need to be discussed

9. Evaluation
   a. Child's vital signs are within normal limits
   b. Child has no permanent neurologic sequelae
   c. Family copes with diagnosis and management of health problem

C. Reye syndrome

1. Description
   a. An acute metabolic encephalopathy of childhood; fatty degeneration of the liver leads to liver dysfunction

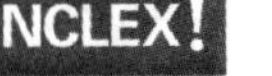

   b. The disease is characterized by five stages
      1) Vomiting and lethargy
      2) Combativeness and confusion
      3) Coma, decorticate posturing
      4) Decerebrate posturing
      5) Seizures, loss of deep tendon reflexes, respiratory arrest
2. Etiology and pathophysiology
   a. While exact etiology is unclear, it usually develops after a mild viral illness such as chickenpox

NCLEX!

   b. Research has linked the development of Reye syndrome to the use of aspirin; following the recommendation that parents use only acetaminophen or ibuprofen, the incidence of Reye syndrome has significantly decreased
3. Assessment
   a. The child presents with an abrupt change in LOC; history reveals the child recovering from a viral disease with sudden onset of vomiting and mental confusion
   b. Liver enzymes and ammonia levels are elevated; blood glucose levels are below normal and prothrombin time is prolonged; bilirubin levels remain normal; liver biopsy shows small fat deposits
4. Priority nursing diagnoses
   a. Risk for injury
   b. Risk for ineffective breathing pattern
   c. Acute confusion
   d. Risk for ineffective family coping
5. Planning and implementation

NCLEX!

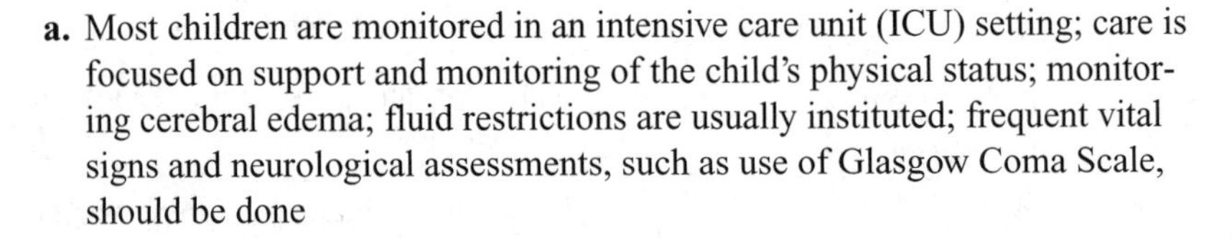

   a. Most children are monitored in an intensive care unit (ICU) setting; care is focused on support and monitoring of the child's physical status; monitoring cerebral edema; fluid restrictions are usually instituted; frequent vital signs and neurological assessments, such as use of Glasgow Coma Scale, should be done

NCLEX!

b. Monitor lab values for elevated ammonia, acidosis, or hypoglycemia; note the child's intake and output

c. Provide all standard nursing measures to prevent complications of immobility

d. Provide emotional support to the family; the sudden onset and rapid deterioration in the child's condition often overwhelm the parents' ability to cope

NCLEX!

6. Medication therapy

a. Controlling cerebral edema is a primary concern; drug management may include corticosteroids to reduce swelling and barbiturates to induce a coma for severe cerebral edema; mannitol (an osmotic diuretic) may be given

b. Phenytoin may be used to control seizures

c. Vitamin K may be given to aid in coagulation

7. Child and family education

a. Parents need explanation of the disease and its causality; the treatment plan must be discussed with the parents as well as the prognosis; explanations about the ICU and medical equipment in use will help the parents cope

b. Discharge planning will include rehabilitative needs of the child as well as followup requirements

c. The public needs to be educated about Reye syndrome and its connection with viral illnesses and the administration of salicylates; the public needs to be aware that if a child displays symptoms, early medical intervention is associated with a better prognosis

8. Evaluation

a. Child demonstrates vital signs within normal limits for age

b. Child demonstrates adequate cerebral perfusion

c. Parents display appropriate coping mechanisms

D. Guillain-Barré syndrome

1. Description

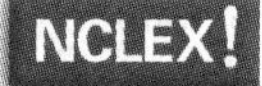

a. An acute demyelinating disease of the nervous system

b. A polyneuropathy with progressive ascending flaccid paralysis

c. Paralytic symptoms are usually preceded by mild flu-like illness or sore throat

2. Etiology and pathophysiology

a. Etiology unknown, but disorder associated with viral illnesses and noninfectious factors such as immunizations, surgery, and trauma

b. Thought to be an immune-mediated disease associated with other viral or bacterial infections; alteration in the myelin surrounding the peripheral nerves

c. Inflammation and edema occurs in spinal and cranial nerves; segmented demyelination and compression of nerve roots in dural sheath; conduction is impaired, resulting in ascending partial or complete paralysis of muscles innervated by involved nerves

d. Nerve involvement may include truncal musculature and cranial nerves leading to respiratory failure or loss of swallow and gag reflexes

e. Progression of paralysis occurs within 1 to 2 weeks

f. The majority of clients recover over 2 to 15 months with no residual disabilities

3. Assessment

a. Muscle weakness, parasthesia, and cramps; paralysis usually ascends from lower extremities; tendon reflexes will be depressed or absent

b. Assess and monitor respiratory function and swallow and gag reflexes

c. Medical diagnosis is confirmed with lumbar puncture and electromyography

1) Lumbar puncture reveals CSF that has increased protein levels and few white blood cells

2) EMG demonstrates an abnormal pattern of nerve conduction

4. Priority nursing diagnoses

a. Impaired physical mobility

b. Ineffective breathing patterns

c. Impaired swallowing

d. Self-esteem disturbance

e. Risk for ineffective family coping

f. Diversional activity deficit

5. Planning and implementation

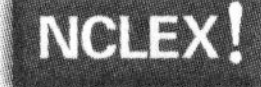

a. Care is supportive and similar to that provided to a quadriplegic client; during initial phase, assess closely for advancement of paralysis to include respiratory area; observe closely for difficulty with breathing or swallowing; place the child on a cardiac monitor and have all emergency equipment accessible to bedside; children with respiratory distress usually require mechanical ventilation

NCLEX!

b. Prevent complications using good postural alignment, frequent change of position, and passive range-of-motion exercises; the recovery period can last from two weeks to several months depending on the degree of paralysis

c. After the recovery period an extensive rehabilitation process begins; while complete recovery is possible, there is the possibility of some permanent disability

d. Emotional support for child and family is an important nursing function; the loss of motor functions and control can be very frightening for a child;

parents need to be encouraged to bring favorite toys from home and provide other comforting activities to help the child feel secure

6. Child and family education

a. Family needs to understand the mechanism of the disease and the treatment strategies being used

b. The parents need to be taught how to provide basic care for their child, the need for good skin care, and turning and positioning

7. Evaluation

a. The child's vital signs are maintained within normal limits for age

b. The child maintains adequate nutritional intake either by mouth, enteral feeding tube, or intravenous line

c. The child is free of potential complications of immobility (i.e., maintaining muscle tone through physical therapy)

d. The child and family cope with the initial loss of function and actively participate in the rehabilitation process

VI. Accidents and Injuries Causing Neurologic Health Problems

A. Head injury

1. Description

a. Any trauma involving the scalp, cranial bones, or structures within the skull; the injury is the result of force or penetration

b. Most common of childhood injuries, with 5 percent being fatal and 20 percent having long-term disabilities related to it

c. Head injury clients often suffer from side effects of the trauma, that is, cerebral edema and increased ICP

d. A minor closed head injury is one in which the client has normal mental status, no abnormal or focal findings on neurologic examination, and no physical evidence of skull fracture at initial exam shortly after injury; client might have had a temporary loss of consciousness (less than one minute), complained of headache, exhibited lethargy, and either vomited and/or had a seizure immediately after the injury, but at the time of exam has the normal findings described

2. Etiology and pathophysiology

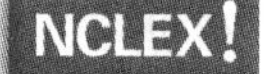

a. Major cause in young children are falls—from changing tables, beds, sofas, and down stairs, especially in walkers; child abuse or shaken baby syndrome is a possible cause in infants under one year of age; other causes include motor vehicle accidents (MVAs), and bicycle, skateboard, snowboard, and skiing accidents, especially where the child did not wear any protective helmet; teenagers may also be injured in alcohol- or drug-related MVAs and sports injuries

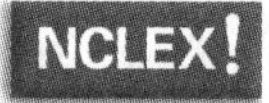

b. Two categories of head injuries

1) *Primary injuries* develop at the time of the trauma when initial tissue damage takes place; this is usually as the result of a direct blow to the

head or acceleration-deceleration movement of brain within the skull (contrecoup injury); at the time of injury, there is an increase in ICP and arterial pressure; apnea and loss of consciousness may occur

2) *Secondary brain trauma* develops as a result of the body's response to the injury; this response can occur from a few hours to a few weeks after the injury; brain damage is usually secondary to hypoxia, hypotension, edema, change in the blood-brain barrier, or hemorrhage; the increased ICP that results can cause irreversible brain damage if left untreated

3. Assessment

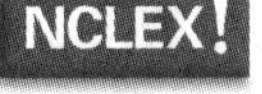

a. Monitor vital signs and neuro signs frequently; changes can indicate hypoxia, decreased perfusion, shock, or increased ICP; **Cushing's triad** is a late sign of increased ICP, characterized by increased systolic blood pressure, bradycardia, and irregular respirations

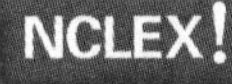

b. Monitor neuro signs, cranial nerves, and LOC using the Glasgow Coma Scale to detect changes in child's condition

4. Priority nursing diagnoses

a. Altered cerebral tissue perfusion

b. Impaired gas exchange

c. Ineffective airway clearance related to decreased level of consciousness

d. Acute confusion related to cerebral injury

e. Risk for ineffective family coping

f. Risk for altered growth and development related to motor, cognitive, and perceptual deficits

5. Planning and implementation

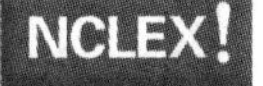

a. To maintain cardiopulmonary function, monitor breathing patterns, check color, and LOC; monitor oxygen saturation with a pulse oximeter; it is critical to prevent brain damage, and that oxygen saturation remain over 95 percent; any decrease in oxygenation should be reported to the physician immediately; maintain seizure precautions; monitor for any signs of increased ICP and report to physician

b. To prevent complications, use good positioning, maintain a quiet environment, and control body temperature

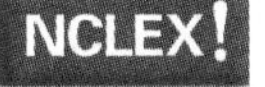

c. To promote optimal recovery, begin rehabilitation while the child is still hospitalized; efforts are coordinated between physical, occupational, and speech therapy; teach parents any strategies being used so that they can continue therapy at home; provide emotional support to the family

d. Coordinate services and resources for discharge; children with major head injury (Glasgow Coma Score less than or equal to 8) have poor outcomes and significant physical disabilities

6. Medication therapy: for the child who requires hospitalization because of the severity of the head injury, mannitol may be used to decrease ICP; control of cerebral edema has been shown to be a significant variable in determining the outcome for a child with a major head injury

7. Child and family education

NCLEX!

a. For even minor head injuries, parents need information about how to care for the child with a head injury; they need to know what behaviors to expect from the child and symptoms to monitor for should complications develop

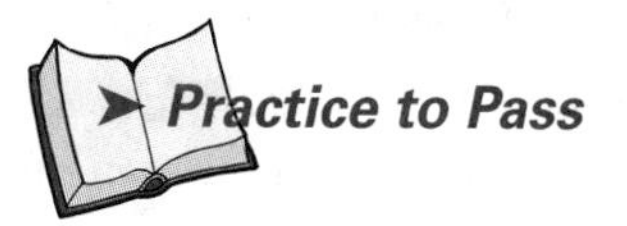

The level of growth and development of a child has a direct relationship to the common injuries that occur during that age. Identify the implications of growth and development for head injuries.

b. Parents need to know that during the recovery period of up to 6 weeks, many children may tire easily, have memory loss or forgetfulness, be easily distractible, have difficulty concentrating, difficulty following directions, irritability or short temper, and need help starting and finishing tasks

8. Evaluation

a. The child's vital signs remain within normal limits for age

b. The child maintains adequate cerebral perfusion

c. The child participates in rehabilitation to attain optimal recovery

d. The family copes with the possible long-term disability

B. Skull fractures

1. Description: fracture to any of the eight cranial bones

2. Etiology and pathophysiology

a. A fracture is caused by a considerable force to the head; any area of the skull with swelling or hematoma should be evaluated as a possible fracture

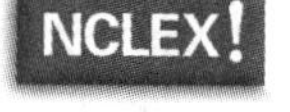

b. Types of skull fractures

1) Linear fracture is a break in the continuity of the skull, and it is usually asymptomatic unless other injury accompanies the fracture

2) Depressed skull fracture occurs when a fragment of the skull bone separates from the rest of the skull and is pushed downward into the brain; requires surgical elevation to prevent brain damage; often accompanied by seizures

3) Basilar fracture involves a fracture at the base of the skull; common symptoms include leakage of CSF from nose or ears, periorbital ecchymosis (raccoon eyes) and bruising behind the ears (battle sign); because of concern about the development of meningitis, the child is placed on antibiotics

3. Assessment: Diagnosis is made by inspection, palpation, x-rays, and CT scans

4. Priority nursing diagnoses

a. High risk for altered cerebral perfusion

b. Risk for infection

NCLEX!

5. Planning and implementation

a. Linear fractures usually heal on their own without intervention; depressed and compound fractures usually require surgical intervention to repair

b. Routine postoperative care similar to any craniotomy (see craniosynostosis presented earlier)

c. Monitor for signs of cerebral edema, damage to cranial nerves and infection

6. Medication therapy: often antibiotics are given to prevent infection postoperatively and if the scalp was also lacerated a tetanus booster might be indicated

C. Contusion

1. Description: bruising of the brain tissue as a result of blunt trauma or coup/contrecoup injuries; it is rare in children under the age of one year
2. Etiology and pathophysiology: injury usually involves damage to parenchyma with tears in vessels or tissue, pulling, and subsequent areas of necrosis or infarction
3. Assessment: symptoms will vary depending on the site of injury; the child may have decreasing LOC
4. Priority nursing diagnoses
   a. Risk for altered cerebral tissue perfusion
   b. Risk for injury (seizures)
5. Planning and implementation
   a. Monitor the child for signs of complications
   b. Observe for any complications
   c. Can have sequelae related to the area of injury
6. Child and family education
   a. Teach parents symptoms of complications that may occur after discharge
   b. Provide written instructions as well as explicit information about when to seek medical care to promote appropriate follow-through
7. Evaluation: child recovers without sequelae

D. Concussion

1. Description: concussion or "mild traumatic brain injury" involves some transient loss of consciousness, usually the result of blunt head trauma
2. Etiology and pathophysiology: brain injury is usually related to stretching, compression, or shearing of nerve fibers; post-concussion syndrome occurs after the initial head injury; poor concentration and problems with memory may be noted at school; the child may complain of headache, dizziness, and photophobia; the parents may report a subtle change in personality
3. Assessment: symptoms include amnesia of the event, headache, and nausea; clients are neurologically intact with a Glasgow Coma Score of 13 to 15; there are three levels of concussion severity
   a. Grade 1: the child has transient confusion with no loss of consciousness and a duration of abnormal mental status for less than 15 minutes
   b. Grade 2: the child has transient confusion with no loss of consciousness and a duration of abnormal mental status for more than 15 minutes
   c. Grade 3: the child has loss of consciousness, for a few seconds or several minutes or longer

4. Priority nursing diagnoses
    a. Altered tissue perfusion, cerebral
    b. Ineffective individual coping secondary to postconcussion syndrome
5. Planning and implementation
    a. Treatment is supportive with close observation for 24 hours in an emergency room or at home under certain circumstances
    b. Children who had loss of consciousness for greater than 5 minutes or amnesia of the event are usually admitted for observation to rule out any other potential injuries
6. Child and family education: child may be discharged home with parents, who have received instructions to continue monitoring the child and what steps to take if complications arise; information about postconcussion syndrome should be shared

E. Subdural hematoma

1. Description: one of two major sites for bleeding or hemorrhage with a head injury in children; a **subdural hematoma** is bleeding between dura and cerebrum; it is more common than **epidural hematoma** (bleeding between the dura and the cranium) and is most frequently seen in infants
2. Etiology and pathophysiology
    a. Subdural hematoma develops slowly, spreads thinly and widely; often results from a fall, birth trauma, or violent shaking
    b. Can be acute (more rapid onset) or chronic (delayed symptoms)
3. Assessment

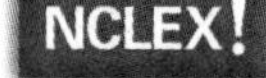

    a. Presenting symptoms are caused by increased ICP and include seizures, vomiting, drowsiness, increased head circumference, bulging fontanels, irritability, and other personality changes

NCLEX!

    b. Older child may complain of headaches
    c. Acute subdural hematoma is usually symptomatic within 48 hours of the injury
    d. Chronic subdural hematoma may take up to 2 weeks before symptoms are observed
    e. Diagnosis is confirmed by computed tomography (CT) scan
4. Priority nursing diagnoses
    a. Risk for injury
    b. Altered tissue perfusion, cerebral
    c. Risk for ineffective breathing pattern
    d. Risk for acute confusion
5. Planning and implementation

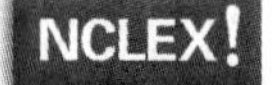

    a. Monitoring of child's vital signs and LOC is critical for early recognition and intervention following a head injury

b. A small subdural hematoma may reabsorb itself

c. Larger acute subdural hematomas require evacuation through burr holes

d. Craniotomy may be required to evacuate a solid clot

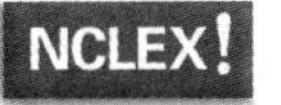

e. Postoperative nursing care requires continued monitoring of vital signs and LOC

6. Child and family education

a. Explain to the parents why monitoring their child is important following a head injury

b. Prepare the parents for the surgical procedure; remind the parents that ecchymosis of the eyes will occur following a craniotomy

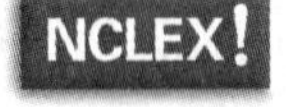

c. Discharge instructions will include monitoring the child for signs of increased ICP

7. Evaluation

a. Child has early recognition of subdural hematoma

b. Child and parents verbalize that they understand the planned surgical procedure

c. Parents restate discharge instructions

F. Epidural hematoma

1. Description: epidural hematoma bleeding with accumulation between dura and skull; not as common as subdural hematomas

2. Etiology and pathophysiology: accumulation of blood applies force or pressure down onto the brain; since bleeding is usually arterial, onset is rapid

3. Assessment

NCLEX!

a. Classic symptoms include irritability, headache, and vomiting, but may have a symptom-free period; symptoms usually appear within minutes to hours of the head injury

b. Can be diagnosed on CT

c. If left untreated, can be fatal

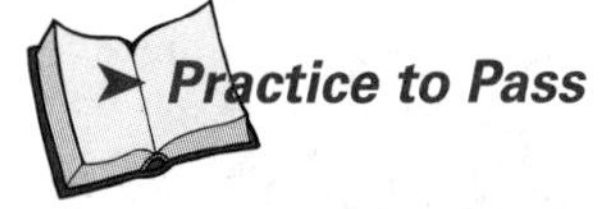

The Glasgow Coma Scale is often used to determine prognosis from a head injury. Compare components of the Glasgow Coma Scale to their relationship with the common symptoms of the minor and major head injury.

4. Priority nursing diagnoses

a. Risk for injury

b. Altered tissue perfusion, cerebral

c. Risk for ineffective breathing pattern

d. Risk for acute confusion

5. Planning and implementation

a. Evacuation may be through burr holes or a craniotomy may be required

b. Rapid recognition and treatment leads to a better prognosis

c. Nursing care is the same as for other types of head injuries and surgical procedures

6. Child and parent education: education for the child with an epidural hematoma is the same as for other head injuries and cranial surgeries; children with neurologic sequelae will need rehabilitation with parents actively involved in the care
7. Evaluation: early recognition and intervention of the epdirual hematoma occurs; child recovers without sequelae

Case Study

A 2-week-old white female is admitted to the hospital for high fever and irritability. She is a full-term, vaginal birth to a Gravida 2 para 2 mother. The infant is diagnosed with meningitis. Her parents both work full time and have health insurance. She has a 3-year-old brother. The family does not have any relatives living closer than a 3-hour drive.

❶ What specific physical parameters should the nurse monitor?

❷ Which nursing interventions would have priority during the first 48 hours of her care?

❸ What would be the usual medical treatment for this health problem?

❹ What developmental implications are there for providing family-centered care for the infant?

❺ In planning for discharge, identify specific areas of support for or teaching with the family.

For suggested responses, see pages 408–409.

Posttest

1 A 3-month-old infant has been admitted with a diagnosis of encephalitis. The first nursing priority would be to assess:

(1) Pupillary reaction.
(2) Level of consciousness.
(3) Ability to maintain airway.
(4) Blood glucose level.

2 The nurse places the young child scheduled for a lumbar puncture in a side-lying position with head flexed and knees drawn up to the chest. The mother asks why the child has to be positioned this way. The nurse explains the rationale for the positioning is that:

(1) Pain is decreased through this comfort measure.
(2) Injury to the spinal cord is prevented.
(3) Access to the spinal fluid is facilitated.
(4) Restraint is needed to prevent unnecessary movement.

3 An 18-month-old child is observed having a seizure. The nurse notes that the child's jaws are clamped. The priority nursing responsibility at this time would be:

(1) Start oxygen via mask.
(2) Insert padded tongue blade.
(3) Restrain child to prevent injury to soft tissue.
(4) Protect the child from harm from the environment.

4 **The nurse conducts Denver II screenings at a community center for infants and young children. The nurse explains that the purpose of these screenings is to:**

(1) Reverse degenerative processes that have occurred.
(2) Recognize early infection in order to prevent spread to individuals in close contact with the child.
(3) Recognize a disorder early so strategies can be developed to promote optimum development.
(4) Measure intelligence and readiness for school.

5 **The nurse is providing client education for a family whose child has cerebral palsy and is receiving baclofen epidural therapy to control spasticity. Which of the following is most important for the nurse to include in the discussion?**

(1) The drug acts to inhibit the neurotransmitter GABA.
(2) The child should be able to run with normal gait after insertion of the pump.
(3) Parents must bring the child back to the clinic on a regular basis to have more medicine added to the pump.
(4) Parents can be taught to regulate the dosage on a sliding scale.

6 **A 10-year-old client presents with weakness in legs and history of the flu. The medical diagnosis is Guillain-Barré syndrome. It would be imperative that the physician be informed if the nurse observes:**

(1) Weak muscle tone in feet.
(2) Weak muscle tone in legs.
(3) Increasing hoarseness.
(4) Tingling in the hands.

7 **The nurse is providing discharge instructions for a child who has suffered a head injury within the last four hours. The nurse will recognize the need for additional teaching when the mother states:**

(1) "I will call my doctor immediately if my child starts vomiting."
(2) "I won't give my child anything stronger than Tylenol for headache."
(3) "My child should sleep for at least 8 hours without arousing after we get home."
(4) "I recognize that continued amnesia about the injury is not uncommon."

8 **The Glasgow Coma Scale is used to measure neurological functioning. Which of the following criteria would indicate the lowest level of functioning for an infant or young child?**

(1) Confused
(2) Irritable, cries
(3) Eyes open only to pain
(4) No response to painful stimuli

9 **Upon performing a physical assessment of a 7-month-old child, the nurse notes an abnormal finding that could suggest cerebral palsy. The finding suggestive of cerebral palsy is that the child has:**

(1) No head lag when pulled to a sitting position.
(2) No Moro or startle reflex.
(3) Positive tonic neck reflex.
(4) Absence of tongue extrusion.

10 **A 4-year-old child is being evaluated for hydrocephalus. An early indication of hydrocephalus in this child would be:**

(1) Bulging fontanels.
(2) Rapid enlargement of the head.
(3) Shrill, high-pitched cry.
(4) Early morning headache.

See pages 155–156 for Answers and Rationales.

Answers and Rationales

Pretest

1 **Answer: 2** ***Rationale:*** Brudzinski's sign indicates meningeal irritation. As the head and neck are flexed toward the chest, the legs flex at both the hips and the knees in response. Brudzinski's sign may be seen in the other options because of the meningeal irritation.
Cognitive Level: Application
Nursing Process: Analysis; ***Test Plan:*** PHYS

2 **Answer: 1** ***Rationale:*** Increased intracranial pressure in infants is characterized by lethargy, irritability, bradycardia, tachycardia, apnea, bulging fontanels, setting-sun eyes, vomiting, and hypertension. Myelomeningocele refers to a neural tube defect, which is obvious on the back. Skull fractures indicate injury to the head and may be asymptomatic or may be accompanied by other pathology that could lead to increased intracranial pressure. Hypertension does not display symptoms of setting-sun eyes.
Cognitive Level: Application
Nursing Process: Analysis; ***Test Plan:*** PHYS

3 **Answer: 3** ***Rationale:*** The most common mechanisms for the development of hydrocephalus include decreased reabsorption (communicating hydrocephalus) and obstruction to the flow of CSF (noncommunicating). Obstruction may result from congenital anomalies, inflammation, external blockage, and other causes.
Cognitive Level: Analysis
Nursing Process: Analysis; ***Test Plan:*** PHYS

4 **Answer: 2** ***Rationale:*** Most children with spina bifida cystica (myelomeningocele included) have the level of their defect at a point which does affect the innervation to both the colon and anal sphincter. The result is constipation and incontinence. Any lack of mobility increases the risk for constipation, and all children need a pattern of regular bowel movements.
Cognitive Level: Analysis
Nursing Process: Implementation; ***Test Plan:*** PHYS

5 **Answer: 3** ***Rationale:*** Clients are considered contagious until the causative organism is determined and antibiotic therapy has been initiated. Children are usually placed in respiratory or droplet isolation. Twenty-four hours of antibiotic therapy usually eliminates the necessity of isolation.
Cognitive Level: Application
Nursing Process: Planning; ***Test Plan:*** SECE

6 **Answer: 4** ***Rationale:*** The child with meningitis will hyperextend the neck and head in an arching position referred to as opisthotonic. The child does this to relieve discomfort from the meningeal irritation. Decerebrate posturing is a symptom of dysfunction at the level of the midbrain and is characterized by rigid extension and pronation of arms and legs. Decorticate posturing is a symptom of a dysfunction of the cerebral cortex and characterized by adduction of the arms at the shoulders, the arms flexed on the chest with hands in fists and wrists flexed, lower extremities extended and adducted. Jacksonian seizure is a simple motor seizure characterized by clonic movements that begin in a foot, hand, or face and then spread to include sometimes the entire body.
Cognitive Level: Application
Nursing Process: Implementation; ***Test Plan:*** PHYS

7 **Answer: 3** ***Rationale:*** Turning the head to one side can occlude the flow of CSF, increasing the ICP. Oxygen can serve as a vasodilator, decreasing the ICP. Keeping the head of the bed slightly elevated also promotes flow of CSF. Diuretics are often part of the medical treatment to decrease ICP.
Cognitive Level: Analysis
Nursing Process: Implementation; ***Test Plan:*** PHYS

8 **Answer: 1** ***Rationale:*** Epidural hematomas are characterized by arterial bleeding. Onset of symptoms occurs within minutes to hours. Other types of bleeding are often venous, which has a slower onset of symptoms.
Cognitive Level: Application
Nursing Process: Analysis; ***Test Plan:*** PHYS

9 **Answer: 3** ***Rationale:*** Obtunded indicates a diminished level of consciousness with limited response to the environment. The child will fall asleep unless given verbal or tactile stimulation. Stupor is a diminished level of consciousness with response only to vigorous stimulation. Semicomatose is when a child only responds to painful stimuli; lethargy is when a child sleeps if left undisturbed but is normally alert when awake.
Cognitive Level: Application
Nursing Process: Assessment; ***Test Plan:*** PHYS

10 **Answer: 2** ***Rationale:*** The most common form of cerebral palsy involves spasticity of muscles. Because of the excessive energy expended, these children often need more calories than other children their age and size. Feeding difficulties are often a component of cerebral palsy, but whether a child needs assistance with feedings is dependent upon the muscle groups affected.
Cognitive Level: Application
Nursing Process: Analysis; ***Test Plan:*** PHYS

Posttest

1 **Answer: 3** ***Rationale:*** While all other choices are important to monitor, the priority in assessing any critically ill child follows the ABC rule—airway, breathing, and circulation.
Cognitive Level: Analysis
Nursing Process: Planning; ***Test Plan:*** SECE

2 **Answer:** 3 ***Rationale:*** This position opens the intervertebral spaces and allows easier access to spinal canal. The position does not decrease pain or help to restrain the child. All lumbar punctures are done below L4 (the level of the spinal nerves) so injury to the spinal cord is always avoided.
Cognitive Level: Analysis
Nursing Process: Implementation; ***Test Plan:*** PHYS

3 **Answer:** 4 ***Rationale:*** Never forcibly restrain a child during a seizure or insert a padded tongue blade; both are more likely to add trauma than prevent. Oxygen via mask is of little benefit. Overall, the child must be protected form injury from the environment.
Cognitive Level: Application
Nursing Process: Implementation; ***Test Plan:*** SECE

4 **Answer:** 3 ***Rationale:*** The Denver II is a developmental screening test. The primary reason for doing developmental screenings to find children who might be at risk and refer them for further assessment so that possible delays can be identified and appropriate early intervention initiated. The Denver II is not a measure of intelligence. It has nothing to do with infection control nor is it an intervention to correct degenerative processes.
Cognitive Level: Application
Nursing Process: Implementation; ***Test Plan:*** HPM

5 **Answer:** 3 ***Rationale:*** This therapy involves an implanted pump that must be accessed through the skin to refill the pump. Parents are not taught to refill the pump. Baclofen does inhibit the neurotransmitter GABA; however, it is not the essential data to be shared with the parents. Promising the parents that the child will be able to run with normal gait offers false hopes. The implanted pump's dosage cannot be changed without special equipment.
Cognitive Level: Analysis
Nursing Process: Planning; ***Test Plan:*** PHYS

6 **Answer:** 3 ***Rationale:*** Guillain-Barré is an ascending paralysis. While the child will have increasingly less muscle tone in extremities, the hoarseness could indicate involvement in the muscles of respiration. Serious concern is raised when the respiratory muscles are affected. Sometimes mechanical ventilation is indicated. Tingling is a common sign of Guillain-Barré and not related to respiratory distress.
Cognitive Level: Application
Nursing Process: Assessment; ***Test Plan:*** PHYS

7 **Answer:** 3 ***Rationale:*** Discharge instructions will include the necessity of waking the child to check for neuro status throughout the night. Vomiting could be a sign of increasing intracranial pressure and should be reported. Narcotics are not given after a head injury. Amnesia for the events surrounding the injury may be permanent. It is not a sign of increasing intracranial pressure.
Cognitive Level: Analysis
Nursing Process: Evaluation; ***Test Plan:*** PHYS

8 **Answer:** 4 ***Rationale:*** No eye opening, no verbal response, and no motor response are the lowest criteria on the scale. Confusion is a criterion applicable only for the older child and adult but is comparable to "irritable and cries" for the infant (which is a 4 out of 5 on the verbal response subscale). "Eyes open only to pain" is next to the lowest level on the eye-opening category.
Cognitive Level: Analysis
Nursing Process: Assessment; ***Test Plan:*** PHYS

9 **Answer:** 3 ***Rationale:*** The Moro or startle, tongue extrusion, and tonic neck reflex are all neonatal reflexes that should have disappeared by this child's age. Lack of head lag indicates good motor development. A developmental delay or the presence of a neonatal reflex are some of the earliest clues to cerebral palsy.
Cognitive Level: Application
Nursing Process: Analysis; ***Test Plan:*** PHYS

10 **Answer:** 4 ***Rationale:*** All of the above are symptoms of increased ICP or hydrocephalus. Head enlargement and bulging fontanels would not be seen in the child after closure of the sutures (12 to 18 months). Shrill, high-pitched cry is a late-stage symptom of children. Headache and vomiting on arising would be an early symptom in an older child.
Cognitive Level: Analysis
Nursing Process: Assessment; ***Test Plan:*** PHYS

References

Ball, J. & Bindler, R. (1999). *Pediatric nursing: Caring for children* (2nd ed.). Stamford, CT: Appleton & Lange, pp. 751–815, 1039.

Bergman, D. A., Baltz, R. D., Cooley, J. R., & Coombs, J. B. (1999). The management of minor closed head injury in children. *Pediatrics, 104*(6): 1407–1415.

Bowden, V. R., Dickey, S. B., & Greenberg, C. S. (1998). *Children and their families: The continuum of care.* Philadelphia: W. B. Saunders, pp. 1317–1422.

Broome, M. E. & Rollins, J. A. (Eds.). (1999). *Core curriculum for the nursing care of children and their families.* Pitman, NJ: Janetti, pp. 350, 354–356.

Celano, R. T. (1998). Diagnosing pediatric epilepsy: An update for the primary care clinician. *Nurse Practitioner: American Journal of Primary Health Care, 23*(3): 69, 73–74, 84–86.

Delgado, M. R. & Combes, M. (1999). Management of motor impariment: Approaches for children with cerebral palsy. *Exceptional Parent, 29*(6): 42–45.

Doire, T. L. (1999). Reye's syndrome. *Nursing 99, 29*(12): 33.

Feickert, H., Drommer, S., & Heyer, R. (1999). Severe head injury in children: Impact of risk factors on outcome. *Journal of Trauma: Injury, Infection, and Critical Care, 47*(1): 33–38.

Hirtz, D., Ashwal, S., Berg, A., Bettis, D., Canfield, C., Camfield, P., Crumrine, P., Elterman, R., Schneider, S., & Shinnar, S. (2000). Practice parameter: Evaluating a first nonfebrile seizure in children. *Neurology, 55:* 616–623.

Hoeman, S. P. (1997). Primary care for children with spina bifida. *Nurse Practitioner: American Journal of Primary Health Care, 22*(9): 60–61, 65–72.

McNeils, A., Musick, B., Austin, J., & Creasy, K. (1998). Psychosocial care needs of children with new-onset seizures . . . part 2 of 3. *Journal of Neuroscience Nursing, 30* (3): 161–165.

Myers, F. (2000). Meningitis: The fears, the facts. *RN, 63*(11): 52–57.

Prior, M. J., Nelson, E. B., & Temple, A. R. (2000). Pediatric ibuprofen use increases while incidence of Reye's syndrome continue to decline. *Clinical Pediatrics, 39:* 245–247.

Ward, L. A. C. (2001). Spasticity in kids: An intrathecal option. *RN, 64*(1): 39–41.

Woestman, R., Perkin, R., Serna, T., Van Stralen, D., & Knierim, D. (1998). Mild head injury in children: Identification, clinical evaluation, neuroimaging and disposition. *Journal of Pediatric Health Care, 12:* 288–298.

Wong, D. L., Hockenberry-Eaton, M., Wilson, D., Winkelstein, M., Ahmann, E., & DiVito-Thomas, P. (1999). *Whaley and Wong's nursing care of infants and children.* St. Louis: Mosby, pp. 254, 290–297, 475–558, 1251, 1762–1830, 1964–1978.

Zupanc, M. L. (1999). Advances in the treatment of pediatric epilepsy. *The Exceptional Parent, 29*(10): 66–69.

CHAPTER 7

Renal and Genitourinary Health Problems

Jacqueline B. Arnett, RN, BSN

CHAPTER OUTLINE

OBJECTIVES

- Identify data essential to the assessment of alterations in health of the renal system of the child.
- Discuss the clinical manifestations and pathophysiology of alterations in health of the renal system of a child.
- Discuss therapeutic management of a child with alterations in health of the renal system.
- Describe nursing management of a child with alterations in health of the renal system.

[Media Link]

Use the CD-ROM enclosed with this text, or log onto the address given to access the free, interactive Companion Website created for this series. The CD-ROM and Companion Website accompanying this book offer additional practice opportunities and information—NCLEX Review, Case Studies, Glossary, In Depth with NCLEX, and more.

www.prenhall.com/hogan

REVIEW AT A GLANCE

anuria *complete or almost complete cessation of urine production by the kidneys*

azotemia *retention of excess nitrogenous wastes in the blood*

chordee *ventral curvature of the penis as seen in hypospadias caused by congenital shortness of the ventral skin*

circumcision *operation to remove part or all of the prepuce*

creatinine *substance produced daily in the body; found in blood, muscle, and urine; measurement of its excretion is used to evaluate kidney function*

cryptorchidism *failure of one or both of the testes to descend*

cystitis *inflammation of the urinary bladder*

epispadias *a malformation in which the urethra opens on the dorsum of the penis; frequently associated with exstrophy of the bladder*

exstrophy *congenital eversion of a hollow organ; a congenital gap in the anterior wall of the bladder and abdominal wall in front of it, the posterior wall of the bladder being exposed*

glomerulonephritis *inflammation of the glomerulus of the nephron*

glomerulus *a tuft formed of capillary loops at the beginning of each nephric tubule in the kidney; this tuft with it's capsule (Bowman's capsule) constitutes the corpusculum renis*

hemodialysis *filtering of the blood to remove toxins (nitrogenous wastes)*

hypospadias *a malformation in which the urethra opens on the ventral aspect of the penis; frequently associated with congenital chordee, a fibrous band of tissue that causes ventral curvature of the penis*

micturition *the act of urinating*

nephron *a long convoluted tubular structure in the kidney, consisting of the renal corpuscle, the proximal convoluted tubule, the nephronic loop, and the distal convoluted tubule*

oliguria *a urine output of less than 0.5–1.0 mL/kg/hour*

peritoneal dialysis *filtering the blood to remove toxins via a catheter inserted into the peritoneal cavity*

prepuce *the free fold of skin that covers the glans penis*

pyelonephritis *inflammation of the renal parenchyma, calyces, and pelvis, particularly due to local bacterial infection*

uremia *excess of urea and other nitrogenous waste products in the blood*

ureteritis *inflammation of a ureter*

urethritis *inflammation of the urethra*

Pretest

1 **A newborn is found to have exstrophy of the bladder. The nurse should evaluate the infant for:**

(1) Hypospadias.
(2) Epispadias.
(3) Cryptorchidism.
(4) Acute tubular necrosis.

2 **A child has been admitted to the hospital with a diagnosis of "rule out nephrosis." The nurse would assess the child for:**

(1) Hematuria.
(2) Edema.
(3) Petechial rash.
(4) Dehydration.

3 **The nurse is caring for a toddler who is not toilet-trained. The doctor has ordered intake and output measurement. The nurse will most accurately measure the urine by:**

(1) Estimating output as small, moderate, or large and recording on the child's chart.
(2) Weighing each wet diaper and recording the amount of urine output as the weight of the diaper.
(3) Subtract the weight of a dry diaper from a wet diaper and record this amount.
(4) Determine urine output by the number of diaper changes in each 24-hour period.

4 **The nurse is teaching the parents of a preschooler information about urinary tract infection and means of reducing their recurrence. Which statement by the parents indicates the need for additional teaching?**

(1) "I should try to get her to drink a lot of water and juices."
(2) "I will buy her underwear a little large."
(3) "Soaking in a bubble bath will reduce meatal irritation."
(4) "If I notice her starting to wet the bed again, I need to have her checked for another urinary tract infection."

5 The nurse would include which of the following in the care of a child with acute glomerulonephritis?

(1) Careful handling of edematous extremities
(2) Observing the child for evidence of hypotension
(3) Providing fun activities for the child on bedrest
(4) Feeding the child a protein-restricted diet

6 A urinalysis is ordered for a child with a throat culture positive for *group A beta-hemolytic streptococcus* (strep throat). The mother asks why this test is being ordered. The nurse explains:

(1) The urinalysis will indicate whether an HIV infection is also present.
(2) Urinary tract infections are common with streptococcal infections and need to receive prompt treatment.
(3) Pyelonephritis is a potential complication of antibiotic therapy.
(4) Group A beta-hemolytic streptococcus infections can be followed by the complication of acute glomerulonephritis.

7 An appropriate nursing diagnosis for a toddler with unrepaired exstrophy of the bladder would be:

(1) Disorganized infant behavior.
(2) Sexual dysfunction.
(3) Urinary retention.
(4) Risk for infection.

8 A child has been admitted to the unit with acute glomerulonephritis. The test that would confirm this diagnosis is:

(1) Antistreptolysin-O (ASO) titer.
(2) Urinalysis.
(3) Blood cultures.
(4) White blood cell (WBC) count.

9 The doctor orders a clean-catch urine specimen on a infant who is not toilet-trained. The best means of collecting this urine would be to:

(1) Perform a straight catheterization.
(2) Apply a urine collection bag.
(3) Use diaper analysis.
(4) Perform Foley catheterization.

10 A teenage child is being treated for renal failure. The nurse would ensure that the child follows a:

(1) High-sodium diet.
(2) High-protein diet.
(3) Low-sodium diet.
(4) Low-fiber diet.

See pages 183–184 for Answers and Rationales.

I. Overview of the Anatomy and Physiology of the Renal System

A. Structures of the renal system

1. Kidney
   a. Internal structures: cortex, medulla, pyramids, papilla, and the pelvis
   b. Microscopic structures: key functional unit is a **nephron** that consists of a renal corpuscle, the loop of Henle, and renal tubules; the renal corpuscle consists of the **glomerulus** (a capillary tuft) enclosed within Bowman's capsule
2. Ureter: narrow, long tube with an expanded upper end that lies inside the kidney pelvis; ureters are lined with mucous membrane and drain urine from the kidney pelvis to the urinary bladder
3. Bladder: elastic muscular organ that is capable of great expansion; lined with mucous membrane arranged in rugae, like stomal mucosa; the bladder stores urine before voiding occurs and also initiates voiding

4. Urethra: narrow tube from the urinary bladder to the exterior of the body lined with mucous membrane; the opening of the urethra to the exterior of the body is the urinary meatus; the urethra passes urine from the bladder to outside the body and in the male, reproductive fluid (semen) from the body

NCLEX!

B. Functions of the renal system

1. Is responsible for the formation and the excretion of urine
2. Regulates fluid and electrolyte balance within the body
3. Regulates acid–base balance within the body
4. Regulates blood pressure
5. Stimulates the production of red blood cells in bone marrow
6. Regulates calcium metabolism in the body

C. Renal system differences between the child and the adult

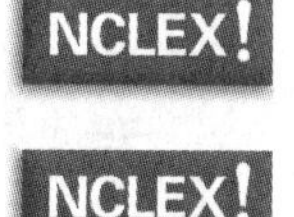

NCLEX!

1. Fluid is more important to the body chemistry of infants and small children because it constitutes a larger fraction of their total body weight

NCLEX!

2. During the first 2 years of life the kidneys are less efficient at regulating electrolyte and acid–base balance; infants are more prone to fluid volume excess and dehydration
3. Bladder capacity increases from 20 to 50 mL at birth to 700 mL in adulthood

NCLEX!

4. Innervation of "stretch" receptors in the bladder wall, which initiates urination and control of bladder sphincters (does not occur before the age of two); children under the age of 2 cannot maintain bladder control
5. The urethra is shorter in children than in adults and may contribute to the frequency of urinary tract infections in children
6. Kidneys are more susceptible to trauma in children because they do not have as much fat padding

Practice to Pass

For each of the six functions of the renal system, name at least two clinical symptoms the client might manifest if that function were impaired.

II. Diagnostic Tests and Assessments of the Renal System

A. Urine specimen: urinalysis for dipstick results, microscopic examination, or for culture; refer to Table 7-1 for normal urinalysis results and to Table 7-2 for significance of color changes

Table 7-1
Normal Urinalysis Results

Macroscopic Exam		Microscopic Exam	
Color	Pale yellow	Red blood cells	0–5/HPF (high-power field)
Turbidity	Clear	White blood cells	0–5/HPF
Odor	Ammonia-like smell	Casts	1 per every 10-20/LPF (low power field)
Specific gravity	1.003–1.030		
pH	4.6–8.0	Crystals	None
Protein	Negative; <10–150 mg/24 hr	Bacteria	<1000 colonies/mL
Glucose	<250 mg/24 hr		
Ketones	Negative		
Bilirubin	Negative		

Table 7-2

Interpreting Changes in Urine Color

Color	Possible Meaning
Pale yellow	Normal
Yellow	Concentrated urine
Amber	Bile in urine
Orange	Alkaline or concentrated urine
Red orange	Acidic urine, medication effect
Red	Blood, menses
Pink	Dilute blood
Burgundy	Laxatives
Tea	Melanin, hematuria
Dark gray	Medications, dyes
Blue	Dyes, medications

1. Clean-catch specimen: urine specimen collected in a clean specimen container following cleansing of the urinary meatus and surrounding tissue; in infants and toddlers, a urine collection bag is used (see Figure 7-1); parental assistance is needed for school-age, toilet-trained children, and specimens are obtained individually by adolescents after careful instruction

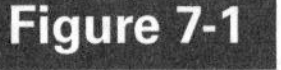

2. Sterile urine specimen: obtained by urinary catheterization only

B. **IVP:** intravenous pyelogram; an x-ray or series of x-rays of the renal pelvis and ureters following injection of a contrast medium; special pre-procedure care may be necessary

C. **KUB:** an x-ray showing the kidneys, ureters, and bladder

D. **Ultrasound:** used to obtain the location, measurement, or delineation of deep structures that may not show up on x-ray; gives a two-dimensional image through transmission of high-frequency ultrasonic waves

E. **Retrograde/antegrade pyelogram:** a ureteral catheter is passed via a cystoscope; contrast dye is injected and a series of x-rays are taken

Figure 7-1

Urine collection bag.

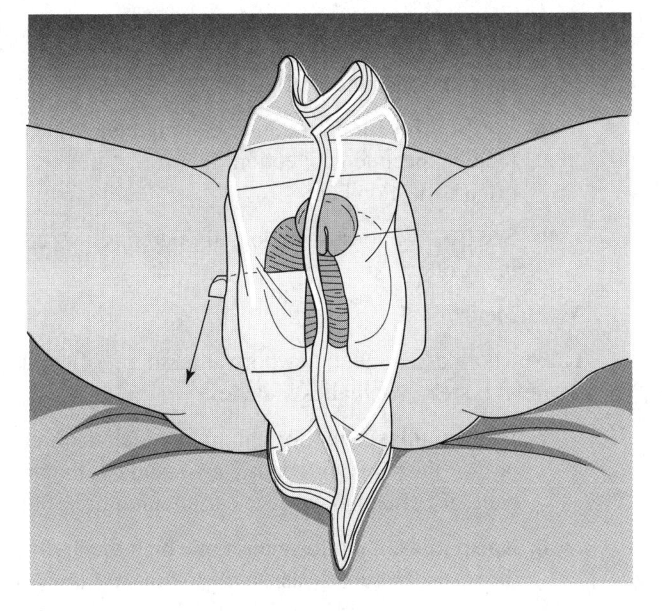

F. **Cystogram:** an x-ray of the bladder only; dye is injected into the bladder via a urethral catheter until the bladder is full; several films are taken and the dye is then drained via the catheter; a final picture is taken when the bladder is emptied

G. **Voiding cystourethrogram:** same process as a cystogram except when the bladder is filled with contrast dye, the urethral catheter is removed; when the client feels the urge to void, he or she is asked to do so; films are taken during bladder filling, during **micturition** (voiding) and after voiding

H. **CT (computed tomography):** visualization of the urinary tract after an oral iodine-containing preparation is taken; the CT scan provides a much more detailed picture than an x-ray

I. **MRI (magnetic resonance imaging):** study based on the reaction of protons and electrons in living tissues to a magnetic field; the images are obtained by measuring the energy utilized by the protons and electrons during the reaction to magnetic field

J. **Serum blood tests**

1. Hemoglobin and hematocrit: clients with alterations in renal health are often anemic; hemoglobin and hematocrit levels are decreased
2. BUN (blood urea nitrogen): measures the amount of urea in the blood; urea is the end product of protein metabolism and is excreted by the kidney; clients with alterations in renal health will have an elevated BUN
3. **Creatinine:** substance produced daily in the body as an end product of metabolism; it is excreted entirely by the kidneys and is therefore directly proportional to renal excretory function; the serum creatinine level should remain normal and constant; in renal impairment, serum creatinine levels increase

NCLEX!

4. Serum electrolytes: measure sodium, potassium, chloride, magnesium, and calcium; the kidneys conserve water and needed electrolytes; children under the age of 2 have immaturely functioning glomeruli, tubules and nephrons, resulting in more water loss in the urine; because of this, infants and toddlers are at greater risk for dehydration and electrolyte imbalances

III. Common Nursing Procedures for Pediatric Clients with Alterations in Renal Health

A. **Urine specimen collection**

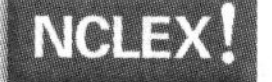

1. Clean-catch specimen collection
   a. See Box 7-1 for directions for applying a urine collection bag for infant and toddler specimen collection; Figure 7-1 illustrates proper application of a urine collection bag
   b. See Box 7-2 for instructions for parent/client education for assisted specimen collection

B. **Assessment**

1. Newborn assessment: newborn assessment often identifies anomalies of the renal system; anomalies include:
   a. **Hypospadias:** a malformation in which the urethra opens on the ventral aspect of the penis; frequently associated with congenital chordee, a fibrous band of tissue that causes ventral curvature of the penis
   b. **Epispadias:** a malformation in which the urethra opens on the dorsum of the penis; frequently associated with exstrophy of the bladder

Box 7-1

Applying a Urine Collection Bag for Infants

- Gather a urine collection bag, soap solution, sterile water, sterile cotton balls and urine specimen container.
- Apply gloves and remove diaper. Clean skin around the meatus. Remove gloves, wash hands.
- Apply new gloves. Using one soapy cotton ball at a time, wipe the genital area three times.
- For males, clean from the tip of the penis towards the scrotum. For females, clean from front to back. Rinse with cotton balls moistened in sterile water. **Use each cotton ball only once and discard.** Dry skin.
- Remove the adhesive backing from the urine collection bag. Place the bag around the labia for females and gently press to skin. Place the bag around the scrotum for males and gently press to skin. Make sure the seal is tight to avoid urine leakage.
- Diaper the infant. Check frequently for urine. Approximately 20 mL is needed.
- When specimen bag is adequately filled, gently pull the bag away from the skin. Fold the opening over and place the entire urine bag in the specimen container. Cap the container tightly and transport immediately to the lab.

c. **Exstrophy:** congenital eversion of a hollow organ (the bladder); a congenital gap in the anterior wall of the bladder and abdominal wall in front of it, with the posterior wall of the bladder being exposed

2. Observation and documentation of voiding patterns: frequent, wet diapers are the norm for well-hydrated children, a change in voiding patterns can indicate dehydration and potential electrolyte imbalances; early identification of abnormal urinary excretion can help prevent serious urinary tract disease, including renal failure

Box 7-2

Client/Parent Education for Obtaining a Clean-Catch Urine Specimen

Females

- Do not touch the inside of the specimen cup or lid.
- Wash hands with soap and water.
- Spread the outer folds of the labia with one hand. Using separate antiseptic towelettes, wipe each side of the labia with a separate towelette. With a third towelette, wipe the urinary meatus in the center; **wipe front to back only.**
- While keeping the labial folds spread apart **(do not let go),** allow the first portion of the urine stream to fall into the toilet.
- **Catch the middle portion** of the urine stream in the specimen cup. **Do not allow specimen cup to touch skin.** Fill one-half full if possible.
- Replace lid (touching outside only) and place container where directed to by healthcare provider.

Males

- Do not touch the inside of the specimen cup or lid.
- Wash hands with soap and water.
- Clean the head of the penis (after pulling back foreskin if not circumcised) three times using a separate antiseptic towelette. Cleaning should move from the urinary meatus outward.
- Begin to urinate into the toilet and then **insert cup into urine stream** and fill approximately one-half full.
- Replace lid (touching the outside only) and place container where directed to by healthcare provider.

C. Catheter care

1. Straight catheterization: most commonly utilized to obtain sterile urine samples; strict aseptic technique must be utilized to avoid introducing harmful pathogens into the urinary tract

2. Indwelling urethral catheters: used postoperatively with children undergoing surgery of the renal system; maintaining a closed drainage system and frequent assessments for catheter patency are mainstays of nursing management; if a child is discharged with an indwelling catheter, parent education and understanding of catheter care and maintenance must be documented

3. Suprapubic catheters: drain urine directly from the bladder, bypassing the urethra

   a. Suprapubic catheters are frequently used postoperatively when surgery is performed on the urethra

   b. In addition to maintaining a closed drainage system and assessing for catheter patency, incision care at the catheter insertion site is another important nursing responsibility

   c. Provide parent education regarding home care of suprapubic catheters for the child who is discharged home with a suprapubic catheter

4. Nephrostomy tubes: inserted directly into the renal pelvis of the kidney; may be unilateral or bilateral

   a. Nursing interventions include maintaining a closed drainage system and frequent assessments for patency and incisional care of the catheter insertion site

   b. Output from nephrostomy tubes must be calculated and documented individually; this helps to quickly identify sources of urinary flow changes

   c. Perform irrigation of nephrostomy tubes only with a physician order, which includes maximum amount of fluid to be used (since the renal pelvis is small, irrigating with too large of a fluid volume can cause serious renal damage)

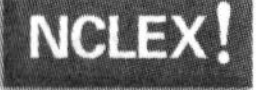

D. Forcing of fluids: implemented after diagnostic tests in which dyes are utilized; encouraging fluids helps to flush the dyes from the urinary tract

E. Fluid restriction: the physician may restrict oral fluid intake in renal system disorders when edema is present or fluid volume excess is a potential complication

F. Intake and output

1. A measurement of fluid and electrolyte balance in the body

   a. Intake: measurement of what is delivered to the child through parenteral or oral routes; measured in cc or mL

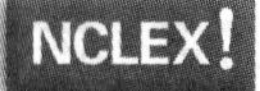

   b. Output: measurement of what is expelled, drained, secreted, or suctioned from the body; is recorded in cc or mL; for infants, counting wet diapers per day (4 to 8/day is normal) is one method of measuring urine output; weighing a dry diaper before it is placed on the infant and then after the infant has voided is another method of measuring urine output for an infant; for each 1g increase in the weight of the diaper, one mL of liquid has been excreted

G. Medication administration

NCLEX!

1. Antimicrobial therapy: specific antibiotics are administered for specific pathogens
2. Pathogens causing urinary tract infections are identified by urine culture and sensitivity
3. The culture identifies pathogens
4. Sensitivity describes what antimicrobials the identified pathogen is sensitive or resistant to
5. Nursing management includes administering antibiotics when scheduled as well as parent/client education regarding the importance of completing entire course of drug therapy even though symptoms may subside

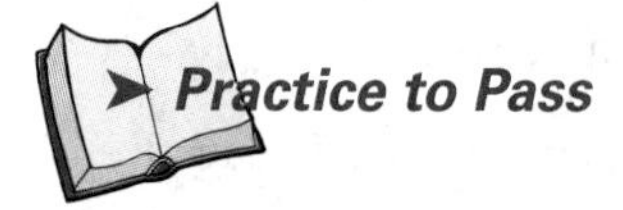

Describe the differences in methods used to collect clean-catch urine specimens from infants, toddlers, school-age children, and adolescents. For each age group, identify developmental factors that impact the method used.

IV. Surgical Interventions for Pediatric Clients with Renal Health Disorders

A. Urinary diversion procedures

1. Ureterostomy: surgical implantation of the ureters to outside the abdominal wall; allows urine to bypass the bladder and drain directly into a collection device
2. Vesicostomy: surgical opening into the bladder in which the bladder wall is brought to the surface of the abdomen
3. Ileal or colon conduit: ureters are removed from the bladder and attached to the ileum or colon, which then acts as a bladder without voluntary control of voiding
   - **a.** The client has a stoma on the abdominal wall and must wear an appliance for urine collection
   - **b.** Urine from an ileostomy may appear cloudy related to secretions from the bowel
   - **c.** Cloudy urine from an ileostomy appliance is not considered a sign of urinary tract infection

B. Issues in psychosocial support for children undergoing surgery of the renal system

1. Implementation of psychological interventions in daily care to address the following concerns of the child or parents
   - **a.** Increased physical care of child, especially if stomas or tubes are involved
   - **b.** Hygiene concerns
   - **c.** Skin problems, especially with urinary diversion procedures

NCLEX!

2. Difficulty leaving child in the care of others
3. Frequent trips to clinic add stress to everyday life
4. Toddlers may be unable to achieve toilet training
5. School-age children suffer from being different and may develop a distorted perception of body image
6. Adolescents may suffer from low self-esteem and have concerns regarding sexuality

C. Priority nursing diagnoses for children undergoing renal surgery

1. Anxiety related to the surgical experience
   - **a.** Provide surgical tour, especially the "wake-up" room
   - **b.** Determine child's words for penis, urination, etc.
   - **c.** Encourage parents to remain with child as appropriate
   - **d.** Provide support and reassurance

NCLEX!

2. High risk for ineffective airway clearance related to poor cough effort associated with post-anesthesia state, postoperative immobility, or pain
   - **a.** Assist child to turn, cough, and breathe deeply; reposition infants frequently
   - **b.** Perform frequent vital signs monitoring
   - **c.** Teach splinting of incision and incentive spirometry preoperatively
3. Pain
   - **a.** Assess and monitor for bladder spasms and incisional pain
   - **b.** Provide analgesics as ordered
4. Risk for fluid volume deficit related to client's age, surgery, catheters and refusal to drink
   - **a.** Regulate IV fluids
   - **b.** Keep accurate intake and output records
   - **c.** Measure daily weights
   - **d.** Record separate output for each drainage tube

NCLEX!

5. Health-seeking behaviors regarding ostomy care
   - **a.** Teach need to keep skin dry and odor free
   - **b.** Demonstrate ostomy care procedures to parents and to child as appropriate to age
   - **c.** Provide written instructions to parents
   - **d.** Provide contact number should problems occur

V. Congenital Renal Health Problems

A. Hypospadias and epispadias

1. Description
   - **a.** Hypospadias: congenital defect in which the urinary meatus is not at the end of the penis but is located on the lower or underside of the shaft (see Figure 7-2a)
   - **b.** Epispadias: congenital defect in which the urinary meatus is not at the end of the penis but on the upper side of the penile shaft; less common than hypospadias (see Figure 7-2b)

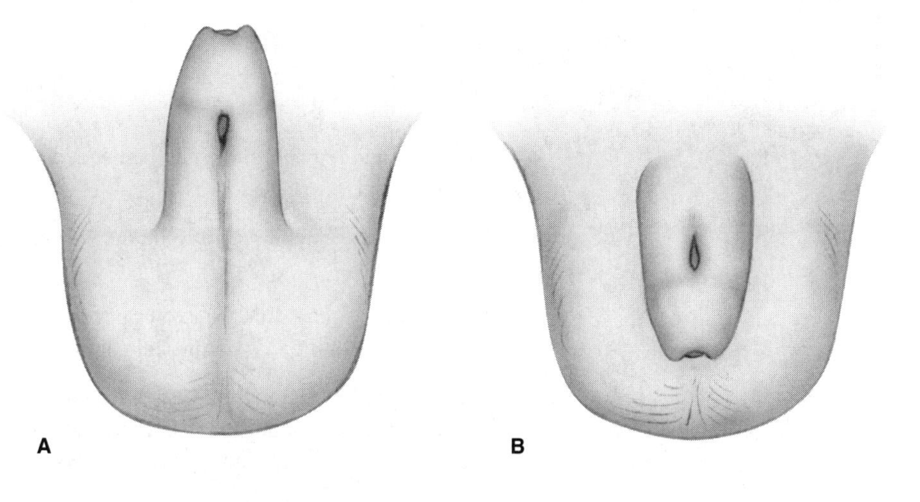

Figure 7-2

A. Hypospadias, B. Epispadias. *Source:* Ball, J. & Binder R. (1999). *Pediatric nursing: Caring for children* (2nd ed.). Stamford, CT: Appleton & Lange, p. 665.

2. Etiology and pathophysiology

- **a.** In hypospadias, opening can be anywhere on the underside of the penis to the base of the penis; in epispadias, the meatal opening can be anywhere along the upper shaft; most frequent anomalies are minor with openings off-center but still on the glans
- **b.** Hypospadias is the more common anomaly, occurring in 1 to 500 newborns
- **c.** Hypospadias is often accompanied by **chordee,** a downward curvature of the penis
- **d.** Epispadias is often associated with exstrophy of the bladder
- **e.** Both males and females can be affected by hypospadias or epispadias; in most instances, the female anomaly does not require surgical correction

3. Assessment: noted on admission to the newborn nursery; the defect does not interfere with voiding but could interfere with reproduction if not repaired before adulthood

4. Priority nursing diagnoses

- **a.** Risk for altered parent/infant attachment
- **b.** Risk for ineffective family coping
- **c.** Anxiety (parental)
- **d.** Body image disturbance (in unrepaired school-age or adolescent child)

5. Planning and implementation

- **a.** Document findings carefully and report to physician
- **b.** **Circumcision** (operation to remove part or all of the prepuce) is delayed as prepuce may be used in the reconstruction
- **c.** If chordee present, curvature of penis may be released before hypospadias repair
- **d.** Surgical correction is usually begun before the age of 18 months

e. Postoperative care

1) The penis may have a urethral stent in place and be wrapped with a pressure dressing

2) Arm and leg restraints may be needed to prevent accidental removal of the stent

3) Encourage increased fluid intake to maintain urine output and stent patency

4) Call physician if no urine output occurs for 1 hour, because there could be kinks in the system or occlusion by sediment

5) Medication therapy includes antibiotics until the stent falls out, acetaminophen (Tylenol) for pain, and anticholinergics such as oxybutynin (Ditropan) for bladder spasms

6. Child and family education

a. Parents need explanation of the disorder as well as information about surgical repair

b. Post-surgical discharge teaching includes double-diapering technique to protect stent, limiting of activity for approximately 2 weeks, restriction of activities that put pressure on the site (riding toys, sitting on lap), medication administration, maintaining adequate fluid intake, monitoring for signs of infection, and to call physician if urine leaks from anywhere but penis (urine will also be blood-tinged for several days)

7. Evaluation: parents show positive infant bonding; parents describe surgical plans

B. Exstrophy of the bladder

1. Description: lower portion of the abdominal wall and anterior bladder wall are missing, resulting in the bladder being open and exposed on the abdomen

2. Etiology and pathophysiology

a. Occurs more frequently in boys than girls and is most frequently associated with epispadias

b. The bladder appears as an angry red mass glistening with urine

c. Continuous drainage of urine from the ureters may lead to excoriation of the skin surrounding the bladder

d. Exstrophy of the bladder can be life-threatening and therefore needs to be corrected as soon after birth as possible

3. Assessment: immediately obvious at birth; the infant should be evaluated for other anomalies

4. Priority nursing diagnoses

a. Risk for infection

b. Risk for altered parent/infant attachment

c. Risk for ineffective family coping

d. Impaired skin integrity

5. Planning and implementation

a. Bladder closure is corrected during the first 48 to 72 hours of life

b. Correction of exstrophy of the bladder is usually a staged surgical correction, with epispadias repair at about 9 months of age (if present) and bladder neck reconstruction with ureteral reimplantation at 2 to 3 years of age

c. Preoperative nursing care involves covering the bladder with sterile plastic wrap and maintaining skin integrity of the surrounding area using skin sealant to protect it from excoriating effects of urine

d. Postoperative nursing care may involve Bryant's traction to facilitate healing, and avoiding abduction of the legs (puts stress on surgical area); change dressings as ordered by the physician; monitor urinary output and characteristics and watch for signs of obstruction, bladder spasms, and urine or blood draining from meatus

e. Emotional support of the infant and parents is important; activities to support bonding as well as helping the parents accept the deformity are a major component of the nurse's activities

6. Child and family education

a. Parents will need an explanation of the anomaly as well as instructions for care

b. As soon as possible, parents should participate in the care of their infant and will need appropriate instructions

7. Evaluation: parents identify positive attributes of their infant and visit their baby often; skin surrounding the bladder remains intact

C. ***Cryptorchidism***

1. Description: a failure of one or both testes to descend from the inguinal canal into the scrotum

2. Etiology and pathophysiology

a. Normal descent of testes occurs in late gestation

b. More frequently seen in premature infants than in full-term infants

c. Failure to descend exposes the testes to the heat of the body, leading to low sperm counts at sexual maturity

d. Undescended testicles are also at greater risk for torsion (twisting of the testes on its blood supply) and trauma; undescended testes have a higher incidence of cancer

e. Frequently associated with an inguinal hernia

3. Assessment: the absence of one or both testes in the scrotal sac may be noted at birth; if testes are not felt on examination, the condition should be monitored as the testes may descend later

4. Priority nursing diagnoses

a. Risk for injury

b. Risk for body image disturbance (in older child with undescended testes)

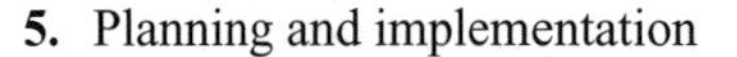

5. Planning and implementation
   - **a.** Often the testes descend on their own during the first year of life
   - **b.** If this does not occur, human chorionic gonadotropin hormone is given to induce descent
   - **c.** If testes remain undescended, an orchiopexy is performed in the toddler years; if testes are damaged or absent, a prosthesis will be placed in the scrotum
   - **d.** Nursing care preoperatively is directed at preparing the child and family for surgery
   - **e.** Postoperatively, nursing care includes putting ice on the surgical area, giving analgesics for pain, and monitoring the child for infection; bedrest is maintained
6. Child and family education
   - **a.** Educate the parents about the surgical process
   - **b.** Since the child will likely go home after recovering from anesthesia, the parents will need instructions on how to care for the child at home
   - **c.** Symptoms of infection should be described
7. Evaluation: the child recovers without signs and symptoms of infection; the parents describe appropriate home care for the child

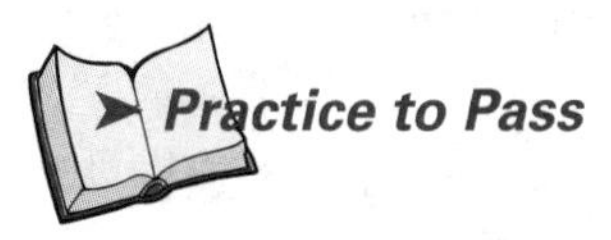

What discharge instructions/parent education should be included for the child being discharged after a urinary diversion procedure?

VI. Acquired Renal Health Problems

A. Acute glomerulonephritis

1. Description
   - **a.** A disease process that affects primarily the glomerulus of the kidney
   - **b.** May be acute or chronic
   - **c.** Post-streptococcal **glomerulonephritis** is the most common form

NCLEX!

2. Etiology and pathophysiology
   - **a.** Acute inflammation of the glomeruli
   - **b.** Acute post-infectious glomerulonephritis is preceded by a streptococcal infection, usually of the skin or respiratory tract
   - **c.** Damage is caused by an antigen-antibody complex that lodges in the glomeruli
3. Assessment
   - **a.** Diagnostic tests include elevated BUN; the elevated erythrocyte sedimentation rate (ESR) indicates inflammation in the body; an elevated antistreptolysin O (ASO) titer indicates a previous streptococcal infection; renal ultrasound shows enlarged kidneys, while urine exams demonstrate gross hematuria, proteinuria, and red blood cell casts; serum samples may also display **azotemia** (retention of excess nitrogenous wastes in the blood), elevated creatinine, and electrolyte imbalance
   - **b.** Nursing assessments include edema, hematuria, lethargy, and anorexia; hypertension can lead to headache, decreased level of consciousness, and convulsions

4. Priority nursing diagnoses
   - **a.** Risk for fluid volume excess
   - **b.** Altered nutrition
   - **c.** Risk for injury related to hypertension and CNS involvement
   - **d.** Activity intolerance
   - **e.** Diversional activity deficit
5. Planning and implementation (see Table 7-3)
   - **a.** Bedrest required during acute period

NCLEX!

   - **b.** Monitor for fluid and electrolyte imbalances; measure intake and output; weigh daily to monitor fluid balance; fluid restrictions are usually ordered; sodium, potassium, and possibly protein intake will be limited; monitor dietary intake to optimize calories consumed
   - **c.** Provide skin care to limit the effects of edema and lethargy

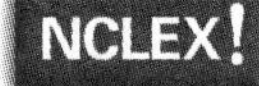

   - **d.** Monitor vital signs including mental status; report increasing hypertension and deterioration of mental status immediately
6. Medication therapy: to treat hypertension and prevent CNS involvement
   - **a.** Antihypertensives, such as hydralazine (Apresoline)
   - **b.** Diuretics, such as furosemide (Lasix)
7. Child and family education
   - **a.** The parents and child will need information about the disease, its treatment, and its prognosis

Table 7-3

Comparison of Features of Acute Glomerulonephritis and Nephrotic Syndrome

Assessment Factor	Acute Glomerulonephritis	Nephrotic Syndrome
Cause	Immune reaction to group A beta-hemolytic streptococcal infection	Idiopathic; possibly a hypersensitivity reaction
Onset	Abrupt	Insidious
Hematuria	Grossly bloody	Rare
Proteinuria	3+ or 4+, not massive	Massive
Edema	Mild	Massive
Hypertension	Marked	Mild
Hyperlipidemia	Rare or mild	Marked
Peak age frequency	5–10 years of age	2–3 years of age
Interventions	Limited activity; anti-hypertensives as needed; symptomatic therapy if CHF occurs	Bedrest during edema stage; corticosteroid administration
Diet	Normal for age; no added salt if child is hypertensive	Nutritious for age; no added salt; small, frequent meals may be desirable
Prevention	Prevention through treatment of group A beta-hemolytic streptococcal infections	None known
Course	Acute 2–3 weeks	Chronic—may have relapses

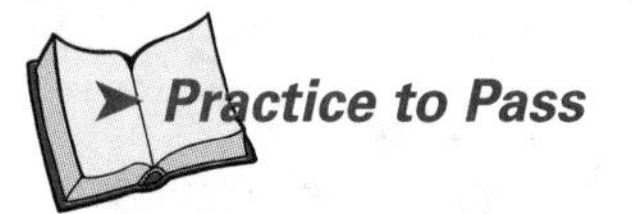

What nursing measures are specific to caring for children with acute glomerulonephritis? What nursing measures are specific to caring for children with nephrotic syndrome? How do they differ?

b. The parents will need information on safely administering medications

c. Instructions may be needed on monitoring blood pressure and weight and how to test the urine for protein

8. Evaluation: parents demonstrate safe administration of medications; parents and child describe necessary home monitoring

B. Nephrotic syndrome

1. Description: clinical state characterized by edema, massive proteinuria, and hyperlipidemia

2. Etiology and pathophysiology

   a. Cause is unknown

   b. Increased permeability of the glomerular membrane allows albumin to pass into the urine; kidneys reabsorb salt and water

   c. Protein deficiency leads to decreased osmotic pressure, allowing fluids to escape into the tissues; massive edema results

   d. Loss of protein leads to decreased immunoglobulins and susceptibility to infection

   e. Hyperlipidemia occurs secondary to liver stimulation by the decreased volume of albumin

   f. Relapses often occur but the frequency of relapses diminish with puberty

3. Assessments

   a. Gradual onset of massive edema, starting as periorbital then shifting to the abdomen and extremities, resulting in dramatic weight gain and abdominal pain

   b. Secondary symptoms of irritability, general malaise, and anorexia occur

   c. Urinalysis reveals proteinuria

4. Priority nursing diagnoses

   a. Risk for infection

   b. Fluid volume excess

   c. Risk for impaired skin integrity

   d. Altered nutrition: less than body requirements

5. Planning and implementation

   a. Monitor weight and intake and output; measure abdominal girth

   b. Promote nutrition by allowing child's preferences; fluids are not usually restricted; diet may be "no added salt"

   c. Promote rest; provide diversional activities as necessary

   d. Prevent skin breakdown: turn and reposition on a regular basis; use special mattresses as needed to help prevent breakdown; keep skin dry and clean

   e. Prevent infection: use careful handwashing; restrict visitors with infectious diseases; children with nephrotic syndrome are often not kept in the hospital after initial diagnosis to reduce exposure to organisms; encourage diet to replace lost protein

f. Refer again to Table 7-3 for comparison of acute glomerulonephritis and nephrotic syndrome according to manifestations, interventions, prevention, and course

6. Medication therapy

a. Intravenous albumin may be administered to reduce the edema; diuretics may also be used for the same purpose

b. Corticosteroids reduce the inflammatory process and reduce the proteinuria

c. Alkylating agents may be used if steroid therapy is unsuccessful

C. Acute renal failure (ARF)

1. Description: sudden onset of diminished renal function

2. Etiology and pathophysiology

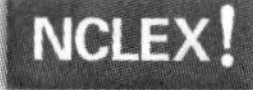

a. Occurs suddenly and is often reversible; generally follows ischemic or toxic trauma to the kidney

b. Three causes

1) Prerenal causes include decreased glomerular filtration secondary to decreases in renal blood flow

2) Intrarenal causes include direct kidney damage or changes caused by toxic substances or infection

3) Postrenal causes include obstruction in the urinary tract (from the renal tubules to the urethral meatus) caused by cancer, calculi, or traumatic interruption

3. Assessment

a. Laboratory findings include hyperkalemia, hyponatremia, and hypocalcemia; BUN and serum creatinine are elevated

b. Clinically the child will be pale and lethargic with edema; hypertension occurs secondarily to fluid volume overload

c. The nursing history may indicate possible causes of the acute renal failure

d. Prognosis depends upon the cause as well as the kidneys' response to therapy

4. Priority nursing diagnoses

a. Altered urinary elimination

b. Risk for altered nutrition: less than body requirements

c. Fluid volume excess

d. Anxiety

e. Risk for ineffective family coping

5. Planning and implementation

a. Medical management depends upon cause

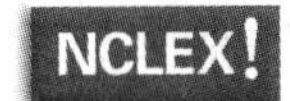

b. Children with ARF are catabolic and at risk for calorie and protein malnutrition related to decreased appetite and fluid restriction; help the child choose a diet for optimal intake of necessary nutrients while restricting sodium, potassium, and phosphorus as needed; initially, parenteral or enteral nutrition may be needed

c. Dialysis may be required during the acute period to correct electrolyte and fluid balances while eliminating wastes

d. Monitor intake and output and weigh the child daily; maintain fluid restrictions, which are calculated to replace insensible losses (one-third daily maintenance requirements); febrile children usually have a 12 percent increase in fluid intake for each 1-degree (Celsius) increase in temperature

e. Monitor blood pressures and report changes to prevent complications

NCLEX!

f. The child will be susceptible to infection so wash hands carefully, protect from infectious people, and promote nutrition

g. Provide emotional support for child and parental anxiety, possible parental feelings of guilt; assist parents and older siblings to participate in care to increase sense of control

6. Medication therapy

a. Antibiotic therapy may be ordered

b. Nephrotoxic drugs (such as aminoglycosides, cephalosporins, sulfonamides, tetracycline, contrast dye with iodine, indomethacin, aspirin, and heavy metals) are usually avoided

7. Child and family education

a. Teach dietary management, including protein, water, and sodium restrictions

b. The parents should learn symptoms of progressive failure and how to monitor weight, intake and output, and blood pressure

c. Discuss with the parents principles of safe and effective drug administration

8. Evaluation: the parents describe symptoms of renal failure and discuss monitoring that will be done in the home; the dietary restrictions are followed

D. Chronic renal failure (CRF)

1. Description: progressive deterioration of renal function

2. Etiology and pathophysiology

a. Etiology of CRF includes congenital abnormalities, damage from disease such as glomerulonephritis, hemolytic-uremic syndrome, infections, and exposure to toxins

b. Gradual loss of functioning nephrons

c. End-stage renal disease refers to a disease where the kidneys can no longer maintain body homeostasis and would lead to death without dialysis

3. Assessment

a. Laboratory test results (rising BUN, creatinine) indicate a failure of the kidneys to cleanse the blood, with resulting **uremia** (excess of urea and other nitrogenous waste products in the blood)

b. Renal biopsy determines the diagnosis and provides a basis for determining treatment

c. Assessment findings will include **oliguria** (urine output less than 0.5–1mL/kg/hour) or **anuria** (complete/almost complete cessation of urine production by the kidneys); sudden weight gain will indicate fluid retention; assess for signs and symptoms of fluid overload; monitor for manifestations of fluid and electrolyte imbalances (see Table 7-4)

d. Assess cardiac, hematological, gastrointestinal, neurological, dermatological, urinary, and skeletal systems for changes secondary to renal failure (see Table 7-5)

4. Priority nursing diagnoses

a. Risk for infection

b. Fluid volume excess

c. Caregiver role strain

d. Altered growth and development

e. Body image disturbance

5. Planning and implementation

a. Medical management is aimed at maintaining fluid and electrolyte balance as close to normal as possible

Table 7-4

Symptoms of Electrolyte Imbalance in Renal Failure

Electrolyte Imbalance	Manifestations
Hyponatremia (decreased sodium)	Headache, muscle weakness, fatigue, apathy, confusion, coma, postural hypotension, anorexia, nausea, vomiting, abdominal cramping, weight loss
Hypernatremia (increased sodium)	Dry mucous membranes, decreased urine output, rubbery skin turgor, excitement, tachycardia
Hypokalemia (decreased potassium)	Anorexia, nausea, vomiting, abdominal distention, lethargy, confusion, depression, weakness, decreased BP while standing, arrhythmias, thirst, increased urine output
Hyperkalemia (increased potassium)	Nausea, vomiting, diarrhea, irritability, weakness, oliguria, numbness, tingling, arrhythmias, sudden death
Hypocalcemia (decreased calcium)	Osteoporosis, fractures, tingling, convulsions, muscle spasms, tetany, calcium deposits in tissue, nausea, vomiting, diarrhea, arrhythmias
Hypercalcemia (increased calcium)	Renal calculi, coma, decreased reflexes, lethargy, arrhythmias, muscle fatigue, bone pain, osteoporosis, fractures
Acidosis (decreased bicarbonate)	Headache, malaise, rapid deep respirations, disorientation, stupor, coma, hyperkalemia

Table 7-5

Clinical Manifestations of Renal Failure

Body System	Clinical Manifestations	Cause of Manifestations
Cardiovascular	Hypervolemia, hypertension, tachycardia, arrhythmias, congestive heart failure, pericarditis	Increased fluid volume, build-up of metabolic wastes, chronic hypertension, change in renin-angiotension mechanism
Hematologic	Anemia, leukocytosis, decreased platelet function, thrombocytopenia	Decreased production of erythropoietin and RBCs, decreased survival of RBCs, decreased platelet activity; blood loss through dialysis and bleeding
Gastrointestinal	Anorexia, nausea, vomiting, abdominal distention, diarrhea, constipation, bleeding	Build-up of uremic toxins, electrolyte imbalances, changes in platelet activity, conversion of urea to ammonia by saliva
Neurologic	Lethargy, confusion, convulsions, stupor, coma, sleep disturbances, behavioral changes, muscle irritability	Uremic toxins, electrolyte imbalances, cerebral swelling caused by fluid shifts
Dermatologic	Pallor, pigmentation, pruritus, ecchymosis, excoriation, uremic frost	Anemia, decreased activity of sweat glands, dry skin, phosphate deposits on skin
Urinary	Decreased urine output, decreased specific gravity, proteinuria, casts and cells in the urine	Damage to the nephron
Skeletal	Osteoporosis, renal rickets, joint pain	Decreased calcium absorption, decreased phosphate excretion

b. Dialysis will be used to maintain the child when renal function is no longer able to maintain homeostasis

c. Chronic renal failure is permanent; kidney transplant may be indicated

d. Renal replacement therapy

1) **Hemodialysis:** filtering of the blood with a dialyzer to remove toxins (nitrogenous wastes) using a special machine; requires vascular access site with frequent monitoring for potential infection; hemodialysis involves a 4- to 6-hour treatment approximately three times a week and is the most effective dialysis treatment in clearing nitrogenous wastes from the blood

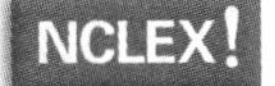

2) **Peritoneal dialysis:** filtering of the blood to remove toxins via a catheter inserted into the peritoneal cavity (see Figure 7-3); peritoneal dialysis is continuous and relatively easy to learn for home dialysis treatment; it is the most widely used renal replacement therapy in children; however, clients are at increased risk for peritonitis

NCLEX!

3) Renal transplantation: kidney transplantation with a kidney from a cadaver (organ donor) or a living relative donor kidney; donation of a kidney from a family-related donor that is histocompatible (has HLA system match) improves the survival rate of the graft; transplantation is considered to be the optimal renal replacement therapy because it provides for normal homeostasis and offers optimal chance for normal growth and development; disadvantages include rejection episodes and complications of immunosuppression

e. General nursing care involves monitoring the child's intake and output, weight, vital signs; watch for signs of electrolyte imbalances; support good nutrition while maintaining the dietary and fluid restrictions

Figure 7-3

Peritoneal dialysis.

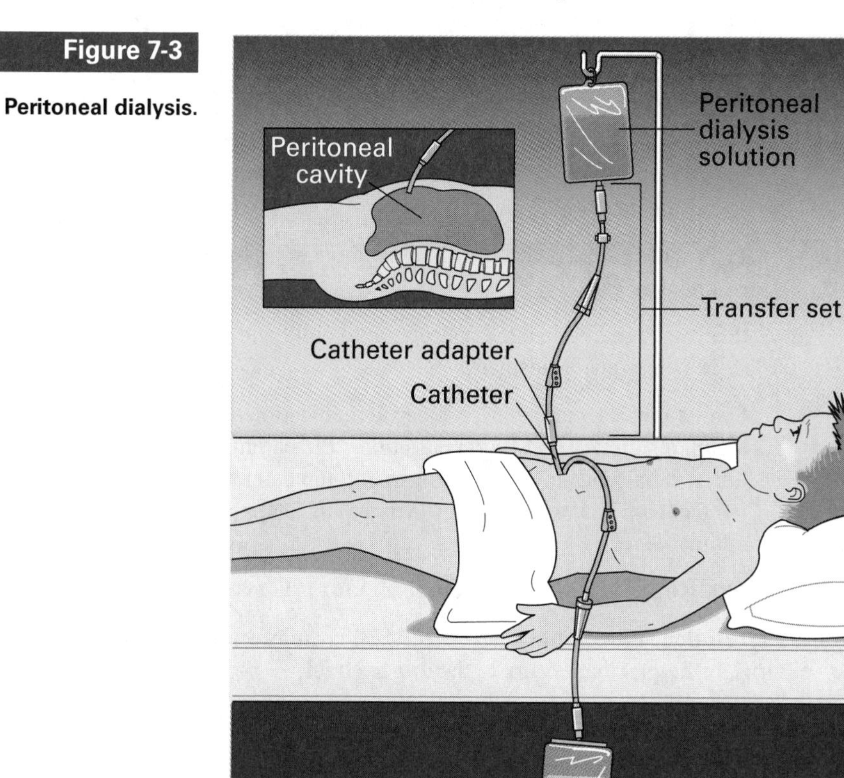

NCLEX!

f. Nursing care of the child receiving peritoneal dialysis includes carrying out dialysis procedure and using aseptic technique to prevent *peritonitis* (noted by fever, vomiting, diarrhea, abdominal pain, tenderness, and cloudy dialysate)

NCLEX!

g. Nursing care of the child receiving hemodialysis includes monitoring for complications that can suddenly occur, including hypotension (nausea and vomiting, abdominal cramping, tachycardia, and dizziness), rapid fluid and electrolyte shifts (muscle cramps, nausea and vomiting, and dizziness), and disequilibrium syndrome (restlessness, headache, blurred vision, altered level of consciousness, nausea and vomiting, muscle twitching)

h. Both child and parents will have emotional needs related to the chronic nature of the disease, ongoing life-sustaining treatment, and the possibility of death; assist with physical and emotional preparation for dialysis and renal transplant

5. Medication therapy

a. Sodium bicarbonate may be needed for severe metabolic acidosis

b. Diuretics are given to promote fluid elimination

c. Vitamins are necessary because of dietary deficiencies; vitamin D and calcium supplements may be ordered

d. Erythropoietin (epoietin alpha, Epogen) may be given to stimulate red blood cell production

e. Antihypertensives may be necessary

6. Child and family education

   a. Teach the parents and child to manage the child's disease at home, including dietary restrictions and needs

   b. Teach parents safe and effective administration of medication and potential side effects of these drugs

   c. Provide parents with information about symptoms of electrolyte imbalances

   d. Provide individualized instruction to child and parents about dialysis and possible renal transplant

7. Evaluation: the parents describe safe medication administration; the child maintains dietary and fluid restrictions; the parents and child describe preparation for dialysis and/or renal transplant; the parents demonstrate adequate coping mechanisms; the child's growth and development is maintained at an optimal level

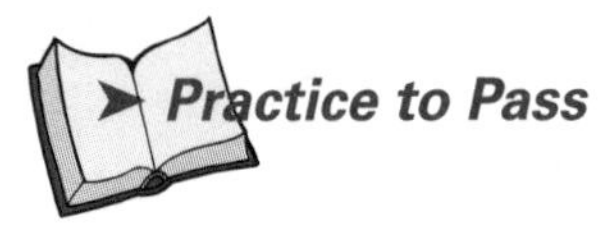

What are the three types of renal replacement therapy? For each type, describe one advantage and disadvantage for the child with renal failure.

VII. Infectious Renal Health Problems: Urinary Tract Infections

A. **Description:** urinary tract infection (UTI) is an infection caused by bacteria, virus, or fungus that occurs in the urinary tract

B. **Etiology and pathophysiology**

1. The site of infection within the urinary tract determines the consequences of an infection within it

   a. Infections of the upper urinary tract, which include **pyelonephritis** (inflammation of the renal parenchyma, calyces, and pelvis, particularly due to local bacterial infection) or **ureteritis** (inflammation of a ureter), are associated with or may result in permanent renal damage or scarring

   b. Infections confined to the lower urinary tract, such as **cystitis** (inflammation of the urinary bladder) and **urethritis** (inflammation of the urethra), may be followed by recurrent episodes, but they have not been associated with long-term sequelae

NCLEX!

2. Acute pyelonephritis is the most commonly occurring bacterial infection documented in young children, with *Escherichia coli* being responsible for approximately 85 percent of UTIs in infants and young children, followed by *Klebsiella* and *Proteus* organisms

3. UTIs are more common in girls than boys (girls have a shorter urethra) and occur most commonly in the 7 to 11 age group

C. **Assessment**

NCLEX!

1. Urinalysis: microscopic urinalysis shows large numbers of white blood cells (greater that 10 WBC/mm^3) as well as large numbers of bacteria

   a. Obtain catheter or urine bag specimens in infants and young children without urinary control (refer back to Box 7-1)

   b. Obtain clean-catch specimens from toilet-trained children (refer back to Box 7-2)

2. Urine culture: *Escherichia coli* is the most frequently found organism after 48 hours of growth

3. Signs and symptoms
    a. Infants: fever, weight loss, failure to thrive, vomiting, increased voiding, foul-smelling urine, and persistent diaper rash
    b. Older children: urinary frequency, pain during micturition, onset of bedwetting in a previously "dry" child, abdominal pain, hematuria, fever, chills, and flank pain

D. Priority nursing diagnoses

1. Pain
2. Altered urinary elimination
3. Risk for injury

E. Planning and implementation

1. Monitor intake and output; renal function should be 1mL/kg/hr; obtain daily weights
2. Encourage frequent voiding in toilet-trained child
3. Encourage increased fluid intake
4. Acidify the urine with ascorbic acid or cranberry juice

F. Medication therapy

1. Give antibiotic therapy
    a. Must continue to give/take doses for full course of therapy to prevent recurrent infection
    b. Untreated lower UTIs can ascend further into the urinary system and lead to acute pyelonephritis
2. Give antipyretic therapy as needed for temperature control

Box 7-3

Child and Family Education for Preventing Urinary Tract Infections in Children

- Encourage complete bladder emptying and explain the need for this as age permits. "Standing urine" in the bladder is susceptible to the growth of pathogens.
- Remind children to void frequently. The bladder flushes away organisms by ridding itself of urine; this prevents organisms from accumulating and invading nearby structures. The convalescent bladder is less resistant to invasion than is a healthy bladder.
- Suggest avoidance of hot tubs, whirlpool baths, water softeners or bubble baths. Oils in these products are known to irritate the urethra and can be potential sources of infection.
- Teach girls the importance of wiping themselves after toileting from front to back to avoid contamination of the urethra with *Escherichia coli,* which is found in stool. Have girls demonstrate this technique on a doll.
- Encourage the use of showers rather than tub baths to help prevent infection.
- Explain the need for cotton underwear, which is more absorbent than nylon or other synthetic materials.
- Suggest apple or cranberry juices to maintain acidity of urine; acidifying the urine decreases the rate of bacterial multiplication; an acid-ash diet consisting of meats, cheese, prunes, cranberries, plums, and whole grains is also beneficial.
- Recommend frequent pad change for menstruating girls and proper genital cleansing during menses. Old, pooled blood fosters growth of organisms.

G. Child and family education

1. Teach parents ways to reduce UTIs (see Box 7-3): avoid bubble baths, tight underwear
2. Encourage the child to void frequently and to drink plenty of liquids
3. Teach parents to administer medications and to complete therapy

H. Evaluation: parents describe ways to reduce UTIs; parents describe safe administration of antibiotics

Case Study

A school-age child with end-stage renal disease (ESRD) is evaluated for renal replacement therapy. Please answer the following questions regarding the child's nursing management in terms of the type of replacement therapy prescribed, as well as general management principles.

❶ What type of diet (including fluids) is prescribed for the child with ESRD? Why?

❷ What type of renal replacement is considered to be the most effective for a child with ESRD? Why?

❸ What are the potential complications of hemodialysis? What are the advantages of hemodialysis over peritoneal dialysis?

❹ Why is peritoneal dialysis more widely used in the treatment of children with ESRD?

❺ What psychosocial concerns need to be addressed with the child with ESRD?

For suggested responses, see page 409.

Posttest

1 **The most important nursing activity in managing a young child diagnosed with urinary tract infection (UTI) is to:**

(1) Provide adequate nutrition to prevent dehydration.
(2) Prevent enuresis.
(3) Administer ordered antibiotics on schedule.
(4) Restrict fluids to provide kidney rest.

2 **When reviewing a urinalysis report of a client with acute glomerulonephritis, the nurse would expect to note:**

(1) Decreased creatinine clearance.
(2) Decreased specific gravity.
(3) Proteinuria.
(4) Decreased erythrocyte sedimentation rate (ESR).

3 **While a child is receiving prednisone (Deltasone) for treatment of nephrotic syndrome, it is important for the nurse to assess the child for:**

(1) Infection.
(2) Urinary retention.
(3) Easy bruising.
(4) Hypoglycemia.

4 **Which of the following interventions will help obtain accurate urinalysis data?**

(1) Force fluids to 1000 mL prior to specimen collection.
(2) Cleanse the specimen container with povidone-iodine (Betadine) prior to collecting the specimen.
(3) Allow the urine to cool to room temperature before taking it to the lab.
(4) Provide client/parent education for specimen collection before the specimen is obtained.

5 **The parents of a child diagnosed with upper urinary tract infection (UTI) ask the nurse why the child needs a daily weight. In formulating a response, the nurse includes that it is important because a daily weight will:**

(1) Determine if the child's caloric intake is adequate.
(2) Indicate the need for dietary restrictions of sodium and potassium.
(3) Keep track of possible loss or gain of fluid retained in body tissues.
(4) Track the amount of fluid ingested orally each day.

6 **A child has been diagnosed with acute renal failure secondary to an infectious organism. The nurse would question the medical order for:**

(1) Aqueous penicillin.
(2) Gentamicin (Garamycin).
(3) Antihypertensives.
(4) Corticosteroids.

7 **The newborn has been diagnosed with cryptorchidism. The physician has ordered human chorionic gonadotropin (HCG) to be administered to the baby. The mother asks the nurse why the baby is receiving this drug. The nurse's best explanation would be the drug will:**

(1) Maintain an adequate temperature around the testes.
(2) Prevent infections in the undescended testes.
(3) Prevent the development of cancer.
(4) Promote descent of the testes.

8 **The nurse admits children with the following diseases to the unit. Which disease places the child at risk for the development of acute renal failure (ARF)?**

(1) Leukemia
(2) Cryptorchidism
(3) Nephrotic syndrome
(4) Phenylketonuria

9 **A child has recurrent nephrotic syndrome. The mother reports to the nurse that she is overwhelmed with the care of her child. After the nurse discusses options with the mother, which statement by the mother indicates continued coping difficulties?**

(1) "I joined a support group like you suggested. I hope it does some good."
(2) "I'm going to ask my mother-in-law to come on a regular basis to allow me an afternoon out."
(3) "My husband has agreed to help me manage my son's medication."
(4) "We're going to skip his dietary restrictions one day a week to allow us both some relaxation."

10 **A child returning to the unit after an intravenous pyelogram (IVP) has an order to drink extra fluids. When the mother asks the purpose of these fluids, the nurse responds that increased fluid intake will:**

(1) Overhydrate the child.
(2) Increase serum creatinine levels.
(3) Make up for fluid losses from NPO status before tests.
(4) Flush any remaining dye from the urinary tract.

See pages 184–185 for Answers and Rationales.

Answers and Rationales

Pretest

1 **Answer: 2** ***Rationale:*** Epispadias is a frequent anomaly associated with exstrophy of the bladder. The other conditions listed are not.
Cognitive Level: Analysis
Nursing Process: Assessment; ***Test Plan:*** PHYS

2 **Answer: 2** ***Rationale:*** Edema is the major clinical symptom of nephrosis. The child may gain twice his or her normal weight in severe cases.
Cognitive Level: Application
Nursing Process: Assessment: ***Test Plan:*** PHYS

3 **Answer: 3** ***Rationale:*** Diapers are weighed on a gram scale before using them and after removal (1 g = 1 mL). The weight of the dry diaper is then subtracted from the wet diaper to determine urine output.
Cognitive Level: Application
Nursing Process: Implementation; ***Test Plan:*** PHYS

4 **Answer: 3** ***Rationale:*** Bubble baths are irritating to the meatus and increase the incidence of urinary tract infections.
Cognitive Level: Application
Nursing Process: Evaluation; ***Test Plan:*** PHYS

5 **Answer: 3** ***Rationale:*** Although children with acute glomerulonephritis may feel well, they are confined to bed until hematuria resolves. This can lead to boredom, making it important for the nurse to provide activities that are fun for the child to help pass the time.
Cognitive Level: Application
Nursing Process: Implementation; ***Test Plan:*** PHYS

6 **Answer: 4** ***Rationale:*** Urinalysis allows for early diagnosis and treatment of acute glomerulonephritis, which is a serious complication that can follow group A beta-hemolytic streptococcal infection.
Cognitive Level: Analysis
Nursing Process: Implementation; ***Test Plan:*** PHYS

7 **Answer: 4** ***Rationale:*** The open bladder allows bacteria to enter the urinary system, and urinary tract infections are common. At this age, sexual dysfunction would not be an appropriate diagnosis. The unformed bladder does not hold urine, so urinary retention would not be an appropriate diagnosis.
Cognitive Level: Analysis
Nursing Process: Planning; ***Test Plan:*** PHYS

8 **Answer: 1** ***Rationale:*** The ASO titer indicates a preceding infection with *group A beta-hemolytic streptococcus.* The urinalysis would show hematuria, but this alone would not be diagnostic of acute glomerulonephritis. Blood cultures may be negative as the infection preceded the illness by 1 to 3 weeks.
Cognitive Level: Analysis
Nursing Process: Analysis; ***Test Plan:*** PHYS

9 **Answer: 2** ***Rationale:*** Clean-catch urine specimens are not sterile urine samples; therefore, catheterization is not necessary. The urine does need to be obtained at the time of voiding.
Cognitive Level: Application
Nursing Process: Implementation; ***Test Plan:*** PHYS

10 **Answer: 3** ***Rationale:*** With the inability to secrete urine, electrolytes will build up in the blood, including sodium and potassium. The child should be on a low-sodium, low-potassium diet with restricted fluids and proteins.
Cognitive Level: Analysis
Nursing Process: Implementation; ***Test Plan:*** PHYS

Posttest

1 **Answer: 3** ***Rationale:*** Urinary tract infections are ascending in nature; an untreated UTI can lead to acute pyelonephritis with resulting kidney scarring and damage. Early diagnosis and prompt antimicrobial therapy will prevent or minimize permanent renal damage.
Cognitive Level: Analysis
Nursing Process: Implementation; ***Test Plan:*** PHYS

2 **Answer: 3** ***Rationale:*** Proteinuria (presence of protein in urine) is a prime manifestation of acute glomerulonephritis. The other options are inconsistent with this diagnosis.
Cognitive Level: Analysis
Nursing Process: Assessment; ***Test Plan:*** PHYS

3 **Answer: 1** ***Rationale:*** Prednisone is a synthetic corticosteroid that depresses the immune response and increases susceptibility to infection. Steroids mask infection; therefore, the child must be assessed for subtle signs and symptoms of illness.
Cognitive Level: Application
Nursing Process: Implementation; ***Test Plan:*** PHYS

4 **Answer: 4** ***Rationale:*** Specimens collected utilizing proper technique will minimize contamination of the urine sample ensuring accurate urinalysis results. It is unnecessary to force fluids prior to specimen collection. The specimen container is not cleansed, although the urinary meatus is. The specimen should be sent to the lab immediately after collection to prevent urine degradation.
Cognitive Level: Application
Nursing Process: Implementation; ***Test Plan:*** SECE

5 **Answer: 3** ***Rationale:*** With infectious or inflammatory processes of the upper urinary tract, the kidneys' ability to filter and reabsorb salt and water is altered, resulting in edema. Weights can be an easy and effective measure to determine fluid loads.
Cognitive Level: Application
Nursing Process: Implementation; ***Test Plan:*** PHYS

6 **Answer: 2** ***Rationale:*** Gentamicin is an aminoglycoside antibiotic that is nephrotoxic. Nephrotoxic drugs should be avoided in a child with acute renal failure.

The other options do not represent drug groups that are particularly nephrotoxic.
Cognitive Level: Application
Nursing Process: Implementation; ***Test Plan:*** PHYS

7 **Answer: 4** ***Rationale:*** HCG is given to induce the descent of testes if testes have not descended during the first year of life. The other reasons listed are incorrect rationales.
Cognitive Level: Application
Nursing Process: Implementation; ***Test Plan:*** PHYS

8 **Answer: 3** ***Rationale:*** Nephrotic syndrome is an inflammatory reaction in the kidneys. The other diseases pose minimal risk of developing acute renal failure.
Cognitive Level: Analysis
Nursing Process: Assessment; ***Test Plan:*** PHYS

9 **Answer: 4** ***Rationale:*** The parents must understand the need for compliance with medical orders to promote the child's health. Relaxation should be accomplished without harming the child.
Cognitive Level: Analysis
Nursing Process: Evaluation; ***Test Plan:*** PSYC

10 **Answer: 4** ***Rationale:*** The additional fluids will increase urinary output, causing greater urine volume and more frequent voiding, thus flushing the dye from the urinary system. The other options do not describe the correct rationale for this intervention.
Cognitive Level: Application
Nursing Process: Implementation; ***Test Plan:*** PHYS

References

Ball, J. & Bindler, R. (1999). *Pediatric nursing: Caring for children* (2nd ed.). Stamford, CT: Appleton & Lange, pp. 33, 40, 660–707.

Burg, F., Ingelfinger, J., Wald, E., & Polin, R. (1998). *Gellis and Kagan's current pediatric therapy* (16th ed.). Philadelphia: W. B. Saunders, pp. 842–902.

Monahan, F. & Neighbors, M. (1998). *Medical-surgical nursing: Foundations for clinical practice* (2nd ed.). Philadelphia: W. B. Saunders Company, pp. 1329–1426.

Stedman, T. (1995). *Stedman's medical dictionary* (26th ed.). Baltimore, MD: Williams & Wilkins.

CHAPTER 8

Endocrine Health Problems

Nancy H. Wagner, MSN, RN

CHAPTER OUTLINE

OBJECTIVES

- Identify data essential to the assessment of endocrine health problems in a child.
- Discuss the clinical manifestations and pathophysiology of conditions related to endocrine health problems of a child.
- Discuss therapeutic management of a child with alterations in health of the endocrine system.
- Describe nursing management of a child with alterations in health of the endocrine system.

[Media Link]

Use the CD-ROM enclosed with this text, or log onto the address given to access the free, interactive Companion Website created for this series. The CD-ROM and Companion Website accompanying this book offer additional practice opportunities and information—NCLEX Review, Case Studies, Glossary, In Depth with NCLEX, and more.

www.prenhall.com/hogan

Review at a Glance

constitutional delay *delayed growth in which the serum gonadotropins are normal, but the bone age is mildly delayed and there is history of small stature in the family*

epiphyseal growth plate *the cartilaginous end of the long bones allowing bone growth*

estrogen *female hormone that is secreted by the ovary and promotes secondary sexual characteristics*

exophthalmos *protrusion of the eyeballs*

follicle stimulating hormone (FSH) *secreted by the anterior pituitary gland and stimulates the secretion of estrogen*

glucagon *a hormone produced by the pancreas that helps release stored glucose from the liver*

hypothalamus *an endocrine gland located in the brain that secretes gonadotropin-releasing hormone*

hypotonia *lack of muscle tone that may be seen in babies that have congenital hypothyroidism*

insulin *a hormone released from the beta cells of the pancreas that aids in energy metabolism*

islets of Langerhans *cells of the pancreas involved in energy metabolism*

karyotype *a picture of the cell during division allowing identification of the chromosomes*

ketoacidosis *a state when glucose is unavailable to the cells for energy and that source of energy is provided by free fatty acids; it is a serious complication of diabetes mellitus*

Kussmaul respirations *deep, pauseless respirations that are characteristic of metabolic acidosis*

luteinizing hormone (LH) *a hormone secreted by the anterior lobe of the pituitary that stimulates the secretion of androgens in males and progesterone in females*

phenylalanine *an essential amino acid found in most natural protein foods*

polydipsia *excessive thirst—a symptom of diabetes mellitus*

polyphagia *excessive hunger—a symptom of diabetes mellitus*

polyuria *passage of a large amount of urine—a symptom of diabetes mellitus*

testosterone *hormone responsible for the production of sperm and the development of male sex characteristics*

thyroid-stimulating hormone (TSH) *a hormone produced by the anterior pituitary gland that stimulates thyroid hormone secretion*

thyroxine (T4) *secreted by the thyroid gland; stimulates cellular growth rate*

thyrotoxicosis *excessive amount of thyroid hormone in blood causing rapid heart rate, tremors, and elevated basal body temperature*

Pretest

1 **A mother tells the nurse that her child has been diagnosed with hypertrophy of the thyroid gland. The mother states the doctor called it something else and asks the nurse what the other name for this is. The nurse's reply should be:**

(1) Glandular enlargement.
(2) Goiter.
(3) Lymphadenopathy.
(4) Thyrotoxicosis.

2 **An infant was born 24 hours ago. The nurse has been instructed to collect blood by heel stick for neonatal screening for congenital hypothyroidism before the baby is discharged. The nurse discusses options with the pediatrician knowing that 24 to 48 hours after birth is not the optimal time to collect this specimen because:**

(1) At 24 hours, the T4 level will be extremely low.
(2) There is an immediate rise in the TSH after birth.
(3) The baby needs to digest formula before a blood sample can be taken.
(4) A thyroid scan should be done first.

3 **The nurse is administering propylthiouracil to a 12-year-old female recently diagnosed with Graves' disease. The child has been receiving the drug 3 times a day for 3 weeks. She suddenly complains of a severe sore throat. What would be the appropriate nursing action?**

(1) Continue to give the medication or she will continue to exhibit signs of Graves' disease.
(2) Offer lozenges for the relief of the sore throat.
(3) Hold that dose and report the complaint to the physician since a sore throat is a common side effect.
(4) Assume that she is complaining in order to avoid going to the school room in the hospital.

4 A 10-year-old diabetic client told the nurse that he had some early signs of hypoglycemia while attending school. What would be the best action for the child to take?

(1) Take an extra shot of regular insulin.
(2) Drink a glass of orange juice.
(3) Skip the next dose of insulin.
(4) Start exercising.

5 The nurse is teaching an adolescent client about the different types of insulin. The client takes NPH insulin at 8:00 A.M. The nurse would instruct the client that he could possibly expect an insulin reaction at what time of the day?

(1) While working out at 9:00 A.M.
(2) While taking a test at 10:00 A.M.
(3) While eating lunch at noon.
(4) While golfing after school at 3 P.M.

6 A teenage mother arrives at the clinic with her new baby who has recently been diagnosed with congenital hypothyroidism. When instructing the mother about administering levothyroxine medication, the nurse would include the information that she should:

(1) Crush the medication and place in a full bottle of formula or juice to disguise the taste.
(2) Administer the medication every third day.
(3) Give the crushed medication in a syringe or in the nipple mixed with a small amount of formula.
(4) Understand that the medication will not be needed after age 5.

7 A new mother of an infant diagnosed with phenylketonuria (PKU) meets with the nurse who informs her that PKU follows autosomal recessive inheritance. The mother states that is a relief since she now knows her next baby will not have the disease. What additional information does the mother need?

(1) With autosomal recessive inheritance, each baby has a 25 percent chance of having the disease.
(2) Only female babies will have PKU.
(3) The mother passes the gene only to male offspring.
(4) Since she already has one baby with the disease, the next one will probably be a carrier for the disease.

8 A 4-month old infant has been diagnosed with PKU. The child has eczema and sensitivity to the sunlight. The mother asks the nurse why her child's skin is so sensitive. An appropriate explanation by the nurse would be:

(1) "Some children just have sensitive skin."
(2) "Your child will outgrow his sensitivity when he is 5 years old. Just use sunscreen for now."
(3) "Your child has a deficiency in melanin because of decreased tyrosine. You will always have to take special care of his skin."
(4) "The phenylketones in your baby's blood concentrate the sun's rays, making burning more likely. Children with PKU can never be in the sun."

9 The nurse was working with a group of parents of children with phenylketonuria. The nurse has completed family teaching on the dietary restrictions. The parents are given sample menus to choose a meal for their child. Which menu choice indicates understanding of the dietary instructions?

(1) A hamburger and a diet soda sweetened with aspartame.
(2) Steak and mashed potatoes with orange juice.
(3) A large bowl of cereal with strawberries and apple juice.
(4) Milkshakes and grilled cheese sandwich.

10 Mothers in the waiting room of the endocrine clinic are discussing their children's illnesses. The mothers of children with phenylketonuria and congenital hypothyroidism recognize there is a common goal in the early treatment of their children. That goal is the avoidance of:

(1) Mental retardation.
(2) Fever.
(3) Obesity.
(4) Protein foods.

See page 211 for Answers and Rationales.

I. Overview of the Anatomy and Physiology of the Endocrine System

A. Thyroid gland

1. Structure

a. Reddish-brown soft mass with right and left pear-shaped lobes that extend from the sides of the thyroid and cricoid cartilage to the sixth tracheal cartilage just below the larynx

b. A narrow isthmus connects the right and left lobes

2. Thyroid gland functions

a. Regulates and accelerates the cell function of all cells including protein, fat, and carbohydrate catabolism; it has a major role in controlling the basal metabolic rate

b. Helps maintain cardiac output, respiratory rate, and utilization of oxygen and carbon dioxide

c. Regulates body heat production and mechanisms of control

d. Aids in growth hormone secretion and skeletal maturation

e. Metabolizes substances as nutrients

1) Maintains appetite

2) Regulates calcium utilization by decreasing the calcium concentration

3) Aids in the utilization of glucose and cholesterol; promotes sensitivity to insulin

3. Thyroid hormones

a. Thyroid hormones include **thyroxine (T4),** triiodothyronine (T3), and thyrocalcitonin

b. The secretion of the thyroid hormones is controlled by the **thyroid-stimulating hormone (TSH);** this hormone is secreted by the anterior pituitary gland; TSH is regulated by thyrotropin-releasing factor (TRF)

c. Hypothyroidism or hyperthyroidism may occur because of deficient levels of thyroid hormone or may be caused by a malfunction of the secretion of TSH or TRF

B. Pituitary gland

1. Structure

a. A round, pea-sized gland that is 1/2-inch in diameter; it is supported by the sella turcica, a bony depression of the sphenoid bone and is attached to the **hypothalamus** (an endocrine gland located in the brain)

b. The pituitary gland is composed of an anterior lobe and a posterior lobe; the anterior pituitary is considered to be the "master gland"

2. Anterior pituitary hormones and functions

a. Somatotropin or growth hormone (GH) promotes somatic growth and maintains blood glucose levels; it promotes growth of bone and soft tissues

b. **Follicle stimulating hormone (FSH)** stimulates the secretion of **estrogen** (a female hormone secreted by the ovary) and progesterone in females; stimulates the seminiferous tubules to produce sperm in males

c. **Luteinizing hormone (LH)** stimulates ovulation in females; stimulates the secretion of **testosterone** (reproductive or sex hormone) in males

d. Luteinizing-releasing hormone stimulates the release of FSH and LH by the pituitary gland

e. Gonadotropins stimulate gonads to mature and produce sex hormones and germ cells

f. Adrenocorticotropic hormone (ACTH) stimulates the adrenal cortex to convert cholesterol into adrenal steroids

g. Prolactin maintains milk production after childbirth

h. Thyroid stimulating hormone (TSH) stimulates the thyroid gland to synthesize and release thyroxine

i. Melanocyte-stimulating hormone promotes the pigmentation of the skin

3. Posterior pituitary hormones and functions

a. Antidiuretic hormone (ADH or vasopressin) stimulates the distal loop of kidney to reabsorb water and sodium

b. Oxytocin stimulates uterine contractions and the let-down reflex in breast-feeding women

C. Ovary

1. Structure

a. Female gonads located in the pelvis behind and below the Fallopian tubes

b. Size and shape of large almonds

2. Ovarian hormones and functions

a. Estrogen stimulates overall cellular RNA and protein synthesis, breast development during puberty and pregnancy, the growth of pubic and axillary hair, pelvic enlargement, and growth of mammary glands; it promotes the epiphyseal closure of bones and stimulates water and sodium retention in the renal tubules

b. Progesterone prepares the uterus for the fertilized ovum; promotes the growth of breasts; during pregnancy, progesterone keeps the uterine smooth muscle calm; it also promotes salt and water retention

D. Testes

1. Structure

a. Lobular male gonads that are composed of tiny tubules called seminiferous tubules, implanted in tissue containing interstitial cells

b. Two testes are located in the scrotum; each is located in a compartment with ducts emerging from the top of the gland to join the head of the epididymis

2. Testes hormones and function

   a. Testosterone stimulates testes to produce spermatozoa; promotes secondary sex characteristics and closure of bone epiphyses; it accelerates protein synthesis for growth of long bones, muscle development, external genitalia enlargement, and growth of body hair

E. Islets of Langerhans/pancreas

1. Structure: the pancreas is a fished-shaped organ that extends from the duodenal curve to the spleen
2. Islets of Langerhans hormones and function

   a. **Islets of Langerhans** are ductless clusters of cells located in the pancreas, consisting of alpha, beta, and delta cells

   b. The alpha cells secretes the hormone **glucagon,** which increases blood glucose by accelerating liver glycogenolysis; glucagon acts as an antagonist to the hormone insulin

   c. The beta cells produce **insulin,** which promotes glucose, protein, and fatty acid transport into the cells; it accelerates the movement of potassium and phosphate ions through the cell membranes with the glucose, thereby decreasing the blood glucose and increasing glucose utilization

   d. The delta cells produce somatostatin, which inhibits the secretion of both insulin and glycogen

II. Congenital Endocrine Health Problems

A. Hypothyroidism

1. Description

   a. A condition present from birth in which the thyroid gland does not produce enough thyroid hormone to meet the metabolic needs of the body; it occurs in 1 in 4,000 live births and is twice as common in girls as in boys; it is less prevalent in African-Americans

   b. Untreated congenital hypothyroidism leads to mental retardation

2. Etiology and pathophysiology

   a. Usually caused by a spontaneous gene mutation, an autosomal recessive genetic transmission of an enzyme deficiency, iodine deficiency, or a failure of the central nervous system-thyroid feedback system mechanism to develop

   b. When these hormones are not available for stimulation of specific target cells, growth delay and mental retardation usually develop

3. Assessment

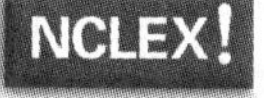

   a. Routine neonatal screening by state mandate is done prior to discharge from the hospital to evaluate the levels of thyroid hormones, although optimal testing occurs at 2 to 6 days after birth since an early test may show the TSH as falsely high

      1) Neonatal screening for congenital hypothyroidism: a filter-paper blood-spot thyroxine (T4) evaluation is taken by a heel-stick blood sample on a newborn between 2 and 6 days of age; some specimens are taken

within the first 24 to 48 hours along with other metabolic screenings; if the specimen is obtained too early, it may result in a false interpretation caused by an immediate rise in the TSH shortly after birth; if the T4 values are low, a sample of the thyroid-stimulating hormone (TSH) is measured; if the TSH level is increased, the result indicates that the hypothyroidism originates in the thyroid gland and not in the pituitary; this test is mandatory in all 50 states

2) Serum measurement of T4, triiodothyronine (T3), resin uptake, free T4, and thyroid-bound globulin may be needed for further testing for potential causes of congenital hypothyroidism

3) If client is discharged prior to 24 hours of life, a home-care nurse may make a home visit to assess the baby and perform the neonatal screening at that time; the screening may be done at a health care facility also

b. If an infant has a T4 level under 3µg/100mL and a TSH level greater than 40µg /mL, he/she would be considered to have primary hypothyroidism

c. If diagnosed with congenital hypothyroidism, serial measurements of height, weight, and head circumference are performed at each follow-up visit to assess signs of inadequate growth; screening should also be done to assess developmental milestones

NCLEX!

d. Signs and symptoms include lethargy, prolonged jaundice, constipation, feeding problems, being cold to touch, excessive sleeping, hoarse cry, large tongue, **hypotonia** (lack of muscle tone), and distended abdomen; the child is often described as "a good baby" because crying is infrequent; the baby may appear puffy and pale

4. Priority nursing diagnoses: Risk for injury; Altered nutrition: less than body requirements; Hypothermia; Constipation; Fatigue; Risk for altered health maintenance

5. Planning and implementation

a. Teach the family about the disorder and its treatment; refer to genetic counseling if it is genetic in origin

b. Monitor growth and development of the infant

c. Provide ongoing client/family education including ongoing medication administration

d. Provide information to family regarding infant stimulation programs or special education centers if the child has cognitive problems; assess for retarded physical growth and slow intellectual development; if mental retardation has already occurred, provide support to the parents and family

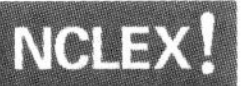

6. Medication therapy: thyroid hormone replacement (Synthroid or Levothroid) therapy is used to eliminate all signs of hypothyroidism, this will establish normal physical and mental growth and development; it is imperative to evaluate blood levels of thyroxine periodically to ensure the appropriate dosage and optimal outcome

7. Child and family education

a. Instruct client and family regarding the importance of daily administration of medication; drug therapy is needed for life; noncompliance can lead to mental retardation and slow growth and development

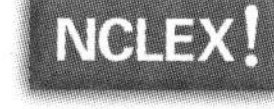

NCLEX!

b. The medication can be crushed and added to formula, food, or water; it can be offered through a syringe or a nipple mixed with formula

c. The medication should never be put in a whole bottle of formula in case the infant does not finish the formula

d. Signs of overdose including irritability, rapid pulse, dyspnea, sweating, and fever; include instructions on taking a pulse in the teaching plan

e. Signs of ineffective treatment are fatigue, constipation, and decreased appetite

8. Evaluation: The client is free of signs of hypothyroidism or hyperthyroidism (from excesive medication); physical and developmental growth is within normal parameters; the parents/caregivers verbalize the importance of daily administration of thyroid hormone and administer as ordered

> ***Practice to Pass***
>
> An infant client was discharged from the newborn nursery prior to having the newborn screening done for congenital hypothyroidism. How should the public health nurse respond if the mother of the client refuses to have the blood drawn on the first home visit?

B. Hyperthyroidism

1. Description

a. Occurs when the thyroid hormone levels are increased (**thyrotoxicosis**), with an accompanying enlarged thyroid gland and exophthalmos

b. Graves' disease is one cause of the disease; the incidence is highest in adolescent girls, but may be present at birth when mothers have Graves' disease

2. Etiology and pathophysiology

a. Graves' disease is an autoimmune disorder; the body produces an autoantibody, thyroid-stimulating immunoglobulin (TSI), that attacks the cells of the thyroid gland; the serum thyroid-stimulating immunoglobulin causes oversecretion of the thyroid hormones

b. There is evidence of familial association; the female to male ratio is 4:1

3. Assessment

a. Serum measurement of T4 and T3 levels: if elevated may indicate the diagnosis of hyperthyroidism; if elevated, a TSH level may need to be obtained

b. Graves' disease is diagnosed by serum blood test results of elevated T3 and T4 levels and a decreased TSH level; the autoantibodies are noted as positive also

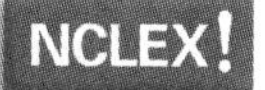

c. Signs and symptoms include: tachycardia, tremor, excessive perspiration, irritability, weight loss, diarrhea, increased appetite, muscle weakness, and fatigue; **exophthalmos** (protrusion of eyeballs) may occur

d. Findings will include a non-tender, enlarged thyroid gland (goiter); exophthalmos may be present in children with accompanied blurring vision

e. The incidence may go undetected for 1 to 2 years prior to diagnosis

f. School work may be affected as changes in behavior will be exhibited

g. Pulse and blood pressure may be elevated

4. Priority nursing diagnoses: Risk for injury; Altered nutrition: less than body requirements; Ineffective thermoregulation (elevated); Fatigue; Body image disturbance; Ineffective management of therapeutic regimen

5. Planning and implementation

   a. Be aware of signs of the disorder such as weight loss, inability to sit still in school, academic problems, short attention span, fatigue, fine motor problems, and exophthalmos

   NCLEX!

   b. Once diagnosed, give instruction to parents/family members and school personnel as appropriate regarding signs and symptoms, dietary requirements, medication therapy, and pre- and postoperative care, since management may include antithyroid drug therapy, radioactive iodine therapy, or surgery

   c. Offer ongoing support to client and family

   NCLEX!

   d. A rare complication of hyperthyrodism is thyrotoxicosis or thyroid storm; thyroid storm is characterized by sudden onset of tachycardia, restlessness, and severe irritability caused by the sudden release and subsequent high level of thyroid hormones; it can be fatal; the nurse must monitor the child for this condition following surgical treatment or during periods of stress and infection

6. Medication therapy: the goal of medication therapy is to decrease the secretion of the thyroid hormone; the following medications may be used:

   NCLEX!

   a. Propylthiouracil (PTU) or methimazole (MTZ, Tapazole) may interfere with the biosynthesis of thyroid hormone by preventing the incorporation of iodine into tyrosine; these medications are usually given three times per day and may take 6 to 12 weeks to produce the full effect; they must be taken as directed and doses should not be skipped; severe leukopenia may occur; sore throat, cervical lymph node enlargement, GI disturbances, fever, skin rashes, itching, and jaundice should be reported to the physician immediately; the medication may alter the taste of foods, so extra seasoning may be needed; sources of iodine (iodized salt, shellfish, turnips, cabbage, and kale) may need to be omitted from the diet

   b. Ablation with radioiodine (131I-iodine) is usually not recommended for the pediatric client because of the potential for carcinoma or genetic damage

   c. A beta adrenergic blocking agent (propranolol) may be indicated after thyrotoxicosis or thyroid storm to reduce the symptoms of adrenergic hyperresponsiveness; it might be needed for 2 to 3 weeks

Practice to Pass

An adolescent client has recently been diagnosed with Graves' disease. She continues to have periods of fatigue, especially during school hours. She has decided that she doesn't want to go to school. As a school nurse, how would you approach this issue to meet her health and school needs?

7. Child and family education

   a. If drug therapy is needed, instruct the client to take the medication as directed; missed doses may cause signs of hyperthyroidism to occur

   b. Teach the parents to offer frequent rest periods for the client; school attendance may be possible, but physical education classes should be discontinued until the thyroid hormone levels have returned to normal levels

   c. Explain the need for consumption of healthy foods versus "junk" foods

   d. Parents should be aware of signs of hypothyroidism caused by overdosage of the drug regimen

   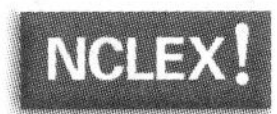

   e. Instruct the parents to provide ventilation and a cool environment for the client until the symptoms subside

f. Provide preoperative education if a thyroidectomy is indicated; emotional support for distress caused by the diagnosis, the client's emotional lability, and/or surgical intervention are essential for the client and family

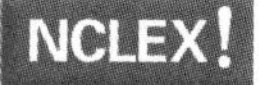

g. Prepare the child for the surgical dressing and a possible endotracheal tube after surgery; teach the child how to support the neck when sitting up

8. Evaluation: the child is free of symptoms of hyperthyroidism; the child grows at an age-appropriate rate; bowel movements are normal; family demonstrates compliance with medication regimen as ordered; family and child describe the side effects of the medication

C. Phenylketonuria (PKU)

1. Description

a. An inherited disorder that affects the body's protein utilization caused by the abnormal metabolism of the amino acid **phenylalanine**

b. It is inherited as an autosomal recessive trait or a mutation affecting 1 in 10,000 to 25,000 live births; it affects mostly white children; PKU is rare in blacks, Japanese, and the Jewish population

2. Etiology and pathophysiology

a. Phenylalanine is an essential amino acid found in most natural protein foods

b. In PKU, there is a deficiency in the liver enzyme phenylalanine hydoxylase, which normally breaks down the amino acid phenylalanine into tyrosine; as a result, phenylalanine metabolite levels increase in the blood, leading to musty body and urine odor caused by the excretion of phenol acids, seizures, hyperactivity, irritability, vomiting, and an eczema-type rash

c. Decreased levels of tyrosine cause a deficiency of the pigment melanin, causing most children with PKU to have blond hair, blue eyes, and fair skin that is prone to eczema

d. Decreased levels of the neurotransmitters dopamine and tryptophan, which affect protein synthesis and myelinization, cause degeneration of the gray and white matter in the brain; mental retardation and seizures occur if the level of phenylalanine is not decreased

3. Assessment

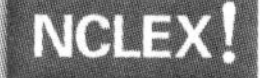

a. Many infants with PKU appear normal at birth; if treatment is not started to lower the phenylalanine level immediately, the infant's IQ can drop as many as 10 points within the first month and will continue to decline

b. Compulsory newborn screening is done by use of the Guthrie blood test by all 50 states at 48 hours after birth

1) The Guthrie blood test is a bacterial inhibition assay for phenylalanine in the blood; *Bacillus subtilis* is present in the blood if increased levels of phenylalanine are present; normal value is 1.6 mg/dL

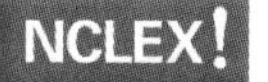

2) The infant should ingest adequate protein (usually 24 hours of normal feedings of breast milk or formula) prior to the test being performed

3) Heel blood should be used for the specimen; the heel stick sample should be collected after the first 24 hours but no later than 7 days after birth

4) A normal level is < 2 mg/dL; the Guthrie test will detect levels greater than 4 mg/dL; if the level is elevated, a repeat Guthrie test is performed to validate the original results

5) If the infant is discharged prior to 48 hours, the test should be performed within 1 week after discharge from the hospital or birthing center by a public health nurse, pediatrician, or pediatric nurse practitioner

NCLEX!

c. Although the child will appear normal at birth, symptoms will develop as the levels of phenylalanine metabolites rise; symptoms of the disease include failure to thrive, vomiting, irritability, and unpredictable behavior in the infant; the urine will have a musty odor; the child may experience myoclonic or grand mal seizures

4. Priority nursing diagnoses: Risk for injury; Altered growth and development; Risk for altered nutrition; Altered family processes; Altered role performance (child)

5. Planning and implementation

a. Mental retardation can occur if condition is left untreated; ensure that the Guthrie blood test has been done correctly and results have been received; repeat blood test if phenylalanine levels are elevated on first test

b. Phenylalanine is an essential amino acid and is thus required; phenylalanine is maintained at a level that allows for normal growth but does not allow the buildup of phenylalanine metabolites; the child must be monitored closely for levels of phenylalanine; it is allowed in the diet based on the weight of the child and usually at a level of 20 to 30 mg of phenylalanine per kilogram of body weight or the amount prescribed by the physician; consult with registered nutritionist to aid in food calculations

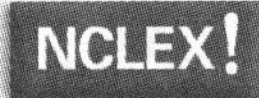

c. The child is placed on a protein-restricted diet; some protein is allowed to provide the phenylalanines essential to life; careful control of the levels of protein in the diet is essential; encourage the use of mature breast milk or modified protein hydrolysate formula with the phenylalanine removed as a source of nutrition for the infant in order to keep the phenylalanine level at 2 to 6 mg/dL; special protein foods are used that are free of phenylalanine; the dietary restrictions may be lifted after maximum brain growth has occurred (around age 8); more recent information may indicate the need to continue the restrictions for life

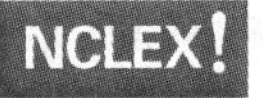

d. Serum phenylalanine levels should be measured periodically throughout the child's life; the restricted phenylalanine diet should be maintained at least through adolescence; children of women with phenylketonuria may be born with congenital defects including mental retardation unless the woman resumes a low phenylalanine diet before conception

e. In young children who were not adequately screened after birth and who develop phenylketonuria, modification of the diet at the time of diagnosis will usually provide benefits in terms of behavior and other symptoms; retardation that has occurred will not be reversed, but further damage may be prevented

f. In the beginning, the parents may be overwhelmed by the diagnosis and the dietary restrictions; emotional support is essential; genetic counseling may be suggested because each child born to this couple may have a 1 in 4 chance of having the disease

6. Medication therapy: anti-seizure medications may be needed if the client is having seizures; a modified protein hydrolysate formula with the phenylalanine removed is used for infant nutrition and as a supplement in childhood

7. Child and family education

   a. Support parents and teach them the disease and its management

   b. Instruct parents that the Guthrie test may need to be repeated if the initial test was done before 24 to 48 hours of age or if the test was positive initially

NCLEX!

   c. Review the low phenylalanine diet with the parents and offer written instructions to validate teaching; specifically review the preparation of the low phenylalanine formula; teach the family to avoid giving the child high protein foods (meats and dairy products) and products containing aspartame as they contain large amounts of phenylalanine

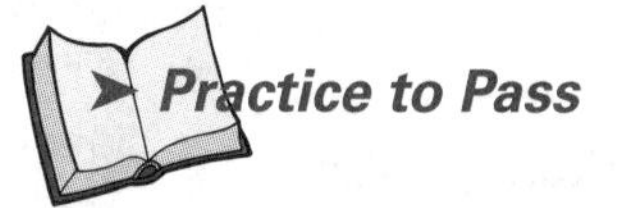

An infant client with phenylketonuria (PKU) arrives in the pediatric clinic with a severe sunburn. Her mother informs you that they attended a baseball game the day before and the baby got a little too much sun. What advice would you give to this mother to avoid future sunburns?

   d. If teaching an adolescent with PKU, encourage the resumption of the low phenylalanine diet, especially if the child is having difficulty with attention span, concentration, and school tasks

   e. Offer emotional support and refer the older child and parents to a support group dealing with the issues and problems related to chronic illness

8. Evaluation: the parents identify dietary restrictions and requirements for their child; the child's growth and development remains within normal limits; the family complies with follow-up blood testing of phenylalanine levels

III. Acquired Endocrine Health Problems

A. Diabetes mellitus

1. Description

   a. A metabolic disease causing a malfunction of carbohydrate, protein, and fat metabolism

   b. Most children have Type 1 diabetes, formerly called insulin-dependent diabetes mellitus (IDDM)

   c. Some children may have Type 2 diabetes, formerly called non-insulin-dependent diabetes mellitus; this disease is usually acquired as an adult, but it may be prevalent in overweight adolescents; it also used to be referred to as MODY or maturity onset diabetes mellitus

   d. The incidence of Type 1 diabetes mellitus is 15 per 100,000 people in North America; the peak ages of onset are between 10 to 12 years of age in girls and 12 to 14 years in boys; the risk increases if the child or adolescent has a first-degree relative or identical twin with the disease

2. Etiology and pathophysiology

   a. Type 1 diabetes does not show any specific pattern of inheritance but may show a familial tendency; it has been postulated that it may be caused by a genetic component, an autoimmune response, or environmental influences such as viruses; an autoimmune response causes the destruction of the insulin-secreting cells (beta cells) of the pancreas in the islets of Langerhans

b. Because over 90 percent of the insulin-secreting cells of the pancreas are destroyed, there is an absence of insulin available for metabolism of carbohydrates for energy; this in turn causes fats and proteins to be burned for energy; the excess amount of unused carbohydrates causes hyperglycemia when blood glucose levels rise above the normal level of 80 to 120 mg/dL

c. As the blood glucose level exceeds the renal threshold of 160 mg/dL, the kidneys are unable to reabsorb all the glucose, thereby allowing glucose to enter the urine (glucosuria); large amounts of electrolytes and water are lost with the glucose leading to increased urination (**polyuria**) and dehydration; the resulting dehydration leads to excessive thirst (**polydipsia**); hunger (**polyphagia**), fatigue, and weight loss may accompany the other symptoms because of cellular starvation since the insulin cannot enter cells (see Figure 8-1)

NCLEX!

d. Since glucose is unavailable to the cell because of the absence of insulin, the body attempts to break down fats to release glucose for energy use; while converting fats for cellular use, the liver produces ketones, acidic waste products of fat metabolism; the ketones cannot be utilized by the cell in the absence of insulin; therefore, ketones accumulate in the blood (causing metabolic acidosis or **ketoacidosis**), and in the urine, thereby inducing ketonuria (increased ketones in the urine); the respiratory system attempts to rid the body of the excess carbon dioxide by increasing the depth and rate of respirations, called **Kussmaul respirations;** if the acidosis is not corrected, acute renal failure, severe dehydration, coma, and subsequent death may occur

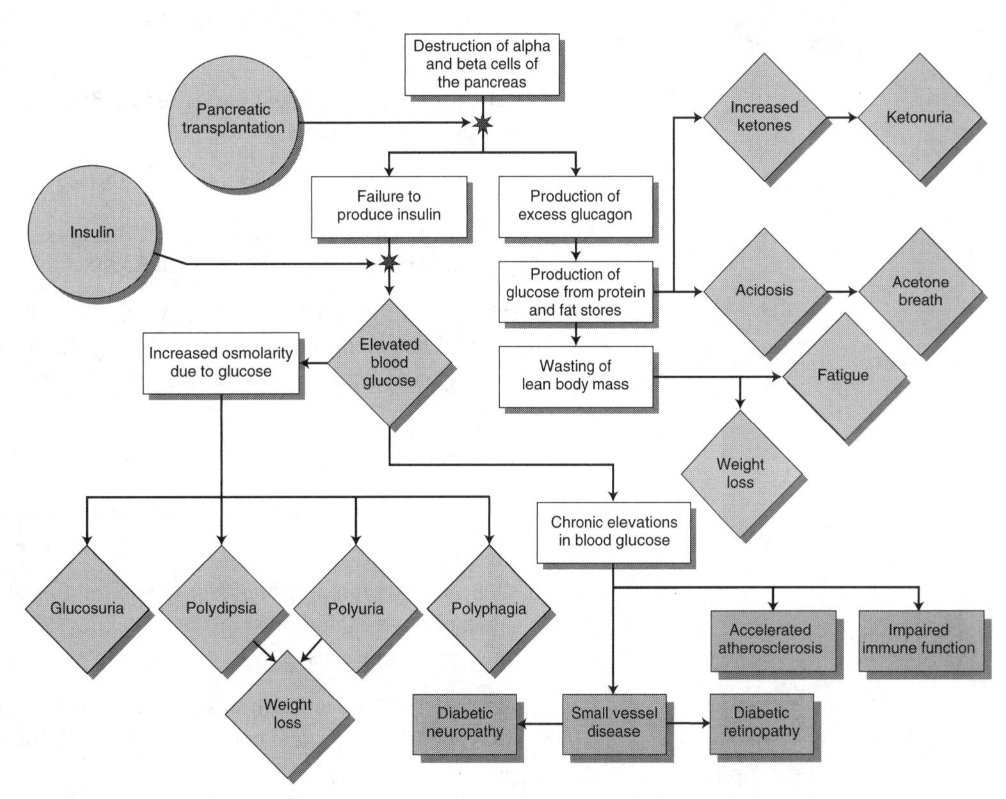

Figure 8-1

Pathophysiology of diabetes mellitus.
Source: Black J. & Matassarian-Jacobs, E. (1997). *Medical surgical nursing: Clinical management for continuity of care* (5th ed.). Philadelphia: W. B. Saunders, p. 1958.

e. About 5 percent of teens who develop diabetes have Type 2 diabetes mellitus, especially those who are overweight; they might need to take an oral hypoglycemic with or without accompanying insulin

f. Long-term complications of diabetes, especially Type 1, include retinopathy, neuropathy, and vascular complications; these are more frequent in the poorly controlled diabetic; the goal of treatment is to prevent long-term complications

3. Assessment

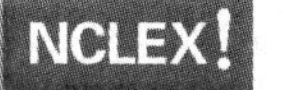

a. The client may present with an elevated serum glucose level (>126 mg/dL for a fasting sample and >200 mg/dL for a random sample), accompanied by classic signs of diabetes: lethargy, confusion, dry skin, thirst, weakness, abdominal pain, fruity breath, and diminished reflexes; ketonuria (ketones in the urine) and glycosuria (glucose in the urine) may be present also

b. Symptoms such as polyuria (enuresis in a toilet-trained child), polyphagia, and polydipsia with accompanying weight loss and fatigue may be reported

c. Dehydration may be present, as indicated by assessment of skin turgor (poor, tenting), mucous membranes (dry), and urine output (low)

d. A complete physical examination, including dietary and caloric intake, and long-term and short-term history is indicated; the history rules out the presence of other illnesses that would cause an elevated blood glucose (stress-related illness, corticosteroid use, fracture, acute infection, cystic fibrosis, pancreatitis, and liver disease)

e. Diagnosis is based on:

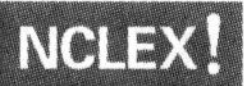

1) Eight-hour fasting blood glucose level, which detects elevated fasting glucose >126mg/dL

2) Ensure that the client has fasted completely for 8 hours or more prior to collection of blood

3) Label blood collection tube as a "fasting sample"

4) Serum electrolytes, pH, PO_2, PCO_2, blood urea nitrogen are used to evaluate state of diabetic ketoacidosis

4. Priority nursing diagnoses: Risk for injury; Risk for fluid volume deficit; Risk for altered nutrition; Impaired skin integrity; Ineffective breathing pattern; Knowledge deficit; Powerlessness; Ineffective management of therapeutic regimen

5. Planning and implementation

a. Provide emotional support to both the child and family, especially if this is a new diagnosis

b. Continuously monitor vital signs, respiratory status, and level of consciousness; monitor hydration status by checking skin turgor, urine output, and mucous membranes

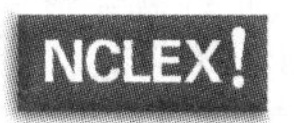

c. Administer intravenous fluids (IV) as ordered that may include electrolytes to regulate acidosis and continuous insulin infusion

d. Keep strict intake and output records

e. Monitor glucose levels with blood or urine testing as appropriate; glucose testing is more accurate and is preferred

1) Test urine for glycosuria and ketones using fresh urine and follow the directions on the package insert; report elevated levels as ordered

2) Test blood for glucose level using the blood chemstrip or blood glucose meter method; report results immediately especially if the blood glucose is >240 mg/dL; it is usually recommended that blood glucose levels be checked before each meal and at bedtime daily

f. When the continuous IV insulin infusion is discontinued, administer insulin subcutaneously as ordered to maintain normal blood glucose levels

g. Diet and exercise work together with insulin to allow normal growth and development

1) The dietary plan includes providing sufficient calories for normal growth and development; the diet is usually low in saturated fat and avoids concentrated carbohydrates

2) Three meals per day and mid-afternoon and bedtime snacks are usually recommended

NCLEX!

3) Exercise makes the body more sensitive to insulin and reduces the insulin requirement; if the child exercises without decreasing the insulin or increasing intake, the child may develop hypoglycemia; exercise is encouraged

4) The importance of exercise must be considered during the initial hospitalization while the child is being stabilized on insulin, but may not be as active as normal; after discharge, when regular activities are resumed, hypoglycemia may occur

NCLEX!

h. A glycosylated hemoglobin is usually performed every 3 months to evaluate longterm control; the hemoglobin A_{1c} is the value tested; the non-diabetic person will have HBA_{1c} levels of 4 to 7 percent, whereas the diabetic client will have higher levels; the higher the value, the poorer the control has been over the last 3 months

6. Medication therapy

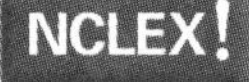

a. For Type 2 diabetes mellitus, oral medications may be used to increase the insulin production in the pancreas; included in this group are sulfonylureas and meglitinides; another group, biguanides, reduces the glucose production from the liver, thus it rarely causes hypoglycemia; insulin sensitizers improve the body's ability to use insulin in the liver and skeletal tissues; another action of these medications involves decreasing the production and release of glucose by the liver; side effects from all oral agents may include headache, dizziness, and edema; liver enzyme levels may increase and must be monitored

b. For Type 1 diabetes mellitus (usually found in children and adolescents), insulin therapy is utilized; in the U.S., U-100 insulin is the standard; the different types of insulin are: rapid-acting, short-acting, intermediate-acting, long-acting, and fixed combinations; the vials of insulin can be kept safely at room temperature (above freezing and below 86ºF) but should be discarded in 1 month after opening, even if refrigerated (see Table 8-1)

1) Most insulins are administered subcutaneously

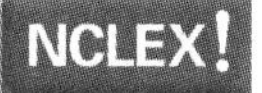

2) Only regular insulin may be administered intravenously

c. Glucagon, a hormone produced by the pancreas that helps release stored glucose from the liver, may be given subcutaneously or intramuscularly to a hypoglycemic client; usually children under 7 years of age will receive 0.5 mg while children over 7 receive 1 mg subcutaneously

NCLEX!

d. Glucose paste or glucose tablets should be available to all diabetic clients, especially those that have documented hypoglycemic events

7. Child and family education

a. Assess family's ability to learn concepts and adjust teaching to level assessed; optimally, offer teaching at least 3 to 4 days after initial diagnosis because of time needed for psychological adjustment of child and family

b. Offer psychological support and provide education and reinforcement of information

c. Keep information sessions limited to 15 to 20 minutes for the child and 45 to 60 minutes for the parents or adults involved; utilize audio-visual methods, books, pictures, and actual diabetic equipment for sensory stimulation to encourage learning

d. Review pathophysiology of Type 1 or Type 2 diabetes as indicated; answer all questions and anticipate unvoiced questions; encourage the parent to purchase a Medic-Alert identification bracelet for the child

NCLEX!

e. Review meal and snack planning; refer to a nutritionist with expertise in diabetes education; familiarize family with carbohydrate, protein, and fat exchange lists; consider periods of rapid growth and levels of growth and development during teaching; discuss issues such as travel, school parties, and holidays; Halloween and Christmas are problem times for these clients

NCLEX!

f. Provide an overview of insulin and specifically instruct the client and family on administration, absorption rates, dosage, storage, injection sites, side effects, and alternatives to the syringe and needle with the syringe-loaded

Table 8-1

Insulin Action (Subcutaneous Route)

Type	Onset	Peak	Duration
Rapid-Acting			
Lispro/Humalog	5–15 minutes	1 hour	≤ 4 hours
Short-Acting			
Regular	Up to 1 hour	2–4 hours	6–8 hours
Intermediate-Acting			
NPH	1–2 hours	6–12 hours	18–26 hours
Lente	1–2 hours	6–12 hours	24–26 hours
Long Acting			
Ultralente	4–6 hours	14–24 hours	28–36 hours

Source: Ball, J. & Bindler, R. (1999). *Pediatric nursing: Caring for children* (2nd ed.). Stamford, CT: Appleton & Lange, p. 886.

injector (Injectease); if the client is receiving short-acting and intermediate-acting insulin at the same time, assure the appropriate mixing technique; teach appropriate disposal of equipment; (see Box 8-1 and Figure 8-2)

g. Teach and supervise blood glucose monitoring using the manual and mechanical blood glucose meter, competence in the manual technique is necessary if the blood glucose meter malfunctions; reinforce teaching with the child if he or she will be performing the testing at home; instruct the family to call the physician if the blood glucose result is above or below their expected parameters; explain that this procedure must be done at least daily to

Box 8-1

Administration of Insulin

Insulin Storage

- Store insulin in a cool room. Do not expose to extreme heat or cold (freezer).
- Do not use an opened bottle of insulin for longer than one month due to loss of potency.

Insulin Administration

If mixing two types: Fast-acting (Regular/Lispro) and intermediate-acting (such as NPH) insulin, follow this procedure:

- Place the two bottles of insulin on a table and read the labels.
- Clean the tops of both vials with alcohol.
- Open the U-100 syringe and draw up air that would equal the amount of intermediate acting insulin (20 μ of air = 20 μ of insulin). Inject the air into the intermediate-acting insulin vial without allowing the needle to touch the liquid insulin. (Keep the vial upright on the table, do not invert)
- Remove the syringe. Draw up the amount of air that would equal the amount of fast-acting insulin and inject that air into the fast-acting insulin vial.
- Slowly invert the bottle of fast-acting insulin and withdraw the ordered amount of insulin.
- Invert the immediate-acting insulin vial, puncture the rubber cap with the needle and slowly withdraw the ordered amount of immediate-acting insulin without injecting any fast-acting insulin into the immediate-acting insulin vial. Some clients may choose to use a syringe-loaded injector (Injectease) or a preloaded pen (Novapen).

Subcutaneous Injection

- Cleanse the site for injection by wiping with an alcohol wipe or washing with soap and water and allow to dry.
- Plan to rotate injection sites to enhance absorption of the insulin. Hypertrophy or atrophy of the area can occur with repeated injections into the same area, slowing insulin absorption by the fat pads that develop in overused areas of injection. Choose an anatomical area and administer insulin in that area six to eight times, with each injection about 1-inch apart. Move to another anatomical area and repeat the process. This aids in more consistent absorption of the insulin since the different sites absorb it at a different rate.
- With the client's one hand, or with help from the parent, gently pinch or bunch up the skin at the site, insert the needle quickly, and inject the insulin at a 90-degree angle. Count to five, release the skin, and withdraw the needle.
- Wipe the site of injection with alcohol.

Continuous Subcutaneous Insulin Infusion

- Requires a portable insulin pump.
- Teach methods of loading the syringe, inserting the catheter, and adjusting the insulin flow according to metabolic needs.

Figure 8-2

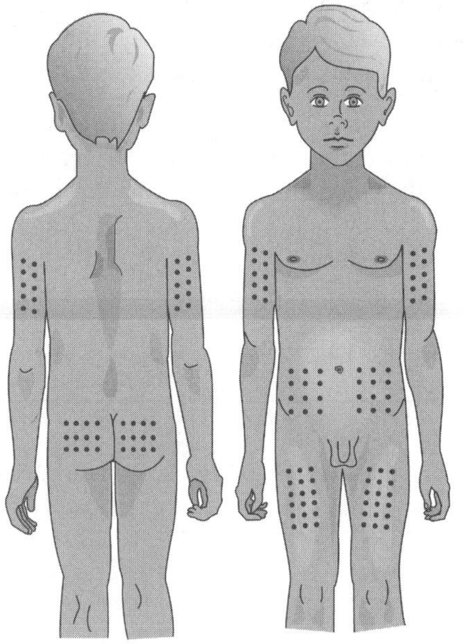

Insulin injection sites. Rotation of sites is important to promote absorption and prevent tissue damage.
Source: Ball, J. & Bindler, R. (1999). *Pediatric nursing: Caring for children* (2nd ed.). Stamford, CT: Appleton & Lange, p. 892.

maintain control of blood glucose levels; many children may need to perform this procedure many times throughout the day; if testing is necessary during school day, offer to teach the school nurse or personnel the appropriate procedure to ensure accuracy (see Box 8-2)

h. Demonstrate the procedure for testing urine for ketones; if the client's blood glucose level is elevated or if there is a sudden onset of infection or illness, urine testing is indicated; daily urine testing for ketones may not be necessary (see Box 8-2 again)

NCLEX!

i. Ensure that the client and family know the signs and symptoms of hyperglycemia and hypoglycemia to avoid complications (see Table 8-2); prior to exercise, less insulin or more food may be needed to avoid hypoglycemia; acute illness, such as gastroenteritis may lessen needs for insulin also

Box 8-2

Glucose Monitoring Techniques

Blood Monitoring
- Use a manual or spring-loaded puncturing device.
- Hold finger under warm water for a few seconds to encourage blood flow to that area.
- Use the side of the finger to avoid repeated discomfort to obtain blood samples and release the puncturing device. Squeeze the finger and apply a droplet of blood to the glucose measuring strip.
- Read blood glucose level displayed on the meter, record on appropriate document, and report as needed.

Urine Testing
- Read instructions on reagent strip bottle.
- Immerse strip into a urine sample and compare strip color with graph on bottle.
- Record results and report as needed.

Table 8-2 A Comparison of Hypoglycemia and Hyperglycemia with Ketoacidosis

	Causes	Symptoms	Treatment
Hypoglycemia	Too much insulin, inadequate intake or missed meals, strenuous exercise without increased intake.	1. Blood glucose levels drop below normal. 2. Diaphoresis, tremors, hunger, weakness, pallor, dizziness, somnolence, coma and convulsions, death.	Depends on the severity of the symptoms but involves the replacement of glucose. Mild or moderate: juice, or regular soda, glucose tablets or gel. Severe: cake frosting available in tube form or glucose paste, parents may be taught to administer glucagon SC.
Hyperglycemia with ketoacidosis	Insufficient insulin. Infection or other illness may contribute to the development.	1. Blood glucose >250 mg/dL. 2. Blood pH of <7.2; bicarbonate <15 mEq/L. 3. Glycosuria and ketonuria, elevated serum potassium and chloride levels. Serum levels of sodium, phosphate, calcium, and magnesium are decreased. 4. Kussmaul respirations, acetone breath, dehydration, weight loss, tachycardia, flushed facial skin, hypotension, and decreased level of consciousness, death. 5. Complaints of stomach ache or chest pain are common, vomiting may occur.	Intravenous insulin. Fluid and electrolytes are replaced as needed in a timely fashion. Normal saline is given IV until glucose decreases to 250–300mg/dL; then solution is changed to D5½ NS to prevent rebound hypoglycemia. Potassium levels are monitored; initial hyperkalemia may change to hypokalemia following fluid and insulin therapy.

j. Stress importance of a regular exercise program and review alternate insulin needs during times of increased activity

k. Teach appropriate record-keeping for blood glucose levels and insulin dosage

l. Consider developmental level when formulating a teaching plan for a child or adolescent client (see Table 8-3); encourage the child to assume responsibility for own care with parental supervision

Table 8-3 Developmental Care Ideas for the Child with Type 1 Diabetes Mellitus

Infants and Toddlers	Preschoolers	School-Age	Teen
Allow the toddler to make choices in food selection while monitoring carbohydrate levels.	Allow the preschooler to make food choices while monitoring carbohydrate levels. Be prepared to substitute snacks at birthday parties and at daycare.	Encourage independence of the school-aged child in food selection and glucose monitoring and insulin injections. Assess level of knowledge.	Assess the teen's body image and sense of identity. Assess compliance with other tasks.
The toddler may wish to help with the finger stick by cleaning his/her finger.	Encourage guided independence during the blood glucose/fingerstick procedure.	Assure that the school personnel will be available and knowledgeable if a hypoglycemic complication should occur during school hours.	Encourage independence with food selection, blood glucose monitoring, and insulin injections. Supervise diabetic tasks if teen is noncompliant.
Monitor temper tantrums as a possible sign of hypoglycemia.	Have appropriate snacks available if needed during sports activities that require a high expenditure of energy.	Encourage exercise but have snacks available for the child. Discourage fast food or snack machine selections.	Discuss future plans with the teen. Include diabetic issues, but promote a normal lifestyle.

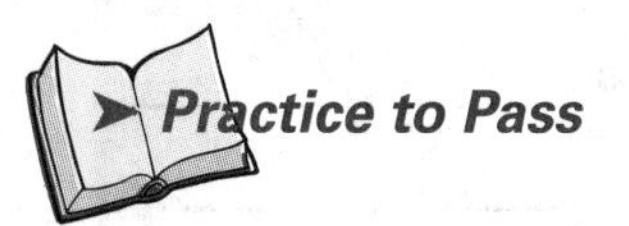

A client's parent informs you that sometimes the parent and child draw up the regular insulin first and other times they draw up the NPH first when combining insulins. They don't understand why the order is important. What would be your response and plan for teaching?

8. **Evaluation:** the client and/or family exhibit specific knowledge of insulin-dependent diabetes mellitus or non-insulin-dependent diabetes mellitus; they demonstrate ability to inject appropriate insulin dosage, perform home glucose monitoring, and identify signs and symptoms of hyperglycemia and hypoglycemia

B. Delayed puberty

1. Description
   a. A condition noted in girls if breast development has not occurred by age 13, pubic hair has not appeared by age 14, or if menarche has not resulted within 4 years after the onset of breast development, usually by the age of 16
   b. In boys, delayed puberty is a concern if there is no testicular enlargement or scrotal changes by 13½ or 14 years of age, pubic hair has not appeared by age 15, or if genital growth is not complete by 4 to 5 years after testicular enlargement
2. Etiology
   a. Delayed puberty can be hereditary; as many family members may have **constitutional delay** (delay of overall growth and puberty)
   b. Delayed puberty may be caused by hypogonadism, where the ovaries and testicles are not secreting their homones—estrogen or testosterone; hypogonadism may be caused by decreased stimulation of the gonads secondary to an abnormality of the pituitary gland or the hypothalamus; the pituitary gland may malfunction as a result of brain tumors, hypothyroidism, anorexia, and other chronic illnesses; there may also be a problem with the testicle itself as exhibited in Klinefelter's syndrome, or with the ovary as in Turner's syndrome; these syndromes are secondary to chromosomal abnormalities and can be evaluated by studying the child's karyotype
      1) Klinefelter's syndrome is manifested by IQ scores below normal range, tall stature, and overly long arms and legs; boys with this disorder have one or more extra X chromosomes, commonly 47 chromosomes with an XXY karyotype; they are usually sterile
      2) Girls who have Turner's syndrome exhibit delayed puberty, short stature, webbed neck, and cubitus valgus (where the forearm deviates laterally); the karyotype demonstrates a female with a missing X chromosome (45XO); these girls are usually infertile
3. Assessment
   a. Assessment of the family growth history is extremely important in the diagnosis of delayed puberty; growth patterns of the parents are of interest to the pediatrician or the pediatric endocrinologist; a complete examination will be done, including measurements of the arm span and (in males) testicular size and penile length; the client may need a bone age, an X-ray of the left hand and wrist that indicates the acceleration of skeletal growth and determines the status of the **epiphyseal growth plate** closure; the beginning of puberty better correlates with the bone age than with the client's chronological age; an MRI or CT scan may be needed to determine a CNS lesion if a brain tumor is suspected
   b. Other tests may include blood levels of FSH (follicle stimulating hormone), LH (leutinizing hormone), and sex hormones; a complete blood count,

thyroid function tests, and a chemistry panel may also be helpful for diagnosis; a **karyotype** (number and types of chromosomes) should be done if Turner's or Klinefelter's syndromes are suspected; the gonadotropin-releasing hormone stimulation test may be used for diagnosis also

c. Many clients with delayed puberty have short stature and may be treated as a child by teachers, coaches, and community members; during the adolescent years, these children and teens may have difficulty in social situations

4. Priority nursing diagnoses: Body image disturbance; Impaired social interaction; Anxiety; Knowledge deficit

5. Planning and implementation

a. Assure children with a constitutional delay and delayed bone age that they usually do not require any treatment as they will eventually begin puberty and go through those stages; medical intervention of low-dose injections of testosterone may be initiated if the adolescent client is over the age of 14

b. If a child has hypogonadism and other conditions have been ruled out, the child may receive hormone therapy to stimulate the development of secondary sexual characteristics; boys receive testosterone enanthate injections, whereas girls take oral ethinyl estradiol with a combination of medroxyprogesterone

c. Provide psychological support to the child especially if he or she has social concerns

6. Medication therapy: boys receive testosterone enanthate injections, girls take oral ethinyl estradiol with a combination of medroxyprogesterone

7. Child and family education

a. Provide information regarding the different stages of puberty and the causes of delayed puberty; gear the discussion to the child's chronological age

b. Instruct the child and family on the administration of hormones if ordered; arrange for home nursing care to provide the injections if needed

8. Evaluation: client and family exhibit knowledge and causes of delayed puberty; adolescent client exhibits evidence of good self-esteem

C. Precocious puberty

1. Description

a. Precocious puberty is a condition that is characterized by the early onset of puberty, usually occurring before age 8 in girls and before age 9 in boys;

b. It is accompanied by the appearance of secondary sexual characteristics and an advanced growth rate and bone maturation; this rapid bone growth will cause early fusion of epiphyseal plates and eventual short stature as an adult

2. Etiology and pathophysiology

a. Most cases of precocious puberty in both boys and girls are idiopathic; some cases are caused by benign hypothalamic tumors, other brain tumors, infection, cranial radiation, and head trauma

b. In normal puberty, the hypothalamus secretes gonadotropin-releasing hormone (GnRH); this hormone stimulates the pituitary gland to secrete leutinizing hormone (LH) and follicle stimulating hormone (FSH) in the male and female

1) In the female, FSH causes the ovary to produce estrogen that causes the development of secondary sexual characteristics

2) In the male, the FSH causes the testes to develop sperm and LH stimulates the production of testosterone causing the development of secondary sexual characteristics

3) During this time, both males and females have accelerated linear and skeletal growth

c. In precocious puberty, the premature secretion of these hormones causes early onset of sexual characteristics; linear and skeletal growth is apparent as these children appear very tall early on, but because of hormone secretion epiphyseal closure occurs, causing short stature as an adult

3. Assessment

a. Signs of precocious puberty in the female include breast development, pubic hair, axillary hair, acne, adult body odor and onset of menstrual periods

b. Signs of precocious puberty in the male include: testicular enlargement, pubic hair, penile enlargement, axillary and chest hair, facial hair, acne, adult body odor, and deepening voice

c. The GnRH stimulation test is helpful in making a diagnosis; synthetic GnRH is given IV, which stimulates the secretion of FSH and LH in the child; blood samples of LH and FSH are obtained every 2 hours to determine levels; if the LH level is higher than the FSH level, puberty has occurred

d. Bone age X-rays will aid in determining epiphyseal maturation and closure; if the bone age is more advanced than chronological age, skeletal growth acceleration is apparent

4. Priority nursing diagnoses: Body image disturbance; Impaired social interaction; Anxiety

5. Planning and implementation

a. Support children with precocious puberty by discussing some of their concerns and issues about body image and sexuality

b. Offer support as the family deals with sensitive issues dealing with premature appearance of secondary sexual characteristics and sexuality

c. Encourage clients to express their feelings about their body changes; role-playing may help with coping with issues of peer teasing

d. Assure children that their friends will go through the same body changes

e. If the synthetic form of luteinizing hormone-releasing factor is used to slow down or arrest the progression of puberty, plan for the monthly or daily injections with the family

6. Medication therapy: a synthetic form of luteinizing hormone-releasing factor (Lupron Depot and other preparations) is used to slow down or stop the progression of puberty and skeletal growth, which will preserve adult height

7. Child and family education

a. Teach the client and parents about the condition and answer all questions or refer to a pediatric endocrinologist

b. If the client is receiving the synthetic luteinizing hormone, instruct the family on the administration of the medication including the technique of either subcutaneous or intramuscular injections; provide the child and family with information about side effects of the drug as per product literature

8. Evaluation

a. The child and family describe the pathophysiology of precocious puberty and their treatment options

b. The child and parents identify the purpose of the medications, describe safe administration, and identify potential side effects

Case Study

A 14-year-old female with Type 1 diabetes mellitus has the flu and stayed home from school today. Her mother reports that she doesn't have much of an appetite and can only get her to eat toast and drink a little tea. You are the nurse in the pediatric office when the mother calls.

❶ What questions will you ask the mother to assure a complete assessment?

❷ What instructions would you give regarding insulin dosage?

❸ What are your priorities when offering dietary instructions?

❹ If urine ketones are present, what advice would you offer the client?

❺ What complications of Type 1 diabetes mellitus would warrant emergency care for this client?

For suggested responses, see page 409.

Posttest

1 **A 12-year-old client was just diagnosed with Type 1 diabetes mellitus. As you are teaching him about his insulin injections, he asks you why he can't take the diabetic pills that his aunt takes. What would be the best response?**

(1) "You will be able to take the pills once you reach adult height."
(2) "You have a different type of diabetes, and the pill won't work."
(3) "We have to test you to see if you can take the diabetic pills."
(4) "You might be able to switch between taking the pills and insulin."

2 **When instructing a client on the best way to check the control of diabetes, you would say:**

(1) "Check your urine glucose three times a week."
(2) "Check the glycosolated hemoglobin every 3 months only."
(3) "Check the blood glucose at least twice a day and the glycosolated hemoglobin every 3 months."
(4) "Don't check anything as long as you feel well."

3 **A mother attends the pediatric clinic with her 10-year-old daughter, who has diabetes. After completing the diabetic teaching, the nurse evaluates the mother's knowledge. Which statement by the mother indicates a satisfactory understanding of diabetes?**

(1) "I worry about my daughter maintaining control since children with diabetes have more complications than adults do."
(2) "My daughter should drink vanilla milkshakes to maintain a high caloric intake."
(3) "Complications from diabetes could include cataracts and kidney stones."
(4) "My child won't need a midafternoon snack since she takes a gym class in the afternoon."

4 **Considering a child's developmental level in diabetic care is essential. The nurse should include which information in teaching the parents of a recently diagnosed toddler with diabetes?**

(1) Allow the toddler to assist with the daily insulin injections.
(2) Prepare meat, vegetables, and potatoes for each dinner. The toddler cannot be allowed any choices in food selection.
(3) Test the toddler's blood glucose every time he goes outside to play.
(4) Allow the toddler to assist with cleaning off his fingers before blood glucose monitoring.

5 **A 2-month-old infant arrives at the pediatric clinic. Upon assessment, the baby exhibits the following characteristics. Which characteristic would be related to the diagnosis of congenital hypothyroidism?**

(1) Open fontanels
(2) Protruding tongue
(3) Tachycardia
(4) Hypertonia

6 **A 10-year-old girl comes to the office of the school nurse after recess. This is the child's first day back in school after hospitalization, where she was diagnosed with diabetes. The child reports she took the dose of insulin as instructed and that it was the same as she took while hospitalized. The nurse notices that she is nervous with hand tremors present. She is pale, sweaty, and complaining of sleepiness. The school nurse would suspect:**

(1) Exercise-induced hypoglycemia.
(2) Hyperglycemia caused by increased intake at lunch.
(3) Ketoacidosis caused by an infection.
(4) The child is avoiding returning to class.

7 **After being diagnosed with Graves' disease, a teenager begins taking propylthiouracil (PTU) for treatment of the disease. What symptom would indicate that the dose may be too high?**

(1) Weight loss
(2) Polyphagia
(3) Lethargy
(4) Difficulty with school work

8 **A 13-year-old male client is being evaluated for delayed puberty. He has had an examination with a pediatric endocrinologist who states that the child has a constitutional delay. What type of follow-up counseling would you offer this client?**

(1) "All of your hormone levels are normal, so no medication is needed at this time. If you want to talk about it, I would be happy to discuss it with you."
(2) "I am worried about your stature. I think you should get another opinion."
(3) "Your father's stature doesn't matter. We just look at your height."
(4) "If you want testosterone shots, I will arrange for them to be given."

9 **A child demonstrates a sudden onset of thyrotoxicosis, exhibited by irritability and restlessness with accompanying hypertension and tachycardia. Besides antithyroid therapy, what other drug therapy does the nurse prepare to administer?**

(1) Antacids
(2) Beta-andrenergic blocker
(3) Muscle relaxants
(4) Cardiac glycoside

10 **Four newborns have had blood drawn for the Guthrie test for phenylketonuria. The nurse would question the results of the baby:**

(1) Whose test is performed at 48 hours of age.
(2) Who was breast-fed for the 24 hours before the test.
(3) Fed glucose water followed by formula for 30 hours.
(4) Tested immediately after birth.

See page 212 for Answers and Rationales.

Answers and Rationales

Pretest

1 **Answer: 2** ***Rationale:*** Hypertrophy or enlargement of the thyroid gland is referred to as a goiter.
Cognitive Level: Application
Nursing Process: Implementation; ***Test Plan:*** PHYS

2 **Answer: 2** ***Rationale:*** Tests done 24 to 48 hours after delivery may be interpreted as high because of the rise in TSH that occurs immediately after birth.
Cognitive Level: Analysis
Nursing Process: Implementation; ***Test Plan:*** HPM

3 **Answer: 3** ***Rationale:*** Sore throat and enlarged cervical nodes are common side effects of the medication. A dosage reduction or withdrawal of the drug should be considered.
Cognitive Level: Analysis
Nursing Process: Implementation; ***Test Plan:*** PHYS

4 **Answer: 2** ***Rationale:*** If a child exhibits signs of hypoglycemia, a source of sugar such as orange juice can elevate glucose levels and prevent further signs of hypoglycemia. A 10-year-old must remember to only take one serving and wait ten minutes for symptoms to be alleviated.
Cognitive Level: Analysis
Nursing Process: Implementation; ***Test Plan:*** PHYS

5 **Answer: 4** ***Rationale:*** The peak action of NPH or Lente Insulin is 6 to 12 hours after administration subcutaneously. During peak times, the client may need a snack to offset potential hypoglycemia.
Cognitive Level: Analysis
Nursing Process: Planning; ***Test Plan:*** PHYS

6 **Answer: 3** ***Rationale:*** Since hypothyroidism is a lifelong condition, the levothyroxine will need to be taken indefinitely. It is important that the infant takes the medication in a small amount of food or liquid and not placed in the bottle since he/she may not receive the full dose if the bottle is not consumed.
Cognitive Level: Application
Nursing Process: Implementation; ***Test Plan:*** PHYS

7 **Answer: 1** ***Rationale:*** In each pregnancy, there is a 25 percent chance of the child having the disease, a 50 percent chance that the child will be a carrier of the gene, and a 25 percent chance that the child will be unaffected. PKU affects both sexes equally.
Cognitive Level: Application
Nursing Process: Analysis; ***Test Plan:*** HPM

8 **Answer: 3** ***Rationale:*** Decreased levels of tyrosine cause a deficiency of the pigment melanin, causing most children with PKU to have blond hair, blue eyes, and fair skin that is prone to eczema.
Cognitive Level: Application
Nursing Process: Implementation; ***Test Plan:*** PHYS

9 **Answer: 3** ***Rationale:*** Foods with low phenylalanine levels include vegetables, fruits, juices, and some cereals and breads. The amount of protein in the diet is restricted based on phenylalanine blood levels.
Cognitive Level: Application
Nursing Process: Evaluation; ***Test Plan:*** PHYS

10 **Answer: 1** ***Rationale:*** Keeping the levels of phenylalanine at a low level in children with PKU and daily administration of levothyroxine in children with congenital hypothyroidism will decrease the

incidence of mental retardation by allowing normal brain growth.
Cognitive Level: Analysis
Nursing Process: Analysis; *Test Plan:* PHYS

Posttest

1 **Answer: 2** ***Rationale:*** Children with Type 1 diabetes must take insulin because they have a total absence of secretion of insulin from their pancreas. Clients with Type 2 diabetes mellitus may produce some insulin so they can take the oral hypoglycemics.
Cognitive Level: Application
Nursing Process: Implementation; *Test Plan:* PHYS

2 **Answer: 3** ***Rationale:*** Checking the blood glucose at least twice a day prevents sustained levels of either high or low glucose readings. The glycosolated hemoglobin measures long term control and is a very important value.
Cognitive Level: Analysis
Nursing Process: Implementation; *Test Plan:* PHYS

3 **Answer: 1** ***Rationale:*** Long-term complications of Type 1 diabetes may include retinopathy, heart disease, renal failure, and peripheral vascular disease. These complications can affect children and adults. The longer the child lives with diabetes, the greater the liklihood of complications. Exercise increases the utilization of glucose, thus an afternoon snack would be very important. Milkshakes contain concentrated carbohydrates that should be avoided.
Cognitive Level: Analysis
Nursing Process: Evaluation; *Test Plan:* PHYS

4 **Answer: 4** ***Rationale:*** The toddler needs to feel some control. Cleaning off his fingers with alcohol, under supervision, will allow some control. Another possibility to promote the toddler's sense of control would be to allow the toddler to choose food selections from options offered.
Cognitive Level: Application
Nursing Process: Planning; *Test Plan:* HPM

5 **Answer: 2** ***Rationale:*** Most babies with congenital hypothyroidism exhibit bradycardia, protruding tongue, and hypotonia. Open fontanels are normal for a 2-month-old infant.
Cognitive Level: Analysis
Nursing Process: Assessment; *Test Plan:* PHYS

6 **Answer: 1** ***Rationale:*** Exercise makes the body more sensitive to insulin, thus metabolizing the glucose faster. While hospitalized, the child was less active. Now that the child has returned to normal activity, the insulin dose is too high or more carbohydrate is required in the diet.
Cognitive Level: Analysis
Nursing Process: Analysis; *Test Plan:* PHYS

7 **Answer: 3** ***Rationale:*** Lethargy may indicate an overdose of the drug, causing the child to exhibit signs of hypothyroidism. The other signs indicate hyperthyroidism.
Cognitive Level: Analysis
Nursing Process: Analysis; *Test Plan:* PHYS

8 **Answer: 1** ***Rationale:*** An adolescent client with delayed puberty may need to talk about issues of low self-esteem. If he has a constitutional delay, puberty will usually follow with time. Hormone therapy is not given until after the age of 14.
Cognitive Level: Application
Nursing Process: Implementation; *Test Plan:* PHYS

9 **Answer: 2** ***Rationale:*** A beta-adrenergic blocking agent provides relief from adrenergic hyperresponsiveness. It is usually needed for 2 to 3 weeks along with antithyroid hormone therapy.
Cognitive Level: Application
Nursing Process: Implementation; *Test Plan:* PHYS

10 **Answer: 4** ***Rationale:*** The screening is done only after an adequate amount of protein has been ingested. Breast milk and formula meet the requirements. The testing is usually done at 48 hours of age.
Cognitive Level: Analysis
Nursing Process: Assessment; *Test Plan:* HPM

References

Ball, J. & Bindler, R. (1999). *Pediatric nursing: Caring for children* (2nd ed.). Stamford, CT: Appleton & Lange, pp. 47, 864–903.

Borgersen, M. (1997). The child with diabetes mellitus. In Ashwill, J. & Droske, S. (Eds.), *Nursing care of children: Principles and practice.* Philadelphia: W. B. Saunders, pp. 1182–1217.

Bottomley, S. (2001). The child with endocrine dysfunction. In Wong, D., Hockenberry-Eaton, M., Wilson, D., Winkelstein, M., & Schwartz, P. (Eds.), *Wong's essentials of pediatric nursing* (6th ed.). St. Louis: Mosby, Inc., pp. 1116–1147.

DiFazio, D. (1998). Health challenge: Alterations in endocrine status. In Bowden, V., Dickey, S., & Greenberg, C.

(Eds.), *Children and their families: The continuum of care.* Philadelphia: W. B. Saunders, pp. 1804–1876.

Estey, D. & Koszarek, K. (1997). Phenylketonuria. In Ashwill, J. & Droske, S. (Eds.), *Nursing care of children: Principles and practice.* Philadelphia: W. B. Saunders, pp. 565–567.

Howie-Stites, J. (1997). The child with endocrine alterations. In Ashwill, J. & Droske, S. (Eds.), *Nursing care of children: Principles and practice.* Philadelphia: W. B. Saunders, pp. 1170–1193.

Kline, N. (1999). The child with endocrine dysfunction. In Wong, D., Hockenberry-Eaton, M., Wilson, D., Winkelstein, M., Ahmann, E., & DiVito-Thomas, P. (Eds.), *Whaley & Wong's nursing care of infants and children* (6th ed.). St. Louis: Mosby, Inc., pp. 1831–1884.

Spratto, G. & Woods, A. (2001). *PDR: Nurse's drug handbook* (2001 ed.). Montvale, NJ: Delmar Publishers and Medical Economics Co., Inc.

Travis, L. (1999). *An instructional aid on insulin-dependent diabetes mellitus* (11th ed.). Austin, TX: Designer's Ink.

Wilson, D. (1999). Health problems of the newborn. In Wong, D., Hockenberry-Eaton, M., Wilson, D., Winkelstein, M., Ahmann, E. & DiVito-Thomas, P. (Eds.), *Whaley and Wong's nursing care of infants and children* (6th ed.). St. Louis: Mosby, Inc., pp. 382–387.

Wilson, D. (2001). Health problems of newborns. In Wong, D., Hockenberry-Eaton, M., Wilson, D., Winkelstein, M., & Schwartz, P. (Eds.), *Wong's essentials of pediatric nursing* (6th ed.). St. Louis: Mosby, Inc., pp. 318–321.

CHAPTER 9

Musculoskeletal Health Problems

Kathleen Peterson-Sweeney, MS, RN, CPNP

CHAPTER OUTLINE

OBJECTIVES

- Identify data essential to the assessment of alterations in health of the musculoskeletal system in a child.
- Discuss the clinical manifestations and pathophysiology of alterations in health of the musculoskeletal system of a child.
- Discuss therapeutic management of a child with alterations in health of the musculoskeletal system.
- Describe nursing management of a child with alterations in health of the musculoskeletal system.

[Media Link]

Use the CD-ROM enclosed with this text, or log onto the address given to access the free, interactive Companion Website created for this series. The CD-ROM and Companion Website accompanying this book offer additional practice opportunities and information—NCLEX Review, Case Studies, Glossary, In Depth with NCLEX, and more.

www.prenhall.com/hogan

Review at a Glance

cartilage *connective tissue that composes most of the skeleton of an embryo and changes to bone through the process of ossification*

clubfoot *congenital malposition of the foot involving bone and soft tissue*

developmental dysplasia of the hip (DDH) *congenital condition where there is improper formation and function of the hip socket*

diaphysis *the long central shaft in long bones that constitutes the major portion of bone*

epiphysis *the rounded end portion of long bones that consists of layers of cartilage, subcondral bone, and sponge-like cancellous bone*

epiphyseal plate *situated between the diaphysis and epiphysis and plays the major role in the longitudinal growth in children*

fracture *discontinuity in the bone caused by force to the bone*

Legg-Calve-Perthes disease *condition in which there is avascular necrosis of the femoral epiphysis in school-age children*

metaphysis *columns of spongy tissue that unite the diaphysis with the epiphyseal plate*

muscular dystrophy *inherited condition where there is progressive weakness and wasting of symmetrical groups of skeletal muscle, with increasing disability and deformity*

ossification *the process of gradual conversion of cartilage to bony structures, which begins in the embryo and continues until 18 to 21 years of age*

osteoblasts *immature bone cells that replace cartilage cells as bones grow*

osteogenesis imperfecta (OI) *inherited disorder characterized by connective tissue and bone defects leading to bones that are fractured by the slightest trauma*

osteomyelitis *infection of the bone, which may be caused by any microorganism, but usually caused by bacteria*

periosteum *thin, tough membrane covering the central shafts of all bones, and that contains blood vessels that nourish the bone*

pseudohypertrophy *enlargement of the muscles as a result of infiltration by fatty tissue that occurs in Duchenne's muscular dystrophy*

scoliosis *lateral curvature of the spine, which may be idiopathic or may be a result of a neuromuscular disease*

slipped capitol femoral epiphysis *a condition where the proximal femoral head displaces posteriorly and inferiorly in relation to the neck of the femur during the rapid adolescent growth spurt*

traction *involves pulling on a body part in one direction against a counter-pull exerted in the opposite direction; used to reduce dislocations and immobilize fractures*

Pretest

1 A 6-year-old child has a cast applied for a fractured radius. The nurse completes an orthopedic assessment on this child. Which of the following symptoms requires immediate attention and should be reported to the physician?

(1) Capillary refill of 4 seconds in the affected hand
(2) Edema in the affected fingers that improves with elevation
(3) Child describing feeling of the affected hand being "asleep"
(4) Skin surrounding the cast is warm

2 Which of the following nursing care measures takes highest priority in caring for a child in skeletal traction?

(1) Assessing bowel sounds every shift
(2) Assessing temperature every 4 hours
(3) Providing adequate nutrition
(4) Providing age-appropriate activities

3 A nurse performs triage in a pediatric orthopedic clinic. Which of the following should the nurse recognize as a symptom of slipped capitol femoral epiphysis?

(1) Pain in the hip of a preadolescent child
(2) Acute onset of knee pain
(3) Presence of a limp in a school aged child
(4) Painful external rotation of the affected leg

4 Which of the following statements made by the parent of a child being discharged with osteomyelitis requires further teaching by the nurse?

(1) "I can stop the antibiotics when I see that my child is feeling better."
(2) "We will make sure that our child has plenty of calcium and protein."
(3) "I will look at the intravenous site for signs of infection a couple of times a day."
(4) "My child won't take physical education at school until allowed by the doctor."

5 **A 5-month-old infant is being assessed for developmental dysplasia of the hip. The nurse will look for a positive:**

(1) Ortolani sign.
(2) Barlow sign.
(3) Allis sign.
(4) Trendelenburg sign.

6 **A newborn is being admitted to the newborn nursery. The nurse would assess the infant for congenital defects. In addition to the abnormal position of the foot, the nurse would note which of the following if clubfoot is present?**

(1) Affected foot is larger and longer.
(2) Affected limb is longer.
(3) There is calf muscle atrophy of the affected limb.
(4) Affected foot is cooler.

7 **A child is admitted with osteogenesis imperfecta (OI). In reviewing laboratory findings, the nurse would expect to find abnormal levels of:**

(1) Calcium.
(2) Phosphorus.
(3) Precollagen type I.
(4) Vitamin D.

8 **Which of the following statements made by a parent of a child with OI needs clarification by the nurse?**

(1) "My child may be able to participate in sports."
(2) "There are no medications available to help this disease process."
(3) "Surgery may be needed to place rods in the bone for stability."
(4) "My child will need to be home schooled to protect him from injury."

9 **Which of the following interventions is inappropriate to incorporate into the plan of care for a child with Duchenne muscular dystrophy hospitalized for a respiratory infection?**

(1) Physical therapy
(2) Vigorous antibiotic therapy
(3) Passive range of motion exercises
(4) Strict bedrest

10 **A 14-year-old adolescent has just been fitted for a Milwaukee brace. Which of the following should the nurse include in teaching about this brace?**

(1) The brace should be worn only when the adolescent is sleeping or in the recumbent position.
(2) The brace should be worn next to the skin.
(3) Exercises to increase pelvic tilt should be done several times per day while in the brace.
(4) The adolescent should experience no pain as a result of wearing this brace.

See pages 239–240 for Answers and Rationales.

I. Overview of the Anatomy and Physiology of the Musculoskeletal System

A. ***Ossification*** is the conversion of **cartilage** (embryonic connective tissue) to bony structures; begins in the embryo and continues until the child is 18 to 21 years old, when skeletal maturation is complete; **osteoblasts** are immature bone cells that replace cartilage cells as bones grow

1. Children's bones are less dense and more porous than adult bones, and therefore they are not as strong and fracture more easily

2. A **fracture** or break in the contour of the bone can result from minor falls or twists

3. Ossification progresses outwardly from the **diaphysis,** which is the hard shaft-like portion that constitutes the major portion of the bone

B. ***Epiphysis:*** located at the end of long bones, consists of layers of cartilage, subchondral bone, and sponge-like cancellous bone

C. ***Epiphyseal plate:*** plays a major role in longitudinal bone growth

1. Situated between the diaphysis and epiphysis

2. Columns of spongy tissue, or **metaphysis,** unite the diaphysis with the epiphyseal plate

3. This is the weakest point of long bones, thus a frequent site of damage

D. ***Periosteum:*** a thin, tough membrane that covers all bones and contains blood vessels that nourish the bone

E. **Tendons and ligaments:** stronger than bone until puberty; as a child grows, muscles increase in length and circumference

NCLEX!

F. **Calcium intake:** during childhood and adolescence it is essential to provide adequate bone density and prevent osteoporosis later in life

II. Congenital Musculoskeletal Health Problems

A. Clubfoot

1. Description

a. In **clubfoot** the foot is twisted and fixed in an abnormal position; may be one or a combination of four deformities

1) Plantar flexion: foot is lower than the heel

2) Dorsiflexion: heel is lower than the foot

3) Varus deviation: foot turns in

4) Valgus deviation: foot turns out

b. Involves bone deformity and malposition with soft tissue contracture

c. One to two of every 1,000 live-born children have clubfoot, with males affected twice as often as females

d. May be unilateral or bilateral

2. Etiology and pathophysiology

a. Exact cause is unknown

b. Abnormal intrauterine position may cause the deformity

c. Neuromuscular or vascular problems may cause deformity

d. Strong familial tendency, with 1 in 10 chance that a parent with clubfoot will have an affected offspring

3. Assessment

a. Foot is twisted in a fixed abnormal position, which is easily recognized at birth; may be recognized on prenatal ultrasound

b. Affected foot is usually smaller and shorter, with an empty heel pad and transverse plantar crease

   c. When the defect is unilateral, the affected limb is usually shorter with possible calf atrophy

4. Priority nursing diagnoses

   a. Impaired physical mobility related to cast wear

   b. Altered parenting related to emotional reaction following the birth of an infant with a physical defect

   c. Risk for impaired skin integrity related to cast wear

   d. Knowledge deficit: deformity, treatment and home care

5. Planning and implementation

   a. Correction is achieved best if it is begun in the newborn period as the small bones in the foot begin to ossify shortly after birth

   b. Manipulation and serial casting is begun immediately and continued for 8 to 12 weeks, with the foot placed in a cast in an overcorrected position; casts are changed every 1 to 2 weeks because of rapid growth

   c. Parents then need to perform passive range of motion (ROM) exercises of the foot and ankle several times a day for several months once cast is off

   d. Infant may need to sleep in Denis Browne splints (shoes attached to a metal bar to maintain position) or wear corrective shoes for up to 1 year

   e. Surgery is performed when not able to achieve full correction with casting; most children have surgery between 4 to 12 months of age, which involves realigning the bones in the foot, held by steel pins, then the foot is casted for 6 to 12 weeks

   f. Nursing care for the child post-casting and post-surgical repair of clubfoot includes:

      1) Neurovascular checks, at least every 2 hours

      2) Observe for any swelling around cast edges

      3) Elevate the ankle and foot on pillows

      4) Monitor drainage in the cast

      5) Pain management

      6) Appropriate distraction

6. Child and family education

   a. Change diapers frequently to prevent soiled diapers from touching the cast and causing the cast to be soiled

   b. Sponge-bathe infant to keep the cast dry

   c. Teach parents that crying episodes must be evaluated carefully, as they may be caused by the tingling sensation of circulatory compression

   d. Reinforce the need for passive ROM exercises several times a day for several months

e. Reinforce use of Denis Browne splints or corrective shoes to maintain correction

f. Discuss options for clothing that accommodates casts

7. Child and family education (see Box 9-1)

Box 9-1

Child and Family Education for a Child in a Brace or a Cast

Perform neurovascular checks

- Observe the fingers or toes for swelling, discoloration, and temperature.
- Check movement and sensation.
- Notify health care professional with any changes in neurovascular status.
- Teach the parents how to blanch the nail bed and watch for capillary refill.

Observe for infection

- Monitor for temperature increase.
- Assess for drainage through the cast/brace.
- Assess for odors coming from beneath the cast/brace.
- Notify healthcare professional for any of the above.

Assess and maintain skin around cast or brace edges

- Perform frequent assessment of the skin around the cast or brace edge for irritation, rubbing, or blistering.
- Keep edges clean and dry, avoiding the use of lotions, powders, or oils near the cast or brace.
- Petal the cast edges as needed.
- Do not allow the child to put anything down the cast.
- If the child is incontinent, protect the cast edges with waterproof tape and plastic.
- Keep the cast or brace clean and dry.

Activity

- Follow the health professional's orders for activity level, restriction of activity.
- Avoid allowing the affected extremity to hang in a dependent position for more than 30 minutes.
- Encourage frequent rest for the first few days following brace or cast application, keeping the injured extremity elevated while resting.
- Keep a clear path for ambulation, removing toys, hazardous floor rugs, pets, or other items over which the child might stumble.
- If in a body cast or brace, assist the child to be mobile with the use of a wagon, cart, or large skateboard.

Comfort

- Assess for discomfort and medicate according to health professional's orders.
- Contact the healthcare provider if pain is not relieved by any comfort measures.

Follow-up

- Encourage compliance with follow-up.
- Take the child to the healthcare professional if the cast becomes too loose, or becomes soft or cracked.

8. Evaluation: the infant has corrected position of affected foot; parents demonstrate knowledge of care of a child with clubfoot

B. *Developmental dysplasia of hip (DDH)* or congenital hip dysplasia

1. Description

a. Refers to a variety of conditions in which the femoral head and acetabulum are improperly aligned; DDH has been referred to as congenital hip dysplasia in the past

b. Occurs in 1 to 2 per 1,000 births, and condition affects females 4 to 6 times more often than males

c. Unilateral in 80 percent of affected children

2. Etiology and pathophysiology

a. The cause is unknown; though certain factors are known to increase the risk of DDH

b. Family history increases the risk tenfold

c. Prenatal conditions may affect the development of DDH

1) Frank breech position

2) Maternal hormones of relaxin and estrogen may cause laxity of the hip joint and capsule, leading to joint instability

3) Twinning

4) Large infant size

d. Sociocultural methods of childrearing, such as the way infants are carried, may promote or decrease the extent of involvement; infants held with hips abducted have decreased involvement

3. Assessment

a. The diagnosis should be made in the newborn period; treatment that is initiated before 2 months of age achieves the highest rate of success

b. During the newborn and infant period, assessment findings of DDH include:

1) Shortening of the affected limb

2) Allis sign: child in supine position, thighs flexed to a 90-degree angle toward the abdomen, unequal knee height

3) Uneven number and placement of skin folds on posterior thighs

4) Restricted abduction of the hips after 6 to 10 weeks of age

5) Wide perineum in bilateral dislocation

6) Positive Ortolani or Barlow signs up to 2 to 3 months of age; to assess for this, lie the infant supine and flex the knees and hips to 90 degrees; place your middle fingers over the greater trochanter and your thumb in the internal side of the thigh over the lesser trochanter; abduct the hips while applying pressure over the greater trochanter and listen for a clicking sound, which would indicate a positive Ortolani's sign; no

sound will be heard with a normal hip; with your fingers in the same position, holding the knees and hips at 90 degrees, apply a backward pressure, and adduct the hips; positive Barlow's sign is present if you are able to feel the hips dislocate; the hips should not be able to be dislocated

c. Assessment findings in an older child include:

1) Affected leg shorter than the other

2) Telescoping or piston mobility of affected leg

NCLEX!

3) History of delay in walking

4) Limp and toe walking

5) Trendelenberg's sign: when the child bears weight on the affected side, the pelvis tilts downward on the normal side instead of upward as it would with normal stability

6) Waddling gait with bilateral dislocation

7) Lordosis with bilateral dislocation

4. Priority nursing diagnoses

a. Knowledge deficit

b. Impaired physical mobility related to restriction of braces and casts

c. Risk for impaired skin integrity related to pressure from casts and braces

d. Risk for altered tissue perfusion (peripheral) related to pressure from casts and braces

e. Risk for altered growth and development related to limited mobility and potential decreased exposure to stimulation

5. Planning and implementation

a. Correction involves positioning the hip into a flexed, abducted (externally rotated) position to press the femur head against the acetabulum and deepen its contour

NCLEX!

b. For infants less than 3 months, the most common treatment is use of a Pavlik harness, an adjustable chest halter that abducts the legs; soft plastic stirrups hold the hips flexed, abducted and externally rotated; may or may not be removed for bathing; usually worn for 3 to 6 months (see Figure 9-1)

c. For infants older than 3 months of age, skin traction followed by spica cast application may be required

d. Correction in the child older than 18 months requires traction, operative reduction, and rehabilitation

6. Child and family education

a. Pavlik harness: proper application, sponge bath, assess skin under straps daily for irritation or redness; t-shirt and knee socks should be worn under the brace to prevent skin irritation; diaper should be placed under the straps and changed without taking the harness off

Figure 9-1

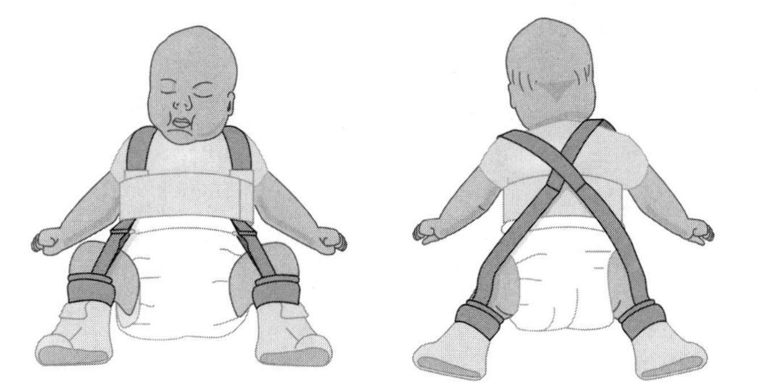

Pavlik harness.
Source: Ball, J. & Bindler, R. (1999). *Pediatric nursing: Caring for children* (2nd ed.). Stamford, CT: Appleton & Lange, p. 827.

b. For all abduction devices: modification of car seat, modification of positioning for nursing and eating

c. Parents need to ensure the child has adequate stimulation with toys and activities at appropriate eye level; encourage activities that stimulate upper extremities

d. Children will catch up with developmental milestones once abduction splint is off

e. Refer back to Box 9-1 for further information

7. Evaluation: the child has normal growth and development; the parent demonstrates care of a child with DDH

C. ***Osteogenesis imperfecta (OI)***

1. Description

a. Characterized by the formation of pathologic fractures resulting from connective tissue and bone defects

b. Occurs in several forms with variable degree of severity

c. Bones are so fragile that fractures result from trauma, but also from simple walking or pressure of birth

d. Occurs in 1 in 30,000 live births and affects boys and girls equally

NCLEX!

e. A child with this diagnosis should not be confused with the child with fractures because of abuse

2. Etiology and pathophysiology

a. Children with OI have normal calcium and phosphorus levels, and abnormal precollagen type I, which prevents the formation of collagen, the major component of connective tissue

b. Bone of children with OI consists of large areas of osseous tissue and increased numbers of osteoblasts

c. Genetically transmitted, generally in an autosomal dominant inheritance pattern, although some types are transmitted in a recessive pattern

3. Assessment

a. Major clinical manifestations include multiple and frequent fractures, some of which may be present at birth

b. As child grows older, multiple breaks tend to cause limb and spinal column deformities, interfering with alignment or growth

c. Other clinical manifestations include blue sclera; thin, soft skin with easy bruising; increased joint flexibility; weak muscles; short stature; conductive hearing loss often by adolescence or young adulthood

d. May have dentinogenesis imperfecta: hypoplastic teeth with opalescent blue or brown discoloration

4. Priority nursing diagnoses

a. Risk for injury related to disease process

b. Risk for altered growth and development

c. Knowledge deficit: disease process and care of child

5. Planning and implementation

a. Keep floors dry; remove objects that could cause falls

b. Handle children gently: avoid lifting by a single arm or leg; use a blanket for extra support when lifting and moving

c. Never hold by ankles when being diapered, but should gently be lifted by slipping a hand under the buttocks

d. Lightweight leg braces, splints, casting, and physical therapy may be helpful

e. Intermedullary rods may be effective in strengthening bones

6. Medication therapy

a. Calcitonin, which aids bone healing, may be used

b. Biphosphonates may be prescribed to increase bone mass

c. Growth hormone may be given to stimulate growth

7. Child and family education

a. Encourage a lifestyle that encourages growth and development, yet minimizes the risk of trauma

b. Teach how to support when bathing, dressing, and moving

c. Encourage exercise, such as swimming, to improve muscle tone and prevent obesity

d. Encourage realistic occupational planning

e. Suggest genetic counseling

f. Educational materials and information can be obtained from the Osteogenesis Imperfecta Foundation (www.oif.org)

8. Evaluation: child has adequate growth and development with minimal fractures

III. Acquired Musculoskeletal Health Problems

A. *Legg-Calve-Perthes disease*

1. Description

a. A self-limiting disorder in which there is aseptic necrosis of the femoral head

b. The disease affects children between the ages of 2 and 12 years, but is most common in those 5 to 7 years of age

c. Occurs in about 1 in 12,000 children

d. Male children are affected 4 to 5 times more often than female children; Caucasian children are affected 10 times more often than African-American children

e. The disease is bilateral in 10 to 15 percent of the cases

2. Etiology and pathophysiology

a. Cause is unknown, though research has shown a familial predisposition with the incidence 20 percent higher in families with a history of this disease; in one-quarter of the cases, the disease is preceded by a mild traumatic injury

b. There is a disturbance of circulation to the femoral capitol epiphysis that produces an ischemic aseptic necrosis of the femoral head

c. Middle childhood is the time when the blood supply to the femoral head is most tenuous, being supplied almost entirely by lateral retinacular vessels; these vessels can become obstructed by trauma, inflammation, coagulation defects, among other causes

d. Affected children may have delayed skeletal maturation and abnormal thyroid levels

e. The pathological events take place in four stages

1) Stage I: avascular stage; aseptic necrosis of the femoral capitol epiphysis with degenerative changes producing flattening of the femoral head

2) Stage II: fragmentation or revascularization stage; old bone absorption and revascularization

3) Stage III: reparative stage; new bone formation

4) Stage IV: regeneration stage; gradual reformation of the femoral head

3. Assessment

a. Mild pain in the hip or anterior thigh and limp that are aggravated by increased activity and relieved by rest

b. Stiffness in the morning or after rest

c. As the disease progresses there is limited range of motion, weakness, muscle wasting, possible shortening of the affected limb, and positive Trendelenburg sign

4. Priority nursing diagnoses

a. Impaired physical mobility related to brace or cast

b. Knowledge deficit: disease process, potential complication

c. Pain related to disease process

d. Diversional activity deficit related to brace or cast

5. Planning and implementation

    a. Prepare the child for an x-ray, as this is the usual diagnostic test; there may be no radiological findings early in the disease, but bone scans and MRIs are helpful to diagnose early disease

NCLEX!

    b. Initial treatment includes rest to reduce inflammation and restore motion

    c. The goal is to keep the head of the femur in contact with the acetabulum, which serves as a mold of spherical shape of the head of the femur

    d. Treatment may be conservative, with rest and avoiding weight bearing on lower extremities, traction and containment with abduction braces, leg casts or leather harness slings

    e. Conservative therapy may be needed for 2 to 4 years

    f. Surgical correction may be done, which returns the child to normal activities in 3 to 4 months

    g. Assist in the selection of suitable activities for a child unable to maintain usual level of physical activity

    h. Ensure compliance with conservative devices

NCLEX!

    i. If surgical treatment is carried out, postoperative care includes frequent neurovascular checks, pain management, and activity based on the surgeon's orders

    j. Assist the family with appropriate activities for the child during treatment

6. Child and family education

    a. Teach the purpose, function, application, and care of the corrective device

    b. Stress the importance of compliance to achieve the desired outcome

    c. Stress the importance of continuing school activities

    d. Promote normal growth and development with appropriate diversional activities

7. Evaluation: the child has normal reformation of the femoral head; the family is able to state the appropriate care for this child

B. *Slipped capitol femoral epiphysis*

1. Description

    a. A condition in which the upper femoral epiphysis gradually slips from its functional position

    b. Incidence is greatest during the rapid growth spurt during adolescence; 13 to 16 years of age for males, and 11 to 14 years of age for females

    c. It is twice as frequent in African-Americans as other races, and twice as frequent in males

2. Etiology and pathophysiology

    a. The etiology is unknown and thought to be multifactorial

b. It is more common in obese or rapidly growing children, suggesting that growth hormone or trauma from excessive weight may have an influence on the etiology

c. There may be a genetic predisposition to the development of this disorder

d. Slippage of the femoral head occurs at the proximal epiphyseal plate, and the femur displaces from the epiphysis; this is usually a gradual process, but may result from trauma

3. Assessment

NCLEX!

a. Onset of symptoms may be gradual, with persistent hip pain that is aching or mild, and can be referred to the thigh and/or knee, along with limp and decreased range of motion and internal rotation of the hip; the child may hold the leg in an externally rotated position to relieve stress and pain in the hip joint

NCLEX!

b. The child with an acute slip presents with sudden, severe pain and cannot bear weight

c. Prepare the client for an x-ray, which will confirm diagnosis

4. Priority nursing diagnoses

a. Pain related to disease process

b. Impaired physical mobility related to non-weight-bearing treatment

c. Altered tissue perfusion (peripheral) related to treatment

d. Altered growth and development related to mobility restrictions of treatment

e. Knowledge deficit: disease process and treatment

5. Planning and implementation

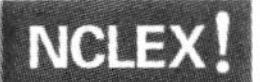

a. As soon as the diagnosis is made, the client should be placed on strict bedrest until surgery; the adolescent may use crutches, as long as the affected leg is non-weight-bearing, but should not sit in a wheelchair, as this may increase the slippage

b. Reinforce initial bedrest, as adolescents often do not see the value of this measure

c. Provide appropriate diversional activities

d. Prepare for surgery with pinning or external fixation to stabilize the femur head

e. Provide postoperative care, including frequent neurovascular checks and pain management

f. Provide adequate nutrition for healing

6. Child and family education

a. Reinforce ambulation and weight-bearing as ordered by the surgeon

b. Contact sports are usually restricted until growth is complete

c. Reinforce compliance with followup visits until epiphyseal plates are closed

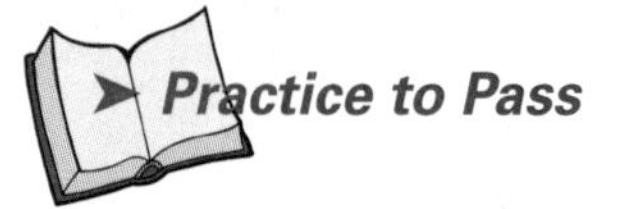

Two male clients have been admitted to the pediatric unit, one with slipped capitol femoral epiphysis, and a second with Legg-Calve-Perthes disease. How will the nursing care be different for these two clients?

7. Evaluation: the adolescent is cooperative with activity restrictions; the adolescent remains free of further injury to the hip

C. ***Scoliosis***

1. Description
   - **a.** Lateral curvature of the spine; may be functional, which occurs as a compensatory mechanism in children who have unequal leg lengths, or poor posture; structural scoliosis is a permanent curvature of the spine accompanied by damage to the vertebrae
   - **b.** Structural scoliosis occurs most often during the rapid growth spurt in adolescence, 11 to 14 years for females, 13 to 16 years for males
   - **c.** The female-to-male ratio is 5:1 for curves greater than 21 degrees
2. Etiology and pathophysiology
   - **a.** 70 percent of structural scoliosis is idiopathic
   - **b.** There is a familial predisposition for structural scoliosis
   - **c.** Scoliosis is common in diseases where there is unequal muscle balance, such as cerebral palsy, muscular dystrophy, and myelomeningocele
3. Assessment
   - **a.** A painless and insidious onset is typical
   - NCLEX! **b.** Parent may first notice that skirts hang unevenly, or that bra straps are adjusted unevenly
   - NCLEX! **c.** On examination there is unequal shoulder heights, waist angles, scapula prominences, rib prominences, and chest asymmetry
   - **d.** Screening by the school nurse begins in the fifth grade as mandated by law in many states
   - **e.** Scoliometer is used to document clinical deformity found on screening
4. Priority nursing diagnoses
   - **a.** Body image disturbance related to bracing
   - **b.** Risk for injury related to brace
   - **c.** Pain related to surgical experience (spinal fusion)
   - **d.** Ineffective breathing pattern related to postoperative discomfort
   - **e.** Impaired physical mobility related to brace wear
   - **f.** Knowledge deficit: diagnosis and treatment
   - **g.** Risk for noncompliance with treatment regimen
5. Planning and implementation
   - **a.** Prepare the adolescent for x-ray, as this will identify the extent of the curvature and give baseline information for followup

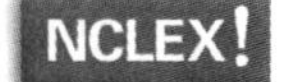

   - **b.** If the spinal curve is less than 15 to 20 degrees, the teen is monitored every 3 to 6 months for change; exercises to improve posture and muscle tone and increase flexibility of the spine are encouraged

c. If the curve is greater than 24 degrees, treatment is rendered by an orthopedic surgeon; if less than 40 degrees, conservative, nonsurgical treatment is warranted, with bracing, such as a Milwaukee brace; this brace, and others like it, are made of leather and plastic; it is worn until the teen's spinal growth stops; see Child and family education

d. Electrical stimulation may be used for mild to moderate curvatures, to cause the muscles to contract at regular and frequent intervals, possibly helping to straighten the spine

e. If the curvature continues to progress or is greater than 40 degrees, surgery is warranted for spinal instrumentation; instruments such as rods, screws, and wires are placed next to the curvature; the spine is then fused in the correct position; bone from the iliac crests may be used to strengthen the fusion

1) See Child and family education section for preoperative teaching

NCLEX!

2) Postoperative care includes range-of-motion (ROM) exercises, log rolling every 2 hours, encouraging coughing and deep-breathing and use of spirometry, NPO, nasogastric tube, strict intake and output, frequent VS and neurological checks, monitoring hematocrit, blood transfusions, pain management, antibiotic administration, antiembolism stockings, and gradual resumption of activity as ordered

f. Halo traction may be used for non-surgical treatment of moderate curves, or postoperatively in severe curves to provide stability for the spine

6. Child and family education

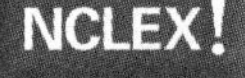

a. Teaching about the use of a Milwaukee or other brace

1) Brace is worn for 23 hours a day

2) Brace is off to shower, bathe, and swim

3) T-shirt should be worn under the brace next to the skin (to protect the skin)

4) Exercises (such as pelvic tilt and lateral strengthening) are done several times a day while in the brace to correct thoracic lordosis

5) Consistent use of brace will provide maximum benefit

6) Slight muscle aches may be noticed when first wearing the brace

7) Encourage teens to be as active as possible while in the brace

b. Preoperative teaching

1) Deep-breathing, coughing, turning every 2 hours, use of spirometry

2) Pain medication

3) Use of nasogastric tube and NPO status

4) Range of motion exercises, activity

5) Possible ICU tour

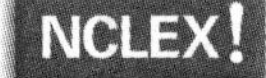

c. Discharge teaching

1) Must not slump in chairs, must not bend or twist the torso or lift over 10 pounds

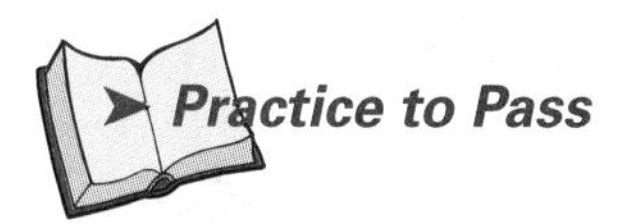

The nurse is caring for a 14-year-old client who is postop day one following a spinal fusion for structural scoliosis. What are the priorities of this client's nursing care?

2) Complying with activity restrictions, which must be followed for 6 to 8 months

3) Addressing self-esteem issues

4) Complying with follow-up visits

7. Evaluation: the spine of the adolescent with scoliosis is stable; the adolescent correctly states activities and care for scoliosis

D. *Muscular dystrophy*

1. Description

   a. Group of disorders that are characterized by progressive degeneration of skeletal muscles (muscles that are under voluntary control)

   b. All muscular dystrophies are inherited disorders

   c. Duchenne's muscular dystrophy (pseudohypertrophic muscular dystrophy) is the most common, inherited as a sex-linked recessive trait, therefore occurs only in boys

   d. Incidence is approximately 1 in 3,500 male births

   e. There is progressive muscle weakness, wasting, and contractures, with loss of independent ambulation by 9 to 11 years of age

2. Etiology and pathophysiology

   a. Lack of dystrophin, the protein that is necessary for muscle contraction

   b. Muscle biopsy shows fibrous degeneration and fatty deposits

   c. The disease ultimately affects the muscles of respiration, allowing pneumonia to develop easily

   d. Death usually occurs at about 20 years of age from respiratory or heart failure

3. Assessment

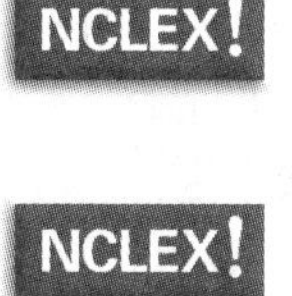

   a. Children generally have a history of meeting motor developmental milestones in the earliest years; symptoms become obvious and acute at 3 years of age

   b. Symptoms often begin with a waddling gait, lordosis, difficulty climbing stairs, running or pedaling a bike

NCLEX!

   c. As the disease progresses, children have difficulty walking on an even surface and rise from the floor only by rolling onto their stomachs, then pushing themselves to their knees, and walk their hands up their legs to stand (Gower's sign)

   d. As the disease progresses, the muscle weakness becomes more pronounced, and ambulation becomes more difficult, necessitating wheelchair use by 11 or 12 years of age

   e. Muscles feel unusually woody on palpation and look enlarged, called **pseudohypertrophy**

   f. Scoliosis of the spine and fractures of the long bones may occur from abnormal muscle tension and lack of muscle support

4. Priority nursing diagnoses

a. Risk for injury related to disease process

b. Anticipatory grieving related to chronic and terminal illness

c. Impaired physical mobility related to wasted muscles

d. Risk for constipation related to poor muscle tone

e. Impaired gas exchange related to accumulation of secretions, lack of mobility

f. Self-esteem disturbance related to debilitating disease process

5. Planning and implementation

a. Care is supportive, with physical therapy to prevent disuse atrophy of unaffected muscles; physical therapy should be instituted when confined to bed with illness, injury, or surgery, if bedrest extends beyond a few days

b. Child should be immobilized for as short a period as possible to help prevent disuse atrophy

c. Frequent rest periods in a recumbent position are helpful to help reduce the incidence of scoliosis

d. Splinting and bracing may help to maintain lower extremity stability and avoid contractures

e. A daily goal for well children should be at least 3 hours of ambulation per day to maintain muscle strength

f. Encourage a low-calorie, high-protein diet to avoid obesity

g. Encourage a high-fiber and high-fluid diet to prevent constipation

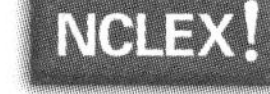

h. Infections become increasingly frequent as the dystrophic process produces a decrease in vital capacity; even minor upper respiratory infections are treated quickly and vigorously with antibiotics and postural drainage

i. Certain surgical techniques allow ambulation longer

6. Child and family education

a. Teach ROM exercises

b. Reinforce diet to prevent obesity and constipation

c. Teach how to achieve the optimal level of activity within the child's limitations

d. Encourage participation in support groups for parents and children

e. Teach self-help skills

f. Provide information on environmental issues that promote mobility and allow for wheelchair use

g. Refer family members for genetic counseling

7. Evaluation: the family states appropriate care of this child to maintain maximum function as long as possible; the child exhibits minimal respiratory infections

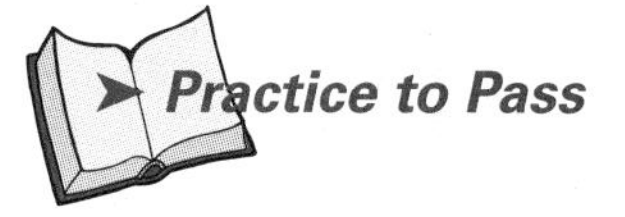

A 15-year-old male is admitted to the adolescent unit with pneumonia. He also has Duchenne's muscular dystrophy. Describe the priorities of his nursing care during this hospitalization.

IV. Infectious Musculoskeletal Health Problems: Osteomyelitis

A. Description

1. **Osteomyelitis** is an infection of the bone
2. Can occur at any age; is most common in children between 1 and 12 years
3. Boys are affected two to three times more often than girls

B. Etiology and pathophysiology

1. May be caused by any microorganism, though usually caused by bacteria; *Staphylococcus aureus* is the offending bacteria most often in older children and *Haemophilus influenza* in younger children
2. Microorganism is carried to the bone site through the bloodstream from another site of infection or by way of a penetrating wound
3. Infective emboli from the focus of infection travel to the small end arteries in the bone metaphysis, where they set up an infectious process
4. An abscess forms, which spreads along the shaft of the bone under the periosteum, possibly extending to and penetrating the bone marrow
5. Edema in the area resulting from the infection reduces the blood supply to the bone, causing death of bone tissue

C. Assessment

1. Generally begins with acute symptoms, systemic malaise, fever, irritability, rapid pulse, and possibly dehydration
2. May be a history of trauma to the bone

NCLEX!

3. Symptoms include pain, tenderness, swelling, and redness in the area of infection; there is also decreased mobility of the affected extremity
4. Blood studies reveal an increased white blood cell count, C-reactive protein, and sedimentation rate; blood cultures will be positive
5. X-ray may not reveal bone changes until 5 to 10 days after the beginning of the infection; computed tomography may show early-stage bone changes

D. Priority nursing diagnoses

1. Pain related to disease process
2. Impaired physical mobility related to disease process
3. Risk for noncompliance related to long course of antibiotics
4. Knowledge deficit: disease process and treatment

E. Planning and implementation

1. Limitation of weight-bearing on the affected extremity; the child may be placed on complete bedrest with immobilization of the affected extremity

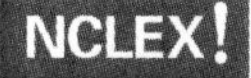

2. Surgery may be needed for incision and drainage; if surgical drainage is carried out, polyethylene tubes are placed in the wound—one tube instills antibiotic solution directly into the wound, while the other provides drainage
3. Strict aseptic technique is used during all dressing changes

4. Diversional activities are important to maintain activity restrictions as the child begins to feel better

5. Physical therapy may be instituted to ensure restoration of optimal function

F. Medication therapy

NCLEX!

1. Intravenous antibiotics for 3 to 6 weeks, initiated in the hospital, and then continued at home; the length of IV therapy is determined by the duration of symptoms, the initial response to treatment, and the sensitivity of the organism

2. Oral antibiotics for 2 weeks following intravenous antibiotics

G. Child and family education

1. Compliance with antibiotic treatment

2. Care and maintenance of intravenous site

3. Activity restrictions that are ordered by the health care professional

4. Providing good food sources of calcium and protein for bone healing

5. Signs and symptoms of infection

H. Evaluation: the family and child comply with antibiotic administration

V. Accidents and Injuries Causing Musculoskeletal Health Problems: Fractures

A. Description

NCLEX!

1. The growth plate or epiphyseal plate is a common place of injury, and can lead to improper growth if not treated correctly; the Salter-Harris classification system is used to describe fractures of the growth plate and is based on the angle of the fracture in relation to the epiphysis (see Figure 9-2)

2. The periosteum of a child's bone is thicker and stronger and aids in rapid healing

B. Etiology and pathophysiology

1. The pliable, more porous bones of children allow them to bend, buckle and break in different ways than those of adults (see Figure 9-3)

2. Fractures may result from trauma—falls, motor vehicle accidents, sports injuries or abuse—or may be a result of bone diseases such as osteogenesis imperfecta or cancer that weakens the bone

3. Adolescents who limit their intake of calories and calcium and who are involved in sports such as distance running or gymnastics are at risk for stress fractures; these fractures may present with chronic pain that changes in intensity

C. Assessment

1. Complaints of children must be taken seriously; they usually only complain when something is wrong

NCLEX!

2. Frequently assess the five "Ps" in the affected extremity

   a. Pain and joint tenderness

   b. Pulselessness distal to the fracture site

Figure 9-2

Salter-Harris classification of fractures. *Source:* Ball, J. & Bindler, R. (1999). *Pediatric nursing: Caring for children* (2nd ed.). Stamford, CT: Appleton & Lange, p. 855.

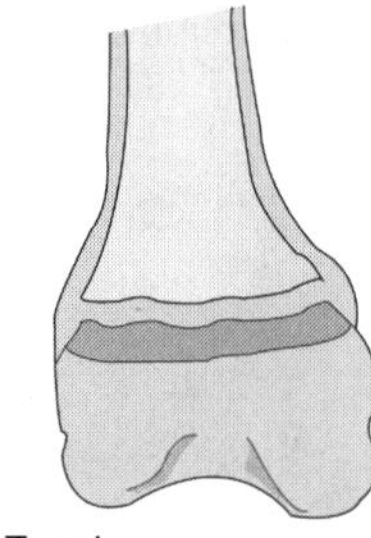

Type I
Common
Growth plate undisturbed
Growth disturbances rare

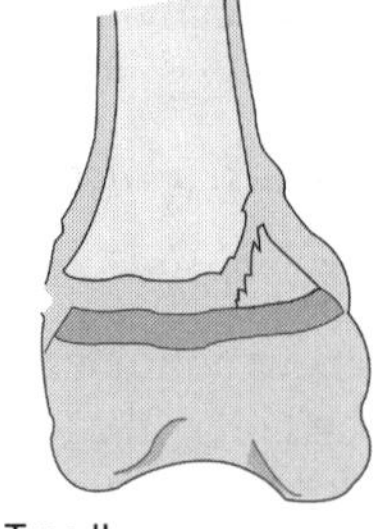

Type II
Most common
Growth disturbances rare

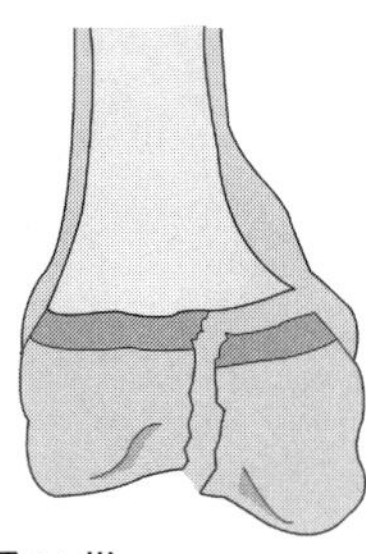

Type III
Less common
Serious threat to growth and joint

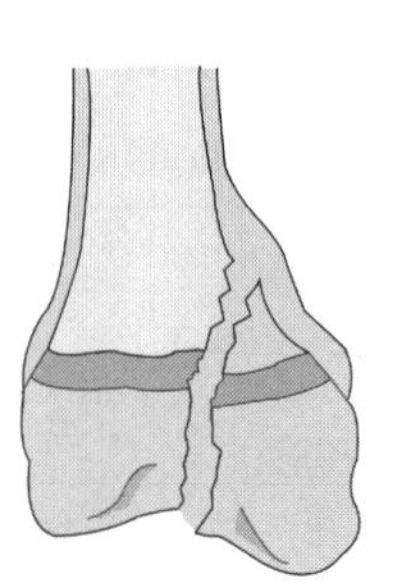

Type IV
Serious threat to growth

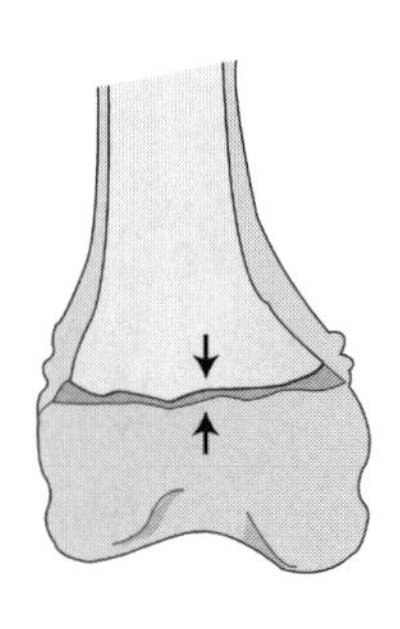

Type V
Rare
Crush injury causes cell death in growth plate, resulting in arrested growth and limited bone length
If growth plate is partially destroyed, angular deformities may result

Figure 9-3

Types of fractures. *Source:* Ball, J. & Bindler, R. (1999). *Pediatric nursing: Caring for children* (2nd ed.). Stamford, CT: Appleton & Lange, p. 854.

Complete (transverse) fracture

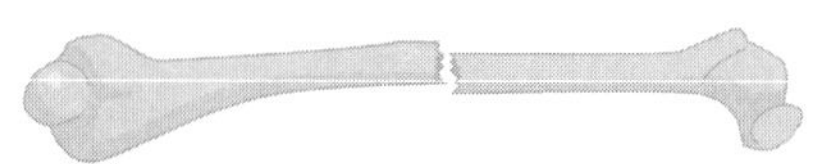

Break across entire section of a bone at a right angle to the bone shaft resulting in two or more fragments

Spiral fracture

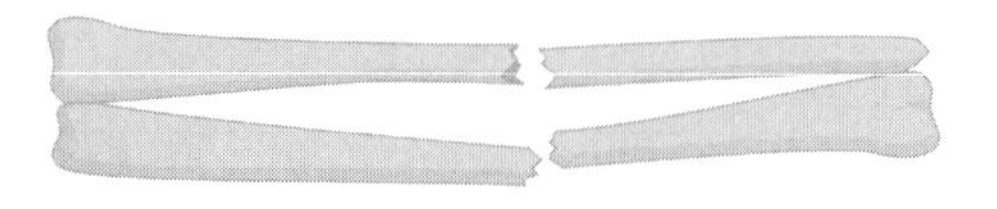

Associated with twisting force; fracture coils around the bone

Open fracture

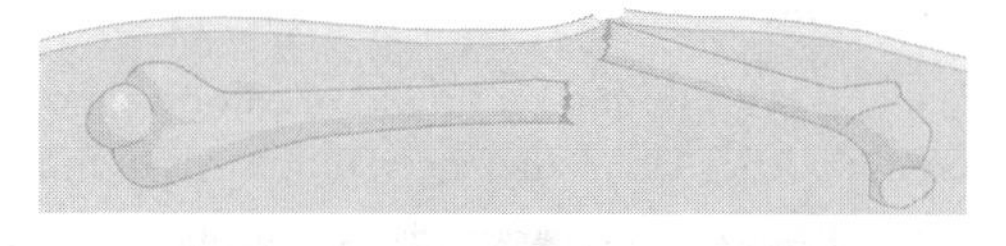

Broken bone protrudes through the skin leaving a path to the fracture site; high risk of infection exists

Greenstick fracture

Caused by compression force; often seen in young children

Closed fracture

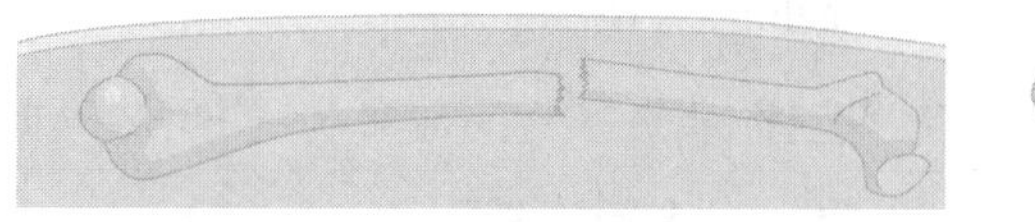

Broken bone does not protrude through the skin

Comminuted fracture

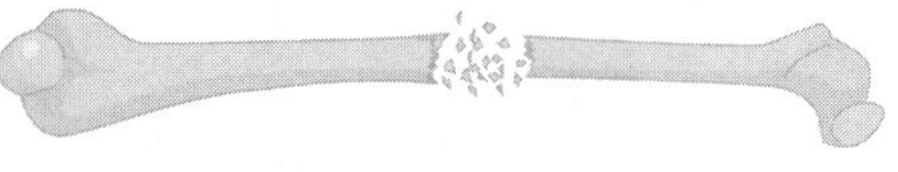

Associated with high impact forces; bone breaks into three or more segments

   c. Pallor

   d. Paresthesia distal to the fracture site

   e. Paralysis or movement distal to the fracture site

3. Assess vital signs, lungs sounds, bowel sounds, and neurological status depending on the cause of fracture

4. Assess blood studies; fracture may cause bleeding or destruction of red blood cells

5. Assess for other associated injuries caused by the trauma that caused the fracture

D. Priority nursing diagnoses

1. Risk for impaired tissue perfusion related to swelling

2. Pain related to injury or muscle spasm

3. Risk for impaired skin integrity related to traction, cast, or splint

4. Risk for infection related to loss of skin integrity

5. Impaired physical mobility related to cast, splint, or traction

6. Knowledge deficit: course of treatment, care of cast, traction

E. Planning and implementation

1. The treatment of a fracture is to realign and immobilize the fractured extremity by **traction** (pulling a body part in one direction with counterpull in another) or closed manipulation and casting until adequate callus is formed

NCLEX!

2. A cast may be applied after closed reduction; a cast may be fiberglass, which dries in 5 to 30 minutes, or plaster, which dries over 24 to 48 hours; various types of casts include short- or long-extremity casts, bilateral long leg cast, shoulder spica cast, single spica, 1½ spica and full spica casts, cylinder cast, bootie cast, and body cast

3. Surgery may be needed for open reduction of the fracture using pins, plates, wires, or screws, in order for healing to occur

4. Children are most frequently hospitalized for fractures of the femur

NCLEX!

5. See Box 9-2 for nursing care of a child in a cast

6. Monitor for complications of fracture reduction: infection with open fractures, neurovascular or vascular injury, malunion or nonunion, and leg length discrepancy

NCLEX!

7. Monitor for deep pain unrelieved by analgesics, which may be a symptom of compartment syndrome; compartment syndrome is considered a medical emergency; the swelling caused by inflammation and casting reduces blood flow to the affected area and can lead to progressive neurological damage; notify the physician immediately

8. Traction is used to reduce dislocations and immobilize fractures; it involves pulling on a body part in one direction against a counterpull exerted in the opposite direction

   a. Traction may be straight or running traction (where the child's body serves as the counterpull), or suspended or balanced traction (where the counterpull is through weights and pulleys)

Box 9-2

Nursing Care of a Child in a Cast

- Assess neurovascular status of involved extremity and compare with unaffected extremity; assess temperature, pallor, pain, tingling sensation, edema, pulse, and capillary refill every 15 minutes for the first hour, hourly for 24 hours, then every 2 to 4 hours.
- Assess the child's ability to move the toes and detect sensation in the affected extremity; compare to the unaffected extremity.
- Report any change in neurovascular status to the physician immediately.
- Assist with proper drying of a plaster cast (takes 24 to 48 hours) by leaving it exposed to air, turning the child every 2 hours and using a fan or cool hair dryer.
- A wet cast is handled only with the palms of the hands to prevent indenting casts and creating pressure areas.
- Relieve edema by elevating limb and applying ice to the outside of the cast.
- Assess pain and institute pain management therapies.
- Provide a well-balanced diet with adequate calories, protein, and calcium.
- Frequently assess skin around the cast edges for redness and breakdown.
- Petal the cast edges if rough or broken down by applying strips of adhesive tape over them.
- Keep the cast dry from water, stool, or urine with the use of plastic wrap.
- Assess for hot spots felt on the cast surface, which indicate infection underneath. Report any hot spots found.
- Assist with mobility with use of wagons, wheeled carts, crutches, or wheelchairs.

b. Skin traction is used when minimal traction is needed; traction is applied to the skin with adhesive materials or straps, foam boots and the skin serve as the counter-pull

c. Skeletal traction is used when a greater strength of traction or a longer period of traction is needed; the pull is directly applied to the bone by pins or wires that have been surgically placed through the distal end of the bone

NCLEX!

d. See Box 9-3 for further information about care for a child in traction

9. The following are various kinds of traction

NCLEX!

a. Bryant's traction: used for children under 3 years of age and weighing less than 35 pounds, who have a fractured femur or congenital hip dysplasia; both legs are placed in skin traction, the hips are flexed at a 90-degree angle, with knees extended, and both buttocks are slightly elevated above the mattress

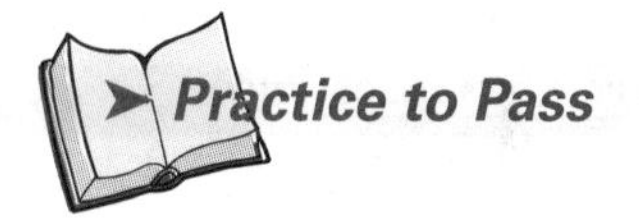

A 23-month-old child is in Bryant's traction for developmental dysplasia of the hip. Describe the nursing care for this child.

b. Buck's traction: used for knee immobilization or for short-term immobilization of a fracture; this running skin traction keeps the leg in extended position without hip flexion

c. Russell's traction: used for fractures of the femur and lower leg; skin traction is placed on the lower leg while the knee is suspended in a padded sling; the hips and knees are slightly flexed; skin care and monitoring of the skin resting in the sling is indicated

d. Dunlop's traction: used for fractures of the humerus; the flexed arm is suspended horizontally; this may be applied as skin or skeletal traction

Box 9-3

Nursing Care of a Child in Traction

Nursing Interventions for All Types of Traction

- Assess neurovascular status of involved extremity and compare with unaffected extremity; assess temperature, pallor, pain, tingling sensation, edema, pulse, and capillary refill every 15 minutes for the first hour, hourly for 24 hours, then every 2 to 4 hours.
- Assess the child's ability to move the toes and detect sensation in the affected extremity, as compared to the unaffected extremity.
- Maintain alignment of affected extremity.
- Ensure that the child is in alignment in bed, and that the head or foot of the bed are elevated as directed for the desired amount of pull and traction.
- Ensure that the prescribed amount of weight is in place and that weights hang freely and are in a safe location.
- Assess pain and institute pain management therapies.
- Provide a well-balanced diet with adequate calories, protein, and calcium.
- Provide diversional activities appropriate to the child's developmental level.
- Check beneath the child for small objects.
- Provide nursing care to prevent complications resulting from immobility.
  - Assess skin surfaces, provide frequent skin care, and include use of trapeze, air mattress, and sheepskin.
  - Assess respiratory status and encourage deep breathing, coughing, incentive spirometry.
  - Assess urinary elimination, monitor intake and output, encourage fluids.
  - Assess bowel function, encourage high-fiber diet.
  - Encourage range-of-motion exercises.
  - Anticipate need for antiembolism stockings on unaffected lower extremity.

Additional Nursing Interventions for Skeletal Traction

- Assess vital signs, especially temperature, every 4 hours or more often if indicated.
- Inspect pin insertion sites at least every 8 hours for redness, swelling, irritation, or drainage.
- Obtain culture of pin sites as ordered.
- Provide pin care according to institution policy.
- Cover the end of pins with protective padding to prevent injury.

Additional Nursing Interventions for Skin Traction

- Replace nonadhesive bandages when permitted or when necessary, ensuring that someone maintains traction on the affected limb during the procedure.
- Assess bandages to ensure that they are correctly applied, neither too loose nor too tight.

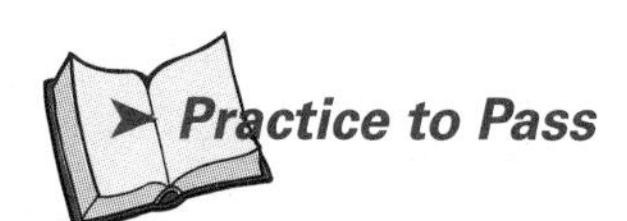

The nurse is caring for a child who had fractures of the tibia and fibula reduced by closed reduction and just had a fiberglass cast applied. What assessments will be done immediately? Which assessment findings would lead the nurse to call the physician?

e. 90-90 traction: skeletal traction used for fractures of the femur or tibia; the hip and knee are positioned at 90-degree angles, and the lower part of the extremity is put into a sling or boot cast; ensure skin care to the area in the boot cast or sling

f. External fixators: attached to the extremity by percutaneous transfixing of pins or wires to the bone; these can be used for simple fractures or for complicated fractures or deformities

F. **Child and family education:** refer back to Box 9-1

G. **Evaluation:** the child's bone heals properly; the child's growth and development is not disturbed by the fracture; the parents state appropriate care of a child in a cast

Case Study

A newborn is found to have developmental dysplasia of the hip prior to being discharged from the birth hospital. You are the nurse caring for this newborn and the new mother prior to discharge.

1. What assessment findings would you expect to find in this newborn?
2. The parents of the newborn ask how this could have happened. How will you respond?
3. What are the priorities of care for this newborn?
4. How will this condition be treated?
5. What teaching needs to be completed with the parents of this newborn prior to discharge?
6. The parents question you about what they can expect regarding long term consequences. How should you respond?

For suggested responses, see pages 409–410.

Posttest

1 Parents of an unborn infant have just learned that, based on ultrasound, their infant has clubfoot. They ask the nurse how clubfoot is treated. Which of the following treatments should the nurse discuss with the parents?

(1) Weekly cast changes with manipulation
(2) Probable surgery on the affected limb
(3) Abduction device to keep the hip in full abduction
(4) Use of a Denis Browne splint to achieve correction

2 An infant is placed in a Pavlik harness for developmental dysplasia of the hip. Which of the following statements made by a parent indicates correct knowledge of the care of this infant?

(1) "The straps of the harness should be placed next to the skin."
(2) "The harness should be worn for 6 hours a day."
(3) "It will take a long time for my child to walk and crawl."
(4) "I can move my child around on a large skateboard."

3 Which of the following nursing diagnoses takes highest priority for the child hospitalized with osteogenesis imperfecta?

(1) Impaired skin integrity related to cast
(2) Pain related to fractures
(3) Risk for injury related to disease state
(4) Body image disturbance related to short stature

4 Which of the following would not be consistent with common assessment findings in a child diagnosed with an acute onset of Legg-Calve-Perthes (LCP) disease?

(1) Swelling and redness of the involved joint(s)
(2) Stiffness in the morning or after rest
(3) Insidious limp after activities
(4) Referred pain to the knee

5 A 12-year-old male is admitted to the adolescent unit with a diagnosis of slipped capitol femoral epiphysis. Which of the following activities should not be allowed prior to surgical correction?

(1) Ambulation with crutches, avoid bearing weight on the affected leg
(2) Sitting in a wheelchair
(3) Moving on a stretcher
(4) Maintaining bedrest

6 Which of the following symptoms is not typical in an adolescent with idiopathic structural scoliosis?

(1) Back pain
(2) Skirts that hang unevenly
(3) Unequal shoulder heights
(4) Uneven waist angles

7 Which nursing diagnosis should take highest priority when working with an adolescent with scoliosis?

(1) Body image disturbance related to treatment of scoliosis
(2) Diversional activity deficit related to treatment of scoliosis
(3) Anxiety related to outcome of treatment for scoliosis
(4) Fear related to treatment and unknown outcomes

8 Postoperative care of an adolescent following a spinal fusion for scoliosis includes:

(1) Oral analgesia for pain.
(2) Logrolling every 4 hours.
(3) Nasogastric intubation.
(4) Straight catheterization every 4 hours.

9 A 3-year-old child is suspected of having Duchenne's muscular dystrophy. Which of the following assessment findings by the nurse would support this diagnosis?

(1) A history of delayed crawling
(2) Inability to ambulate independently
(3) Difficulty climbing stairs
(4) Gower's sign

10 A child is suspected of having osteomyelitis. Which of the following blood values supports this diagnosis?

(1) Decreased white blood cell (WBC) count
(2) Positive blood cultures
(3) Increased hematocrit (Hct)
(4) Increased BUN

See pages 240–241 for Answers and Rationales.

Answers and Rationales

Pretest

1 **Answer: 3** ***Rationale:*** The sensation of numbness or tingling is a sign of neurovascular impairment. Neurovascular impairment can lead to nerve ischemia and destruction, with possible permanent paralysis of the extremity. Any symptom of neurovascular impairment, such as paresthesia, lack of pulses, edema that does not improve with elevation, pallor, and pain, needs immediate attention.
Cognitive Level: Analysis
Nursing Process: Analysis; ***Test Plan:*** PHYS

2 **Answer: 2** ***Rationale:*** The child with skeletal traction has a pin that passes through the skin into the end of a long bone. This procedure provides an entrance for microorganisms. Frequent monitoring of the pin site, pin care according to institutional policy, and frequent monitoring for signs of infection take priority over the other nursing interventions listed.
Cognitive Level: Analysis
Nursing Process: Analysis; ***Test Plan:*** PHYS

3 **Answer: 1** ***Rationale:*** Slipped capitol femoral epiphysis is a slipping of the femoral head that occurs most frequently before or during the rapid adolescent growth spurt. The onset of symptoms is gradual, and include limp, holding the leg in external rotation to relieve pain, restricted and painful internal rotation, and knee and hip pain.
Cognitive Level: Analysis
Nursing Process: Assessment; ***Test Plan:*** PHYS

4 **Answer: 1** ***Rationale:*** The therapeutic management of the child with osteomyelitis includes limiting weight-bearing on the affected part, immobilization,

and administration of antibiotics. Antibiotic therapy may continue intravenously for 3 to 6 weeks, and orally for another 2 weeks, depending on duration of symptoms, response to treatment, and sensitivity of the organism. Discharge teaching needs to include follow-up antibiotic care at home, care of the IV site, and continuing antibiotic therapy even though it may seem as if all the symptoms are gone. Food sources such as calcium and protein should be provided for bone healing.
Cognitive Level: Analysis
Nursing Process: Evaluation; ***Test Plan:*** HPM

5 **Answer: 3** ***Rationale:*** All four of these signs are assessment tests for developmental dysplasia of the hip. Ortolani and Barlow signs disappear after 2 to 3 months. Trendelenburg sign will be seen in the child who is able to stand. Allis sign, shortening of the affected limb on the affected side, is a reliable test at 4 months of age.
Cognitive Level: Application
Nursing Process: Assessment; ***Test Plan:*** PHYS

6 **Answer: 3** ***Rationale:*** Clubfoot is apparent at birth, with the affected foot fixed in an abnormal position. The affected foot is usually smaller, shorter, with an empty heel pad. The affected limb is usually shorter and has some calf muscle atrophy.
Cognitive Level: Analysis
Nursing Process: Assessment; ***Test Plan:*** PHYS

7 **Answer: 3** ***Rationale:*** Children with this disorder have normal calcium and phosphorus and abnormal precollagen type I. This prevents the formation of collagen, the major component of connective tissue. The precollagen remains relatively unstable and unable to undergo final transformation into collagen.
Cognitive Level: Analysis
Nursing Process: Assessment; ***Test Plan:*** PHYS

8 **Answer: 4** ***Rationale:*** The child with mild OI may be able to participate in sports, and many are able to participate in swimming. There are no current medications that stop this disease process. There are a variety of surgical procedures that may be done to help strengthen the bones; one is the insertion of intermedullary rods to provide for stability. The child with OI may participate in schools, though care must be taken to protect this child from injury.
Cognitive Level: Analysis
Nursing Process: Evaluation; ***Test Plan:*** PHYS

9 **Answer: 4** ***Rationale:*** Children with muscular dystrophy quickly suffer from complications of immobility. Therefore, when hospitalized, these children should have physical therapy, range of motion exercises, and bed-to-chair activity as soon as possible. Children with respiratory infections are treated with vigorous antibiotic therapy, as well as postural drainage and cupping.
Cognitive Level: Analysis
Nursing Process: Planning; ***Test Plan:*** PHYS

10 **Answer: 3** ***Rationale:*** The Milwaukee brace is worn for scoliosis, when the degree of curve is greater than 20 but less than 40 degrees. It is worn for 23 hours a day. Exercises to increase pelvic tilt, for lateral strengthening, and to correct lordosis should be done several times a day while in the brace. The brace should be worn over a t-shirt to minimize skin irritation. The adolescent may experience muscle aches resulting from new alignment.
Cognitive Level: Application
Nursing Process: Implementation; ***Test Plan:*** HPM

Posttest

1 **Answer: 1** ***Rationale:*** The initial treatment for clubfoot begins immediately or shortly after birth and consists of weekly cast changes and manipulation. Surgery is completed only if nonsurgical intervention of serial casting is not effective. A Denis Browne splint may be used to maintain correction once it is achieved. Abduction devices are used for hip conditions.
Cognitive Level: Application
Nursing Process: Implementation; ***Test Plan:*** PHYS

2 **Answer: 4** ***Rationale:*** A child in an abduction splint needs to be kept mobile, which can be done with the use of a wagon, large skateboard, or cart. Though diapers should be placed over the straps of a Pavlik harness, a t-shirt should be worn under the straps of the harness. The harness should be worn for 23 hours a day. The child quickly "catches up" once the device is no longer worn if developmental milestones are delayed because of the abduction device.
Cognitive Level: Analysis
Nursing Process: Evaluation; ***Test Plan:*** HPM

3 **Answer: 3** ***Rationale:*** Because of their very fragile bones, children with OI experience countless fractures, and the prevention of injury takes highest priority in this child's care.
Cognitive Level: Analysis
Nursing Process: Analysis; ***Test Plan:*** PHYS

4 **Answer: 1** ***Rationale:*** Swelling and redness of involved joints is a symptom found in juvenile arthritis, not LCP disease. All of the other symptoms listed are consistent with this diagnosis.
Cognitive Level: Analysis
Nursing Process: Analysis; ***Test Plan:*** PHYS

5 **Answer: 2** ***Rationale:*** Once the diagnosis is made, the child should not bear weight on the affected hip, as weight bearing can increase the amount of slippage. Wheelchair use should be avoided, as this also may increase the amount of slippage.
Cognitive Level: Analysis
Nursing Process: Planning; ***Test Plan:*** PHYS

6 **Answer: 1** ***Rationale:*** Back pain is not identified as a symptom of idiopathic structural scoliosis. All the other listed symptoms are.
Cognitive Level: Analysis
Nursing Process: Assessment; ***Test Plan:*** PHYS

7 **Answer: 1** ***Rationale:*** Treatment for scoliosis extends over a long period of time, during the time when a great deal of their psychological identity is formed. Treatment involves a modified lifestyle and being "different" from their peers, so issues of self-image are paramount and should take priority.
Cognitive Level: Analysis
Nursing Process: Analysis; ***Test Plan:*** PSYC

8 **Answer: 3** ***Rationale:*** There is some degree of paralytic ileus following a spinal fusion; therefore, nasogastric intubation is required along with frequent assessment of return of bowel function. The pain experienced by this client is severe and requires intravenous medication, preferably with patient-controlled analgesia (PCA). Logrolling must be done every 2 hours, once allowed, to prevent the accumulation of secretions in the lungs. Urinary retention is common, and an indwelling catheter is used if present rather than repeated straight catheterization.
Cognitive Level: Application
Nursing Process: Implementation; ***Test Plan:*** PHYS

9 **Answer: 3** ***Rationale:*** The child with Duchenne's muscular dystrophy has a history of meeting early developmental milestones. Symptoms usually begin at around 3 years of age and include difficulty climbing stairs, running, and pedaling. As the disease progresses, the child has a difficult time ambulating on even surfaces, and Gower's sign is seen. The child loses the ability to ambulate independently by the age of 10 to 12.
Cognitive Level: Analysis
Nursing Process: Assessment; ***Test Plan:*** PHYS

10 **Answer: 2** ***Rationale:*** Blood studies in a child with osteomyelitis will reveal an increased WBC count, C-reactive protein, and sedimentation rate. The blood culture is usually positive. This disease process does not affect the HCT or BUN.
Cognitive Level: Analysis
Nursing Process: Assessment; ***Test Plan:*** PHYS

References

Ball, J. & Bindler, R. (1999). *Pediatric nursing: Caring for children* (2nd ed.). Stamford, CT: Appleton & Lange, pp. 817–861.

Burns, C. & Brady, M. (2000). Musculoskeletal disorders. In C. Burns, M. Brady, A. Dunn, & N. Starr, *Pediatric primary care: A handbook for nurse practitioners* (2nd ed.). Philadelphia: W. B. Saunders, pp. 1134–1171.

Pillitteri, A. (1999). *Child health nursing: Care of the child and family.* Philadelphia: Lippincott, pp. 538–543, 924–957.

Wong, D., Hockenberry-Eaton, M., Wilson, D., Winkelstein, M., Ahmann, E., & DiVito-Thomas, P. (1999). *Whaley & Wong's nursing care of infants and children* (6th ed.). St. Louis: Mosby, pp. 505–513, 1887–1963, 1995–1998.

CHAPTER 10

Integumentary Health Problems

Vera Dauffenbach, MSN, EdD, RN

CHAPTER OUTLINE

OBJECTIVES

- Identify data essential to the assessment of alterations in health of the integumentary system in a child.
- Discuss the clinical manifestations and pathophysiology of alterations in health of the integumentary system of a child.
- Discuss therapeutic management of a child with alterations in health of the integumentary system.
- Describe nursing management of a child with alterations in health of the integumentary system.

[Media Link]

Use the CD-ROM enclosed with this text, or log onto the address given to access the free, interactive Companion Website created for this series. The CD-ROM and Companion Website accompanying this book offer additional practice opportunities and information—NCLEX Review, Case Studies, Glossary, In Depth with NCLEX, and more.

www.prenhall.com/hogan

Review at a Glance

bulla *fluid-filled lesion greater than 1 cm in diameter*

cellulitis *inflammation of the skin and subcutaneous tissue*

dermis *highly vascular, inner supportive layer of the skin*

eczema *also known as atopic dermatitis; chronic superficial inflammatory skin disorder characterized by dry scaly patches and pruritus*

epidermis *tough, outer layer of the skin*

erythema *diffuse skin redness*

impetigo *highly contagious superficial skin infection caused by group A beta-hemolytic streptococcus or* Staphylococcus aureus

lichenification *large, dry thickened lesions*

macule *discolored spot on the skin that is neither raised nor depressed*

papule *raised lesion*

pediculosis capitus *head lice*

pruritus *itchiness*

pustule *small, blister-like elevation that contains pus*

scabies *skin infestation caused by the scabies mite*

vesicle *small, blister-like elevation that contains serous fluid*

Pretest

1 When bathing a 3-year-old with eczema, the nurse tells the mother to have the bathwater:

(1) As hot as the child can tolerate.
(2) Hot to the touch on the inner wrist.
(3) Tepid.
(4) Cool.

2 The nurse explains to the mother that a child who has begun treatment for impetigo with a topical antibiotic can return to daycare:

(1) Immediately.
(2) After 48 hours.
(3) As soon as crusts are evident.
(4) When crusts fall off.

3 When assessing a child's hair and scalp, the nurse notices what looks like dandruff but it does not flake off easily. The nurse suspects the child has:

(1) Scabies.
(2) Eczema.
(3) *Pediculosis capitus.*
(4) Impetigo.

4 The nurse plans to position a child with a circumferential burn of the right leg:

(1) Flat in bed.
(2) With the right leg dependent.
(3) On the left side.
(4) With the right leg elevated.

5 A 3-year-old child has been diagnosed with eczema. The nurse will assess for:

(1) Pruritus.
(2) Pustules.
(3) Vesicles.
(4) Lichenification.

6 A child has been diagnosed with eczema. While taking the nursing history, the nurse will assess for a family history of:

(1) Scabies.
(2) Cellulitis.
(3) Asthma.
(4) Impetigo.

7 When assessing a child with periorbital cellulitis, the nurse will want to ask the parent about a recent history of:

(1) Otitis media.
(2) Sinusitis.
(3) Dog bite.
(4) Sun exposure.

8 **A child will be treated at home for cellulitis of the left leg. The nurse will include in client education the need for:**

(1) Continuing oral antibiotics until the prescription is completed.
(2) Strict bed rest with the left leg elevated.
(3) Increased fluid intake.
(4) Limiting visitors to prevent spreading infection.

9 **When teaching a mother how to use an anti-lice shampoo, the nurse should include the information that she should:**

(1) Use ample shampoo to cover the hair.
(2) Apply about 2 ounces of shampoo to wet hair.
(3) Leave the shampoo on hair for 20 to 30 minutes before rinsing.
(4) Use hot water for both shampoo and rinse.

10 **The nurse would share which of the following pieces of information to increase treatment compliance in a teenager with eczema?**

(1) The appearance of the skin will improve in a few days.
(2) Avoiding foods with eggs and milk will speed healing.
(3) Scarring is not likely if the treatment plan is followed.
(4) This problem will not likely recur past adolescence.

See pages 261–262 for Answers and Rationales.

I. Overview of the Anatomy and Physiology of the Skin

A. Skin structure

1. Layers (see Figure 10-1)
   - **a. Epidermis:** tough, outer layer of the skin
   - **b. Dermis:** highly vascular, inner supportive layer of the skin
   - **c.** Subcutaneous fat
2. Accessory structures
   - **a.** Hair
   - **b.** Nails
   - **c.** Glands
     - 1) Sebaceous: provide sebum into hair follicle
     - 2) Sweat: provide thermoregulation through sweating

B. Skin functions

1. Sensitivity to pressure, pain, touch, and temperature
2. First line of defense against infectious organisms
3. Thermoregulation through sweating, shivering, and subcutaneous insulation
4. Protects underlying tissues and organs from injury
5. Synthesizes vitamin D
6. Excretes water, salt, and electrolytes
7. Regenerates itself through shedding of old cells and replacing with new cells

Figure 10-1

Layers and structures of skin.
Source: Ball, J. & Bindler, R. (1999). *Pediatric nursing: Caring for children* (2nd ed.). Stamford, CT: Appleton & Lange, p. 909.

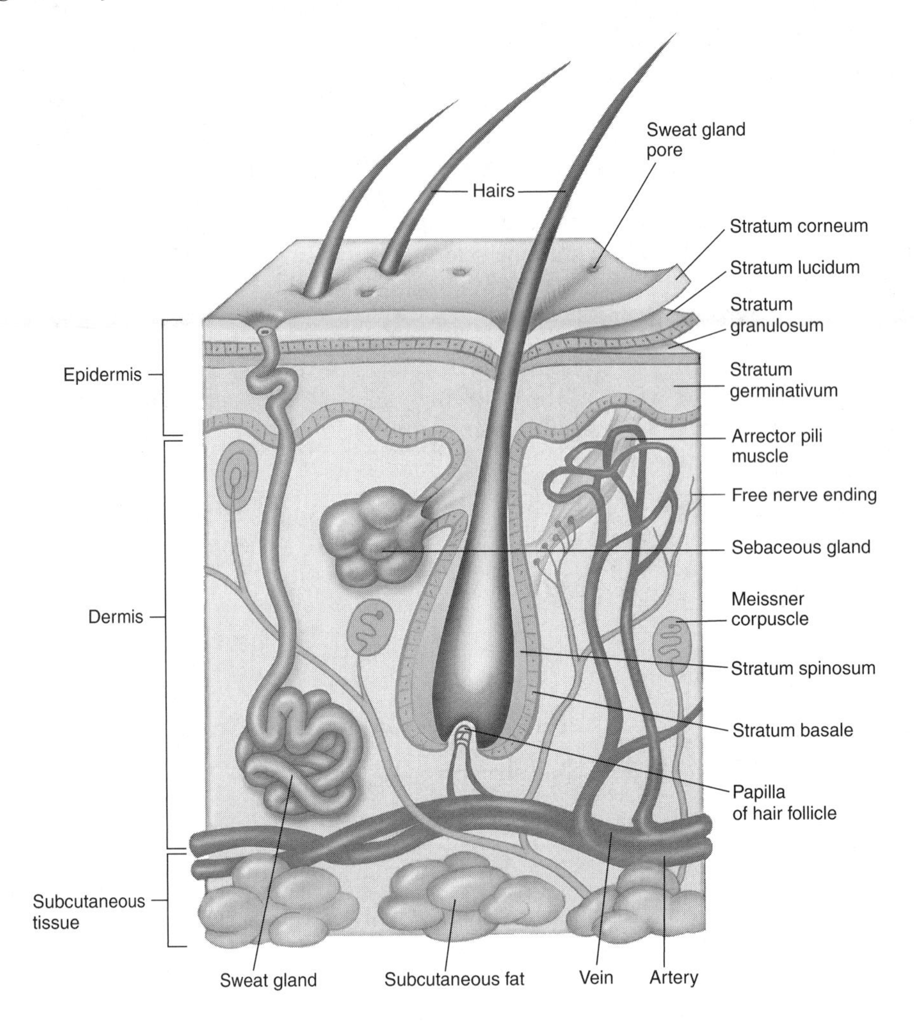

C. Pediatric variations in skin

1. Newborns are covered by lanugo, fine soft hair that is shed in the first month of life

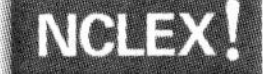

2. Newborns have thin skin with little subcutaneous fat that allows rapid heat loss and problems with thermoregulation
   a. Leads to increased absorption of harmful chemical substances
   b. Sweat glands not fully developed until middle childhood
3. Newborns' skin contains more water than older children
4. Dark-colored areas called Mongolian spots may be present on the sacrum or buttocks of Native American, Asian, African-American, or Latino infants

II. Diagnostic Tests of the Skin

A. **Skin cultures:** noninvasive procedure in which a skin sample is obtained with a sterile applicator; used to identify viral, bacterial, or fungal causes of skin lesions

B. Skin scrapings: noninvasive procedure in which epithelial cells are scraped off and examined microscopically to identify viral, bacterial, fungal, or parasitic causes of skin lesions

C. Skin biopsy: invasive procedure in which a skin sample is removed for histological analysis

NCLEX!

1. Requires informed consent
2. Apply pressure to the site until bleeding stops; suture may be required
3. Used to identify tumors or persistent dermatitis

III. Acquired Integumentary Health Problems: Eczema

A. Description: ***eczema*** is a superficial inflammatory skin disorder

1. Sometimes called atopic dermatitis (having a hereditary allergic tendency)
2. A chronic, superficial inflammatory skin disorder characterized by severe **pruritus** (itchiness)
3. Affects infants, children, adolescents, and adults
4. 60 percent of affected children develop symptoms during infancy

B. Etiology and pathophysiology

1. Unknown etiology but occurs more frequently in children when one or both parents have allergies like asthma, hay fever, or contact dermatitis
2. Infantile eczema frequently related to food allergies
3. Eczema in older children often related to allergies to dust mites
4. Intensified by dry skin, detergents, constricting clothing, or perfumed soaps and lotions

NCLEX!

C. Assessment

1. In infancy, red **papules** (raised lesions) usually appear first on the cheeks and then spread to the forehead, scalp and down extensor surfaces of the arms and legs
2. Characterized by intense pruritus which causes excoriation of the skin that then leads to exudate and crust formation
3. Childhood stage may follow continuously from infancy or eczema may make first appearance in toddler
4. Childhood eczema characterized by dry, scaly, papular patches of skin on wrists, hands, ankles, antecubital and popliteal spaces
5. In adolescence, exudation often caused by external irritation or secondary infection
6. Adolescent eczema characterized by **lichenification** (large, dry, thickened lesions or plaques) on flexor folds, face, neck, back, upper arms, and dorsal aspects of hands, feet, fingers, and toes
7. Diagnosed by family history of allergies and inspection of skin
8. No laboratory test diagnostic for eczema

D. Priority nursing diagnoses

1. Impaired skin integrity
2. Risk for infection
3. Body image disturbance
4. Knowledge deficit

E. Planning and implementation

NCLEX!

1. Bathe or shower daily with tepid water using mild soap only on nonaffected areas
2. Do not use bath additives such as baking soda, bubble bath, or bath oils

NCLEX!

3. Pat, rather than rub, skin dry
4. Immediately after bath, apply emollient such as Eucerin or Lubriderm
5. Avoid use of perfumed or scented lotions
6. Apply wet wraps to severely affected skin after applying topical medications
7. Use antibacterial soaps for handwashing
8. Keep fingernails clean and short
9. Avoid wool or constricting clothing, which can promote itching or trap perspiration

NCLEX!

10. Place cotton gloves or socks over the hands of infants or young children to prevent itching
11. Provide support to the child and family during flare-ups and reassurance that lesions do not produce scars unless excessively scratched and secondarily infected

F. Medication therapy

1. Topical steroids (hydrocortisone 1% or triamcinolone 0.1%) are applied to lesions to reduce inflammation during flare-ups
2. Tar preparations are sometimes used during flare-ups when symptoms are mild
3. Antihistamines used to control itching
4. Oral antibiotics are used only if there is widespread skin breakdown or infection

G. Child and family education

1. Teach appropriate application of creams, ointments, or tar preparations
2. Teach proper application of soaks or compresses

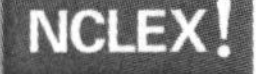

3. Identify foods that exacerbate the rash and avoid them
4. Explain the need to avoid getting sunburns

NCLEX!

5. Teach the need to avoid known or suspected contact allergens, pets, or environmental factors

6. Discuss with family the use of antihistamines before naps or bedtimes if sleep deprivation occurs caused by itching
7. Explain the importance of following the treatment plan to promote healing and prevent infections
8. Discuss the fact that the condition is not contagious
9. With infants, introduce one new food at a time to see if a flare-up occurs

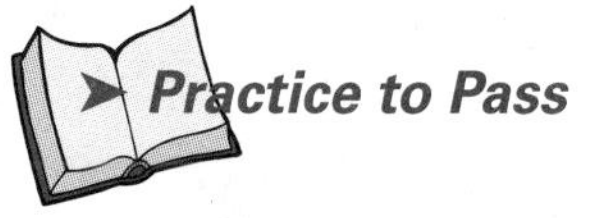

What comfort measures could the nurse suggest to the mother of an 8-month-old with eczema?

H. Evaluation: skin remains intact and free of secondary infection; child and family express positive image and demonstrate understanding of care during and between exacerbations

IV. Infectious Integumentary Health Problems

A. *Impetigo*

1. Description

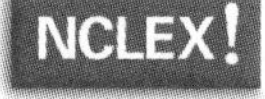

   a. A highly contagious, superficial skin infection caused by staphylococci or streptococci or both
   b. Accounts for almost 10 percent of all childhood skin disorders
   c. Most often occurs on face, neck, arms, hands, or legs

2. Etiology and pathophysiology
   a. Impetigo contagiosa (nonbullous) primarily caused by *group A beta-hemolytic streptococcus* and *Staphylococcus aureus* (*S. aureus*)
   b. Bullous impetigo always caused by *S. aureus*
   c. Causative bacteria are carried in nares and may pass onto skin
   d. Bacteria invade superficial skin in which a break has often occurred
   e. Infection can be spread after scratching an infected site
   f. Infection commonly acquired through contact with infected children who share toys, books, towels, or toiletries
   g. Infection may also be caused by direct skin contact during play or sports

3. Assessment
   a. Lesions are rarely painful but pruritus and burning may be present

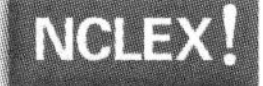

   b. Nonbullous impetigo begins as a single erythematous **macule** (nonraised discolored spot) 2 to 4 mm in diameter that rapidly progresses to a **vesicle** (small, blister-like elevation that contains serous fluid) or **pustule** (small, blister-like elevation that contains pus); vesicle ruptures leaving a honey-colored crust over the superficial erosion

NCLEX!

   c. Lesions rapidly spread to adjacent skin showing linear pattern of child's scratching
   d. Mild regional lymphadenopathy may occur
   e. Bullous impetigo lesions are usually less than 3 cm in diameter with little erythema that erupt on untraumatized skin

f. Characterized by **bullae** (fluid-filled lesions greater than 1 cm in diameter) that rupture and leave a varnish-like superficial erosion with little crusting

g. Tends to spread peripherally

h. Scraping from lesions show strep or *S. aureus*

4. Priority nursing diagnoses

    a. Impaired skin integrity

    b. Risk for infection

    c. Knowledge deficit

5. Planning and implementation

    a. Soak crusts in warm water

    NCLEX!

    b. Gently cleanse with antibacterial soap and remove crusts

    c. Do not touch or pick at lesions

    d. Child should wash hands frequently with antibacterial soap

    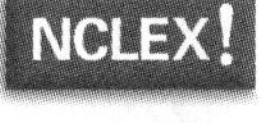

    e. Anyone who touches lesions should wash hands immediately with antibacterial soap

    NCLEX!

    f. Keep fingernails short and clean to prevent spread of infection from scratching

6. Medication therapy

    NCLEX!

    a. Apply topical antibiotic ointment such as Neosporin, Polysporin, Bacitracin, or mupirocin (Bactroban) 3 or 4 times daily for 5 to 7 days or as ordered

    b. Systemic antibiotic may be ordered, such as dicloxacillin (Dynapen), cephalexin (Keflex), cefaclor (Ceclor), or erythromycin, if no response to topical antibiotics in 72 hours

7. Child and family education

    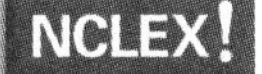

    a. Infection is communicable for 48 hours after antibiotic treatment is begun

    b. Child may return to daycare or school after 48 hours of therapy

    c. Inform school or daycare of infection so other children can be checked and so toys, etc. can be sanitized

    d. Family members and others in frequent contact with child should be checked for lesions

    e. Family members shouldn't share towels, washcloths, or clothes

    f. Linens and clothes of infected child should be washed separately

    NCLEX!

    g. Cleanse lesions and treat with antibiotics (topical and/or oral) for full length of prescription

8. Evaluation: improvement at site is seen within 72 hours; infection does not spread; family and child demonstrate safe and effective administration of ointments and oral antibiotics

B. *Pediculosis capitus* (head lice)

1. Description
   - **a.** Infestation of the hair and scalp with lice
   - **b.** Highly communicable parasite spread through direct contact (body to body, hair to hair) or indirect contact (clothing, brushes, hats, bedding)
2. Etiology and pathophysiology
   - **a.** Lice live and reproduce only on humans
   - **b.** Eggs (nits) are laid on hair shaft near the scalp
   - **c.** This is a common problem in child care centers and schools
   - **d.** Incidence is greatest in school-age children
   - **e.** Incubation period for nits is 8 to 10 days
   - **f.** It is least common among African-American children because of the shape of hair shaft
   - **g.** Lice can survive for up to 48 hours away from human host
   - **h.** Nits can survive for 8 to 10 days away from human host
   - **i.** Lice bites release saliva into the dermis, which causes itching
   - **j.** Severity of symptoms are usually proportional to the degree of infestation
3. Assessment

NCLEX!

   - **a.** Look for presence of whitish nits, about 1 mm in diameter, attached to hair shafts near scalp
   - **b.** Nits are most commonly found behind ears and on crown of head and nape of neck
   - **c.** Adult lice have six legs and range from light beige to black in color; may be seen on scalp
   - **d.** Infestation is characterized by intense continuous pruritus on scalp
   - **e.** Itching may cause erythema, scaling, and skin excoriation
   - **f.** Secondary infection may occur in excoriated areas
4. Priority nursing diagnoses
   - **a.** Health-seeking behaviors
   - **b.** Risk for infection
   - **c.** Pain
   - **d.** Knowledge deficit
5. Planning and implementation

NCLEX!

   - **a.** Apply about 2 ounces of pediculicidal agent onto wet hair and add additional water to make a lather

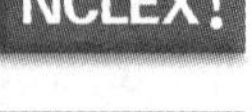

   - **b.** Allow lather to remain on hair for 10 minutes; do not allow to remain longer because of toxicity

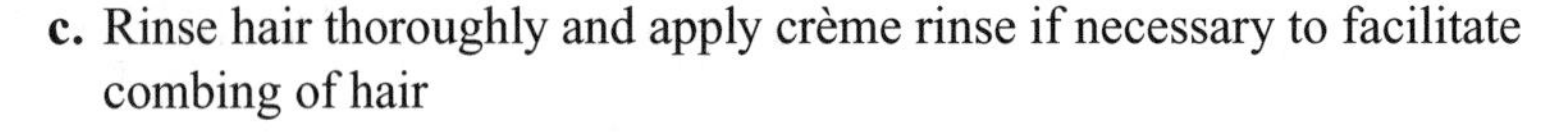

c. Rinse hair thoroughly and apply crème rinse if necessary to facilitate combing of hair

d. Remove nits from damp hair by dividing hair into 1-inch sections and using a fine-tooth comb

e. Begin at crown of head first

f. Pin hair out of the way when a section has been thoroughly combed

NCLEX!

g. Delouse the environment by washing all of child's daily clothes and linens in hot water with detergent and drying for at least 20 minutes in a hot dryer

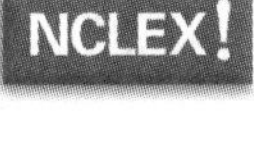

h. Stuffed toys and bedding that cannot be washed should be sealed in plastic bags for 2 weeks to make sure any nits are dead

i. Vacuum all floors, rugs, furniture, and play areas

NCLEX!

j. Combs, brushes, and hair ornaments should be discarded or soaked for 1 hour in a solution made from anti-lice shampoo or Lysol diluted with water

6. Medication therapy

NCLEX!

a. Over-the-counter pediculicidal agents include permethrin (Nix), pyrethrum (Rid), and lindane (Kwell)

b. After initial treatment, one additional treatment may be needed no sooner than 7 days

7. Child and family education

a. Inform the parents to notify child care center or school of lice infestation so other children may be checked

b. Inform parents that child may return to child care center or school following treatment

NCLEX!

c. Explain to parents that all other persons in the household and other contacts should be checked for lice

d. Teach children not to share hats, combs, hair ornaments, towels, etc

NCLEX!

e. Explain to child and family that treatment plan must be followed meticulously or live lice or nits may reinfest the child and others

f. Explain that nit removal is time-consuming and may be uncomfortable for the child, especially those with long or thick hair

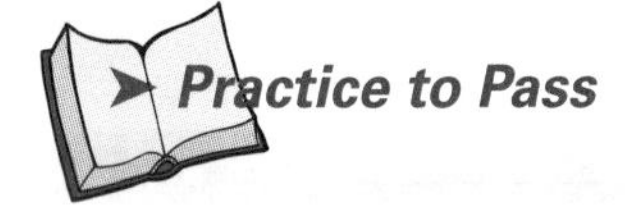

Practice to Pass

What measures should the nurse suggest as important to rid the home of lice and nits?

g. Teach family members how to examine for and identify lice and nits

h. Explain that a second treatment with anti-lice shampoo may be recommended 7 to 10 days after first treatment

i. Explain to family that lice affects children of all socioeconomic levels

j. Provide support and reassurance to family that may be embarrassed by a lice infestation

8. Evaluation: lice infestation is cleared; secondary infection does not develop; family and child demonstrate safe and effective administration of therapy

C. *Scabies*

1. Description

a. Contagious skin condition caused by the human mite *Sarcoptes scabiei*

b. Affects children (and adults) of all ages, socioeconomic levels, and both genders

c. Rash may have various types of lesions (papules, vesicles, or nodules)

d. Pruritus is severe, especially at night

2. Etiology and pathophysiology

a. Transmitted by close personal contact

b. Mite present on an infected child is attracted to odor and warmth of uninfected child

c. Female mite burrows into outer layer of epidermis to lay eggs, 1 to 3 eggs per day for 15 to 30 days before dying

d. Larvae hatch in several days and move toward skin surface

e. After mating the males die and females continue the reproductive cycle of burrowing, hatching, and mating

f. Mite secretions, ova, and feces are highly irritating so itching begins about 1 month after infestation

3. Assessment

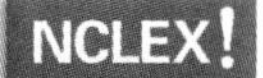

a. Intense pruritus, especially at night and nap times

b. Infants and young children may be irritable, restless, and sleep fitfully

NCLEX!

c. Lesions appear as linear, grayish burrows 1 to 10 cm long ending in a pinpoint vesicle, papule, or nodule

d. Burrows may be obliterated by excoriation from scratching

e. In infants and young children, lesions are often found on palms, soles, and axilla

f. In older children, lesions are often found in the webs of the fingers, body creases, axilla, waistline, and near genitalia

g. Skin scraping from a burrow examined under a microscope may reveal mites, ova, or feces

4. Priority nursing diagnoses

a. Impaired skin integrity

b. Pain

c. Risk for infection

d. Knowledge deficit

5. Planning and implementation

a. Give child a warm soap and water bath

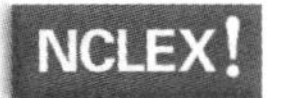

b. Apply scabicidal lotion to cool, dry skin over the entire body from the chin down

c. Leave on for 8 to 12 hours before washing off

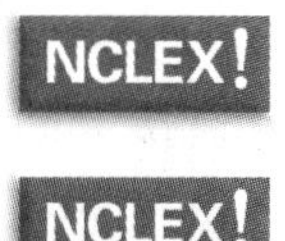

d. Lotion may be applied to the face of children over the age of 2 months if lesions are present

1) Do not apply to entire face of infants, only to scalp and forehead if necessary

2) Special attention should be paid to application of the lotion in the skin folds, between fingers and toes, ears, navel, and under fingernails

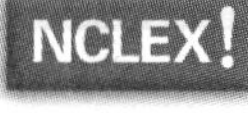

e. All family members and close contacts (playmates and caregivers) should be treated

f. Clothing, bedding, and towels should be changed daily and washed in hot water and dried in a hot dryer

g. Vacuum floors, carpets, and furniture

h. Items that cannot be washed should be sealed in plastic bags for 4 days before use

i. Provide support to family that may be distressed and believe scabies resulted from poor hygiene or unsanitary conditions

6. Medication therapy

a. Scabicidal medications include crotamiton (Eurax), permethrin 5% cream (Elimite), and lindane (Kwell, Scavene); lindane should not be used on infants or young children because of the risk of neurotoxicity and seizures

b. One liberal application should be sufficient

c. Follow directions precisely

d. Oral antihistamines may be prescribed to reduce pruritus in older children

e. Soothing creams or lotions may also be used to reduce pruritus

f. Antibiotics are only prescribed if secondary infection develops

7. Client and family education

a. Not all lesions clear immediately and, along with pruritus, may persist for 2 to 3 weeks until epidermis is replaced by natural shedding

b. Inform child care center or school of scabies

c. Child may return to child care center or school following treatment

d. All persons in the household and close contacts should be treated

e. Treatment plan should be followed meticulously

How will the school nurse differentiate impetigo from scabies?

f. Teach family how to examine for and identify signs of secondary infection

g. Scabies does not result from poor hygiene, unsanitary living conditions, or lack of vigilance on part of parents

h. Explain that children shouldn't share clothes, towels or hygiene items

8. Evaluation: scabies infestation is cleared; secondary infection does not develop; family and child describe care of infestation and environment

D. *Cellulitis*

1. Description

   a. Acute inflammation of the skin involving the epidermis, dermis, and underlying connective tissue

   b. Occurs in all age groups

   c. Most common site is legs but any area can be affected

2. Etiology and pathophysiology

   a. History of trauma, impetigo, recent otitis media, or sinusitis

   b. Infecting agents are usually *group A beta-hemolytic streptococcus* or *S. aureus*

   c. In the skin, these infecting agents produce large amounts of enzyme-spreading factors that break down the fibrin networks that usually contain or localize an infection

   d. Onset and spread may be rapid

   e. Cellulitis around the eye (periorbital cellulitis) usually results from a recent sinus infection

   f. Facial cellulitis in young children usually results from recent episode of otitis media

3. Assessment

   NCLEX!

   a. Children appear ill and are often febrile

   b. **Erythema** (diffuse redness) or lilac-tinged skin at site of cellulitis

   c. Pitting edema is frequently present over affected area

   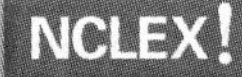

   d. Warmth and tenderness are present over affected site

   e. Reddish areas of "streaking" away from site may be present

   f. Regional lymph nodes are often enlarged

   g. Pain is present at site

   h. Border of affected area is usually indistinct and not elevated

   NCLEX!

   i. White blood count is elevated

   j. Blood cultures will identify infectious agent

   k. Fluid aspirated from lesion can be cultured to identify infectious agent

4. Priority nursing diagnoses

   a. Impaired skin integrity

   b. Pain

   c. Knowledge deficit

5. Planning and implementation

   a. Hospitalization is needed if cellulitis is on face or covers a large area, otherwise home management is preferred

b. Administer antibiotics, systemic if hospitalized or oral if at home

c. Monitor vital signs, especially temperature

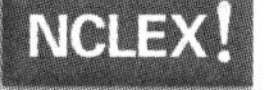

d. Apply warm compresses to affected area

e. Elevate affected limb

f. Maintain bed rest during acute phase

g. Apply non-occlusive dressing if there is a skin tear or rupture in affected area

6. Medication therapy

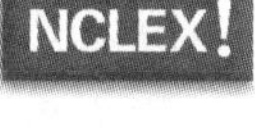

a. Broad spectrum parenteral antibiotics until infection subsides, then switch to oral; frequently prescribed antibiotics are nafcillin (Nafcil), dicloxacillin (Dynapen), or ceftriaxone (Rocephin)

NCLEX!

b. Oral antibiotic usually prescribed for 10 days; frequently prescribed antibiotics are Augmentin, oxacillin, or Bactrim

c. Acetaminophen given for pain or fever

7. Client and family education

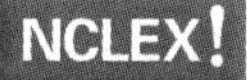

a. Teach the parents to continue antibiotics for full duration of prescription

b. Explain to parents to continue warm compresses as needed

c. Explain to family to contact health care provider if increased temperature, pain, or swelling

d. Explain that marked improvement should be seen in 48 hours

8. Evaluation: infection clears within 10 days; family and child demonstrate safe and effective administration of antibiotics

Practice to Pass

What assessment data will the nurse collect when examining a toddler with what appears to be facial cellulitis?

V. Accidents and Injuries Causing Integumentary Health Problems: Burns

A. Description

1. Injury to the skin and possibly the subcutaneous tissue, caused by thermal, chemical, electrical or radioactive causes

2. Injury can range from mild redness and slight tenderness to massive tissue destruction covering a large surface area

3. Second-leading cause of injury or death in children under age 14

B. Etiology and pathophysiology

1. May be accidental or non-accidental (adult abuse or neglect)

2. Thermal burns: exposure of the skin to flames, scalds, or contact with a hot object

3. Chemical burns: exposure of the skin or mucous membranes to chemical or caustic agents

4. Electrical burns: exposure to electrical current in wires or appliances

5. Radioactive burns: exposure of the skin to sunlight or radioactive substances

6. Classification of burns based on depth of damage (see Table 10-1)

Table 10-1
Classification of Burns

Type of burn	Appearance	Depth	Healing
Superficial partial thickness (first-degree)	Red, dry skin	Epidermis	3–7 days without scarring
Partial thickness (second-degree)	Bright pink or red skin, moist, blisters	Epidermis and dermis	On own; may be grafted to speed healing if large area
Full thickness (third-degree)	Deep red, brown or black skin, may be charred	Epidermis, dermis, and underlying tissue (subcutaneous fat, perhaps muscle)	Requires grafting unless very small injury

7. Local and systemic effects are related to the extent of damage

a. In partial thickness (second-degree) burns substantial edema and capillary damage occur at the site of injury

b. In full thickness (third-degree) burns a systemic response occurs of increased capillary permeability, which causes loss of fluid, electrolytes, and plasma proteins

8. Severity of burns is also related to extent of body surface area affected and size and age of child; the Lund and Browder chart identifies extent of burn

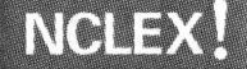

a. Minor burns: partial- and full-thickness burns to less than 10 percent of total body surface area (TBSA) with no other significant injuries; child is more than 5 years old; and no burns on hands, feet, genitalia, face, nor any circumferential burns

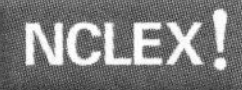

b. Major burns: full thickness burns of more than 10 percent of TBSA; burns of hands, feet, genitalia, face, or any circumferential burns; respiratory tract involvement; fractures or other soft tissue injuries; or deep chemical or electrical burns

9. The extent of injury is further determined by considering the intensity and duration of contact with the burn source (lower burn temperatures and shorter duration of contact can cause a more severe burn in a young child than an older one because of thinner skin)

10. In superficial burns (e.g., sunburn), damaged epithelium peels off in 5 to 10 days without scarring

11. In partial-thickness (second-degree) burns, crusts form in 3 to 5 days, and healing takes place from beneath

12. In full-thickness (third-degree) burns, healing is slow with thin epithelial covering in about a month; scarring is usual

13. Systemic effects of severe burns include asphyxia from smoke inhalation that causes edema of respiratory passages; shock from fluid shifts; renal failure from shock; protein loss from open wound; potassium excess from tissue destruction and renal failure

C. Assessment

1. Calculate TBSA involved

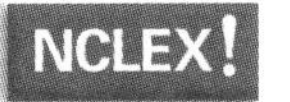

2. Burns covering more than 10 percent TBSA usually require fluid replacement

3. Assess depth of burn injury (refer back to Table 10-1)
4. Assess involvement of body parts

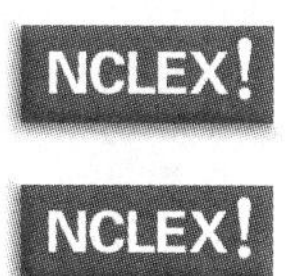

   a. Hands, feet, face, and perineal area burns have higher potential for functional impairment
   b. Circumferential burns (those surrounding an extremity or the trunk) are considered major burns
5. Pain that may be severe is present in superficial and partial-thickness burns

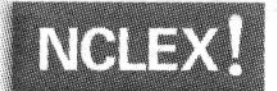

6. Third degree burns have no pain because nerve endings have been destroyed, though may feel pressure
7. Younger children have a higher mortality rate than older children with similar burns
8. Assess renal function and urine output
9. Perform respiratory assessment including rate, breath sounds, wheezing, hoarseness, smoky breath odor, or accessory muscle use; concurrent inhalation injury possible
10. Measure vital signs
11. Record weight, actual or stated

D. Priority nursing diagnoses

Practice to Pass

Describe the clinical manifestations of a second-degree burn.

1. Impaired skin integrity
2. Pain
3. High risk for infection
4. Risk for impaired circulation
5. Risk for fluid volume deficit or excess
6. Risk for altered nutrition
7. Risk for impaired mobility
8. Anxiety
9. Knowledge deficit

E. Planning and implementation

1. Administer analgesics as needed
   a. For major burns, morphine by the intravenous route is usually prescribed
   b. Administer analgesic about 30 minutes before wound care
2. Fluid replacement
   a. Place a large-bore peripheral IV in nonburned skin
   b. Ringer's lactate is the fluid of choice

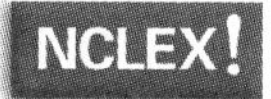

   c. Fluid replacement is based on a formula that considers body weight, body surface area, and maintenance needs
3. Insert Foley catheter; monitor intake and output

4. Monitor vital signs
5. Elevate burn site (if practical) to reduce edema
6. Administer tetanus toxoid unless immunization status is known
7. Keep environment warm to minimize heat loss

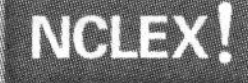

8. Prevent wound infection
   a. Apply topical antimicrobials to small burns
   b. Major burns may use mafenide (Sulfamylon), silver sulfadiazine (Silvadene), or bacitracin as topical antimicrobials
   c. Use medical and surgical asepsis
   d. Infants and young children may need to be restrained
   e. Use systemic antibiotics as needed
9. Monitor bowel function; major burns may cause paralytic ileus or occult bleeding from stress ulcer
10. Give high-calorie, high-protein, high-carbohydrate diet to promote wound healing
    a. Tube feeding or hyperalimentation (total parenteral nutrition) may be needed in major burns
    b. Vitamin and mineral supplements given as necessary
11. Perform active or passive range of motion (ROM) exercises if possible
12. Debride wound every 8 to 12 hours as ordered
13. In major burns, prepare for hydrotherapy to cleanse wound
14. Weigh daily to aid in calculation of fluid replacement, medication dosages, and caloric needs
15. Provide care for skin graft and donor sites as ordered if procedure is necessary
16. Work with health care team to plan for rehabilitation and home care
17. Provide emotional support to child and family who may fear pain and disfigurement

F. Medication therapy

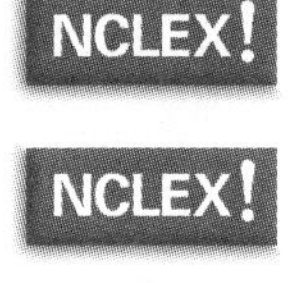

1. Analgesics for pain control; narcotics (morphine sulfate) are the drug of choice for major burns
2. Antibiotics for prevention of infection; systemic antibiotics rarely used unless systemic infection present
   a. Mafenide (Sulfamylon) is applied in thin layer over open wound and covered with dressing

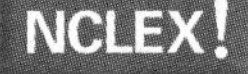

   b. Sulfadiazine (Silvadene) is applied in thin layer over open wound and covered with dressing; use with caution when impaired renal function exists; must be washed off and reapplied every 8 to 12 hours

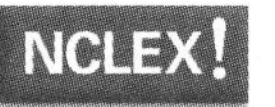

3. H_2-receptor antagonists such as cimetidine (Tagamet), ranitidine (Zantac), or famotidine (Pepcid) are given to prevent stress ulcers in major burns

G. **Evaluation:** pain is controlled; wound infection and systemic complications do not develop; disfigurement is minimized; child and family describe purpose of therapy; child and family describe safe and effective antibiotic administration; child follows through on therapy

Case Study

You are a school nurse. A 7-year-old boy has what looks like impetigo on his right forearm. You call the mother at work at 10:00 A.M. and ask her to come immediately to pick up her son and seek medical attention.

1. What did you see that made you suspect impetigo?
2. Why should the child not be sent home on the bus with a note for the mother?
3. How will the mother be expected to care for her son at home?
4. What are the primary goals in treating impetigo?
5. When do you expect the child to return to school?

For suggested responses, see page 410.

Posttest

1 **A 4-year-old child was just diagnosed with impetigo. What is the most important action the nurse should take to make sure it does not spread?**

(1) Apply bacitracin.
(2) Keep it covered.
(3) Isolate the child at home.
(4) Teach and use good handwashing.

2 **Which of the following would be appropriate home care instructions for a family that has a lice infestation?**

(1) Immerse combs and brushes in boiling water for 30 minutes to kill lice.
(2) Vacuum floor and furniture to remove hair that might have live nits.
(3) Take the child's clothing and bed linens to a dry cleaner for sanitation.
(4) Use commercial anti-lice sprays on furniture and mattresses.

3 **A 10-year-old child sustained partial thickness burns to his right arm and abdomen after tossing gasoline on a fire. What would the nurse expect the appearance of the burn site to be?**

(1) Smooth and bright red
(2) Bright red with numerous blisters
(3) White and waxy
(4) Dark brown and firm

4 **Permethrin 5% (Elimite) is prescribed for a 10-year-old child diagnosed with scabies. What instructions should the nurse provide for the mother?**

(1) Apply the lotion liberally from head to toe.
(2) Wrap the child in a clean sheet after treatment.
(3) Leave the lotion on for 4 to 6 hours.
(4) Apply lotion only after the child has had a bath and dried thoroughly.

5 **When assessing a child with a possible diagnosis of facial cellulitis, the nurse will want to question the parent about a recent history of:**

(1) Otitis media.
(2) Cat scratch.
(3) Sunburn.
(4) Sinusitis.

6 In teaching a group of school children, a nurse would explain that lice on a child can be most easily spread by:

(1) Sitting close to someone who had lice.
(2) Sharing hats at recess.
(3) Riding in the same car.
(4) Riding on the same bus.

7 What would be an appropriate nursing goal for a 10-year-old girl with eczema of the elbows, hands, and face?

(1) Pain will be managed.
(2) Spread of infection will be prevented.
(3) Well-hydrated skin will be maintained.
(4) Dietary restriction will be maintained.

8 A 5-year-old boy was brought to the Emergency Department after being burned trying to put out a fire that started in his closet where he was playing with matches. What should be the priority nursing assessment?

(1) Level of pain
(2) Airway patency
(3) Psychosocial needs
(4) Signs of infection

9 Intravenous morphine is ordered for a 13-year-old boy hospitalized with major burns to 30 percent of his body. What is the rationale for IV morphine?

(1) Longer half-life
(2) Predictable absorption rate
(3) Prevents ileus
(4) Fewest side effects

10 The nurse is providing a teaching session for parents about over-the-counter treatment for head lice. Which of the following will be mentioned as appropriate for treating this problem?

(1) Neosporin
(2) Mafenide (Sulfamylon)
(3) Silver sulfadiazine (Silvadene)
(4) Permethrin (Nix)

See pages 262–263 for Answers and Rationales.

Answers and Rationales

Pretest

1 Answer: 3 ***Rationale:*** Hot water can exacerbate symptoms of eczema and increase pruritus. Tepid water feels more comfortable than cool water.
Cognitive Level: Application
Nursing Process: Implementation; ***Test Plan:*** PHYS

2 Answer: 2 ***Rationale:*** Impetigo remains contagious for 48 hours after antibiotics are begun. The presence or absence of crusts does not address the issue of contagion.
Cognitive Level: Application
Nursing Process: Planning; ***Test Plan:*** SECE

3 Answer: 3 ***Rationale:*** The characteristic appearance of *Pediculosis capitus* (lice) is nits that adhere to the hair shaft about 1/4-inch from the scalp. They cannot be easily brushed off as dandruff. Scabies, eczema, and impetigo do not typically appear on the scalp and present as skin lesions elsewhere on the body.
Cognitive Level: Analysis
Nursing Process: Assessment; ***Test Plan:*** PHYS

4 Answer: 4 ***Rationale:*** The fluid shift that occurs in burns leads to edema, so the burned extremity should always be elevated above the level of the heart.
Cognitive Level: Application
Nursing Process: Implementation; ***Test Plan:*** PHYS

5 Answer: 1 ***Rationale:*** Eczema in a young child tends to be characterized by dry, scaly crusts that are well circumscribed. Pruritus is always present.
Cognitive Level: Application
Nursing Process: Assessment; ***Test Plan:*** PHYS

6 Answer: 3 ***Rationale:*** About 60 percent of children with eczema have a family history of asthma or other allergy. Scabies is caused by contact with a mite; impetigo and cellulitis are bacterial infections.
Cognitive Level: Application
Nursing Process: Assessment; ***Test Plan:*** HPM

7 Answer: 2 ***Rationale:*** Sinusitis frequently precedes periorbital cellulitis. Facial cellulitis may be preceded

by otitis media. A dog bite could cause cellulitis anywhere. Sun exposure causes a thermal injury.
Cognitive Level: Analysis
Nursing Process: Assessment; ***Test Plan:*** PHYS

8 **Answer: 1** ***Rationale:*** The only way to eliminate the infectious agent is to complete the prescribed course of antibiotics. Strict bedrest is not indicated, although the child initially may feel more comfortable resting with the extremity elevated. Fluid intake has no effect on the course of the infection, which is not contagious; therefore, visitors do not have to be limited.
Cognitive Level: Application
Nursing Process: Implementation; ***Test Plan:*** PHYS

9 **Answer: 2** ***Rationale:*** Use water that is a comfortable temperature for the child. Use about 2 ounces of the prescribed shampoo and leave on only as long as directed on the bottle (no more than 10 minutes) because it is toxic.
Cognitive Level: Application
Nursing Process: Implementation; ***Test Plan:*** HPM

10 **Answer: 3** ***Rationale:*** A teenager can and should be part of the treatment plan. If itching is avoided to prevent excoriation and secondary infection, scarring is unlikely. Improvement is often slow, and the problem may persist into adulthood. Food avoidance will not change the course of the disease.
Cognitive Level: Analysis
Nursing Process: Planning; ***Test Plan:*** HPM

Posttest

1 **Answer: 4** ***Rationale:*** Handwashing is always the most important action that a nurse can take to prevent the spread of infection. Merely applying ointment or covering the site does not address the spread of infection, nor does isolation of a child at home. The nurse would teach the family the importance of good handwashing.
Cognitive Level: Analysis
Nursing Process: Implementation; ***Test Plan:*** SECE

2 **Answer: 2** ***Rationale:*** Live nits can hatch up to 8 to 10 days later, so it is important to remove them from the environment. Soaking combs in a Lysol or anti-lice shampoo mixture will kill lice or nits. Dry cleaning is not necessary because home washing and drying on hot settings will be sufficient to kill lice and nits. Use of commercial sprays is not recommended.
Cognitive Level: Application
Nursing Process: Implementation; ***Test Plan:*** SECE

3 **Answer: 2** ***Rationale:*** The characteristic appearance of second-degree burns is bright red skin with blisters of varying sizes. A first-degree burn typically only has pink or red skin. A third-degree burn may be dark in color, from deep red to black.
Cognitive Level: Analysis
Nursing Process: Analysis; ***Test Plan:*** PHYS

4 **Answer: 4** ***Rationale:*** Permethrin is applied to cool dry skin after a bath, but only from the neck down. The child may dress after the lotion is applied. It should be washed off after 8 to 12 hours. A second application is often prescribed for 1 week later.
Cognitive Level: Application
Nursing Process: Implementation; ***Test Plan:*** SECE

5 **Answer: 1** ***Rationale:*** A recent history of otitis media is often present in children with facial cellulitis. Sunburn would present as more diffuse and widespread redness. An insect or animal bite can be a cause of cellulitis, but in the case of a cellulitis on the face the nurse would question a recent history of an ear infection if a bite were not obvious.
Cognitive Level: Analysis
Nursing Process: Assessment; ***Test Plan:*** PHYS

6 **Answer: 2** ***Rationale:*** Lice can only be passed by direct contact because lice do not fly. The usual mode of transmission is sharing of hats, combs, brushes, or hair ornaments. Being close to someone in a classroom, bus, or car does not presuppose direct contact with hair or nits that have been shed on hair.
Cognitive Level: Analysis
Nursing Process: Implementation; ***Test Plan:*** SECE

7 **Answer: 3** ***Rationale:*** Keeping the skin well hydrated will prevent the need to scratch dry skin that can lead to excoriation and secondary infection. Eczema is not infectious, nor is it managed by dietary restrictions. Pruritus, not pain, is associated with eczema.
Cognitive Level: Analysis
Nursing Process: Planning; ***Test Plan:*** HPM

8 **Answer: 2** ***Rationale:*** Because he was in close proximity to the fire and tried to put it out, he is at risk of having inhaled smoke and therefore having a compromised airway. Assessing pain, psychosocial needs, or for infection occurs only after establishing airway patency.
Cognitive Level: Analysis
Nursing Process: Planning; ***Test Plan:*** PHYS

9 **Answer: 2** ***Rationale:*** The predictable rate of absorption makes IV morphine useful in treating severe pain. Side effects, including ileus, are considered secondary to the desired effect of predictability in managing pain. Knowing the half-life is not a rationale for use of IV morphine.
Cognitive Level: Analysis
Nursing Process: Analysis; ***Test Plan:*** PHYS

10 **Answer: 4** ***Rationale:*** Permethrin is the over-the-counter treatment of choice for head lice. Other choices are topical agents, but they would not be used for lice. Option 1 would be used for infection, while options 2 and 3 would be used to treat burns.
Cognitive Level: Application
Nursing Process: Implementation; ***Test Plan:*** HPM

References

Ball, J. & Bindler, R. (1999). *Pediatric nursing: Caring for children* (2nd ed.). Stamford, CT: Appleton & Lange, pp. 908–951, 1724.

Behrman, R. F., Kliegman, B. M., Jenson, H. R. (2000). *Nelson's textbook of pediatrics* (16th ed.). St. Louis: Mosby, pp. 287–293, 1994–1998, 2028–2030, 2043–2046.

Bowden, V. R., Dickey, S. B., & Greenberg, C. S. (1998). *Children and their families: The continuum of care.* Philadelphia: W. B. Saunders. pp. 1728–1783.

Hall, J. C. (1999). *Sauer's manual of skin diseases* (8th ed.). Philadelphia: Lippincott Williams & Wilkins, pp. 30–31, 227–231, 368–370.

Hay, W. W., Hayward, A. R., Levin, M. R., & Sondheim, J. M. (1999). *Current pediatric diagnosis and treatment.* Stamford, CT: Appleton & Lange, pp. 286–287, 347–359.

Hazinski, M. F. (1999). *Manual of pediatric critical care.* St. Louis: Mosby, pp. 629–637.

Hill, D. J., Sporik, R., Thorburne, J., & Hosking, C. S. (October 2000). The association of atopic dermatitis in infancy with immunoglobulin E food sensitization. *Journal of Pediatrics 137* (4): 475–479.

Huether, S. E. & McCance K. L. (2000). *Understanding pathophysiology* (2nd ed.). St. Louis: Mosby, pp. 1091–1139.

Jarvis, C. (2000). *Physical examination and health assessment* (3rd ed.). Philadelphia: W. B. Saunders, pp. 213–265.

Kozier, B., Erb, G., Berman, A. J., & Burke, K. (2000). *Fundamentals of nursing: Concepts, process, practice* (6th ed.). Upper Saddle River, NJ: Prentice Hall, Inc, pp. 541–548.

Lewis, S. M., Collier, I. C., & Heikemper, M. M. (2000). *Medical-surgical nursing: Assessment and management of clinical problems* (5th ed.). St. Louis: Mosby, pp. 482–550.

Wilson, B. A., Shannon, M. T., & Stang, C. L. (2001). *Nursing drug guide 2001.* Upper Saddle River, NJ: Prentice Hall, Inc., pp. 944–947.

Wong, D. (1999). *Nursing care of infants and children* (6th ed.). St. Louis: Mosby, pp. 400, 650–652, 839–845, 1336–1362.

CHAPTER 11

Immunologic Health Problems

Marilyn L. Weitzel, MSN, RN, Doctoral Candidate
Judy E. White, RNC, MA, MSN

CHAPTER OUTLINE

OBJECTIVES

- Identify data essential to the assessment of alterations in health of the immunologic system in a child.
- Discuss the clinical manifestations and pathophysiology of alterations in health of the immunologic system of a child.
- Discuss therapeutic management of a child with alterations in health of the immunologic system.
- Describe nursing management of a child with alterations in health of the immunologic system.

[Media Link]

Use the CD-ROM enclosed with this text, or log onto the address given to access the free, interactive Companion Website created for this series. The CD-ROM and Companion Website accompanying this book offer additional practice opportunities and information—NCLEX Review, Case Studies, Glossary, In Depth with NCLEX, and more.

www.prenhall.com/hogan

Review at a Glance

anaphylaxis *a severe, potentially fatal hypersensitivity reaction; the histamine released leads to respiratory and vascular changes*

antigen *a substance that possesses a unique configuration enabling the immune system to recognize it as foreign; any substance that causes the production of antibodies; antigens are usually large molecular-weight proteins*

antigen-antibody reaction *the attachment of an antibody to an antigen that forms the basis for B-cell-mediated immunity*

antibody *a protein produced by the immune system that binds to specific antigens and eliminates them from the body*

autoimmune disease *a disease process where the body identifies itself or a component of itself as foreign and attacks itself*

differential blood count *a blood test that indicates the percentages of the different types of white cells present in the blood and is sometimes useful in identifying the cause of an illness*

incubation period *the period between exposure to the antigen (bacterial or viral organism) and the formation of the first general symptoms of the disease*

immunity *the resistance of the body to the effects of a harmful organism or its toxin*

immunization *the process of introducing an antigen into the body, allowing immunity against a disease to develop naturally*

period of communicability *the period of time when an illness is directly or indirectly transmittable from one person to another*

prodromal period *the period of time between the initial symptoms and the presence of the full-blown disease*

sepsis *a generalized infection spread throughout the body through the bloodstream*

TORCH *an acronym for a complex of communicable diseases often present at birth; the acronym stands for T = toxoplasmosis; O = other (such as syphilis, hepatitis); R = rubella; C = cytomegalovirus; H = herpes simplex; this group of viruses can cause teratogenic effects to the unborn fetus*

vaccine *the specific medication given to stimulate an immune response*

Pretest

1 A 14-year-old child is receiving intravenous antibiotics for an infection. The physician has ordered gentamycin (Garamycin). Because of the side effects of this drug, the nurse would monitor:

(1) Temperature.
(2) Blood pressure.
(3) Intake and output.
(4) Breath sounds.

2 A 3-year-old child is admitted to the hospital to rule out an infection. Which diagnostic test is likely to differentiate an infection from an allergic response?

(1) Hemoglobin and hematocrit
(2) Red blood cell count
(3) White blood cell count differential
(4) Platelet agglutinization

3 A 2-year-old child has eczema that causes extreme itching. Treatment has not been able to control the rash. It has been determined that the primary allergen is wheat. An appropriate nursing diagnosis for this child would be:

(1) Risk for infection.
(2) Altered nutrition, more than body requirements.
(3) Ineffective infant feeding behavior.
(4) Noncompliance.

4 A child's mother tells the nurse that her child has been on steroids for several months. Which of the following vaccines is contraindicated?

(1) Tetanus toxoid
(2) Measles, mumps, and rubella (MMR) made from egg embryo
(3) Poliovirus vaccine inactivated
(4) Poliovirus vaccine live oral trivalent

5 A child with severe combined immunodeficiency disorder (SCID) is being discharged from the hospital to home. The nursing care goal for the client before and after discharge would be that the child:

(1) Remains well oxygenated.
(2) Remains free of infection.
(3) Maintains hydration.
(4) Avoids contact with other people.

6 **A child is being worked up for allergies. The mother asks how the diagnosis will be made. The nurse's response is based on the knowledge that allergies can be diagnosed based on:**

(1) Medical history of urticaria alone.
(2) IgG levels.
(3) Decreased eosinophil count.
(4) RAST test.

7 **A child is born with microcephaly. Part of his assessment includes a TORCH test. In providing client education, the nurse explains to the mother that TORCH test will assess for:**

(1) Presence of the TORCH virus.
(2) Complications of pregnancy.
(3) Presence of one or more specific viruses.
(4) Evidence of thalidomide poisoning.

8 **A 4-month-old infant has been admitted with a diagnosis of sepsis. The nurse would monitor the child for evidence of:**

(1) Hypothermia.
(2) Rash.
(3) Sunken fontanels.
(4) Glucosuria.

9 **A 12-year-old child with HIV+ antibodies is going home from the hospital. Which of the following are the most important home-going instructions?**

(1) Growth and developmental milestones
(2) Immunization schedules
(3) Lab studies and results
(4) Prevention of the spread of HIV

10 **A 4-year-old child has been exposed to chickenpox. After the nurse has provided information about chickenpox, the nurse asks the mother to repeat the information. The statement by the mother that indicates a need for additional information is:**

(1) "During the prodomal period, my child will have pox all over his body."
(2) "Chickenpox is a viral infection that can be spread to other children."
(3) "I should monitor my child for Reye syndrome, which is a complication of chickenpox."
(4) "My child should not visit my pregnant sister at this time."

See page 284 for Answers and Rationales.

I. Overview of the Anatomy and Physiology of the Immune System

A. Nonspecific *immunity* (the resistance of the body to a harmful organism)

1. Functional at birth
2. First line of defense
3. Reacts similarly to all invaders
4. Includes phagocytosis of foreign material by white blood cells
   a. Polymorphonuclear leukocytes or granulocytes, which include basophils, eosinophils, and neutrophils, are the most common type of white blood cells and are involved in the acute inflammatory process
   b. Monocytes migrate to the tissues where they become macrophages and have great phagocytic ability, functioning to eliminate foreign invaders and other material
   c. Lymphocytes include B lymphocytes (B cells) and T lymphocytes (T cells), which are responsible for the specific immune response as well as NK cells (Natural Killer cells) concerned with viral control as well as autoimmune responses

5. The "inflammatory response" is a nonspecific response to any tissue injury aimed at maintaining the body's homeostasis; chemicals are released from the injured cells, which cause blood vessels to dilate, bringing large numbers of neutrophils and macrophages to the area for phagocytosis of injured cells and foreign material, allowing healing to occur

B. Specific immune response

1. Second line of defense
2. Not functional at birth, must be learned by the body
3. Not fully functional until a child is 6 years old
4. Humoral immunity depends upon the antibody-producing abilities of B-cells
    a. In response to **antigens** (foreign substances that trigger an immune response), B-cells convert into plasma cells and secrete specific **antibodies** (immune system proteins) to assist the body in eliminating foreign proteins
    b. Five classes of antibodies with different functions
        1) IgG is the antibacterial and antiviral antibody found in large quantities in all body fluids; this antibody can cross the placenta; maternal IgG provides passive immunity for the first 6 months of the infant's life
        2) IgA is found in saliva, tears, bronchial secretions, mucous secretions of the small intestine, the vagina and in breast milk; IgA is not present at birth and reaches normal levels at 6 to 7 years of age
        3) IgM is the body's primary antibody response to an antigen; IgM levels are low at birth and reach adult levels by 1 year of age
        4) IgD's role in unknown but seems to be related to B-cell differentiation

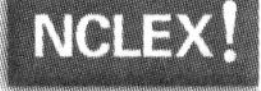

        5) IgE is normally found in very small amounts; IgE is associated with allergic reactions; elevated levels of IgE are associated with allergic individuals and clients infected with intestinal parasites; IgE is not present at birth
5. Cellular response
    a. T cells are produced in the thymus and function to protect the individual from intracellular organisms, viruses, and slow growing bacteria
    b. Responsible for the rejection of foreign grafts
    c. Specialized types of T cells include killer T cells, suppressor T cells, and helper T cells
    d. Killer T cells kill virus infected cells and depend upon IgG being bound to the cell
    e. Suppressor T cells inhibit the activities of other T and B cells
    f. Helper T cells help regulate the actions of B cells
6. Complement
    a. Enzyme that responds to **antigen-antibody reactions** causing inflammation and destruction of foreign cells

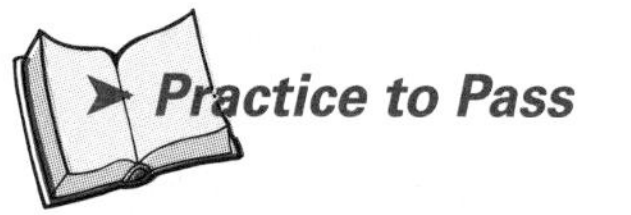

Compare and contrast nonspecific immunity and specific immunity.

b. Plays a role in **autoimmune diseases** (body attacks itself)

c. Levels of proteins lower in newborns than older children and adults

II. Diagnostic Tests and Assessments of the Immune System

A. Bone marrow aspiration: fluid-containing bone marrow cells are aspirated from the iliac crest to provide information about hematologic and immunologic disorders

1. Usually performed under local anesthesia
2. Post-procedure complications include bleeding and infection

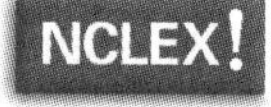

B. White cell differentials (*differential blood count*): compare the percentages of types of white cells against the whole; by evaluating the change in the types of white blood cells, information can be obtained related to the type of infection

1. Neutrophils rise in response to acute infections
2. Elevations in eosinophil counts are associated with allergies and parasitic infections as well as skin diseases such as eczema and psoriasis
3. Basophil counts may rise in response to chronic infection and stress; these white blood cells contribute to the inflammatory process and allergic reactions because they release histamine

C. Allergy testing

1. Determines reactions to specific antigens
2. Four types of allergy tests available

Practice to Pass

Describe the preparation of the client needed prior to bone marrow aspiration, WBC and differential, and allergy testing.

a. Scratch tests can test many antigens at once; although less sensitive than other allergy tests, results can be obtained in about 30 minutes

b. Prick test is similar to the scratch test in that antigens are placed on the skin; tends to be slightly more sensitive than the scratch test

c. Intradermal testing injects the antigen into the dermis; reactions are noted by redness and swelling

d. Radioallergosorbent testing (RAST) looks for allergen-specific IgE antibodies in a blood sample; it is no more sensitive than the other methods but does not involve the risk of **anaphylaxis** or other allergic reactions

III. Common Nursing Techniques and Procedures for the Immune System

1. Immunity from disease can be acquired either from exposure to the disease or by **immunization** (introducing an antigen into the body)

a. Active immunity involves the body's formation of antibodies in response to exposure to an antigen

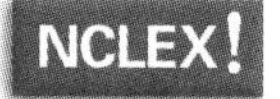

b. Passive immunity is temporary immunity achieved by the administration of antibodies produced by another individual; when antibodies pass from the mother to the fetus, passive immunity is acquired

2. **Vaccines** contain antigens to specific diseases; they cause the body to respond with the development of antibodies and active immunity

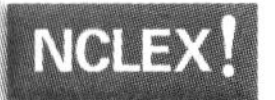

a. Vaccines may contain killed virus, live virus, or toxoids; live vaccines have weakened virus but still carry the risk of infection; killed virus and toxoid vaccines do not carry this risk; live vaccines should be avoided in the immunocompromised or pregnant client

b. Childhood vaccinations are currently recommended for hepatitis B, diphtheria, tetanus, pertussis, hemophilus influenzae B, polio, measles, mumps, rubella, and varicella; vaccinations for hepatitis A are also recommended in certain areas

c. Vaccination schedules allow initial vaccination to occur after passive immunity from the mother has disappeared; some vaccinations do not provide lifelong immunity and should be repeated

d. The American Academy of Pediatrics provides current recommendations on the vaccination schedule (see Chapter 1)

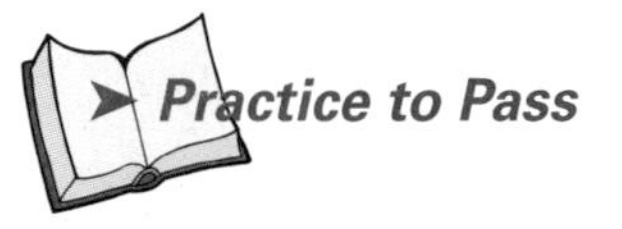

How does the nurse ensure practicing according to the current vaccine recommendations?

e. Prior to administering vaccinations, the absence of allergic reaction history should be verified

f. Instruct parents to maintain the vaccination schedule; if vaccinations are delayed, follow AAP recommendations for completing the vaccination program

IV. Congenital Immunologic Health Problems

A. Severe combined immunodeficiency disease

1. Description

a. Severe combined immunodeficiency disease (SCID) is the most severe of several different congenital disorders of the immune system yielding susceptibility to infections

b. Other forms of immunodeficiency include B cell and T cell deficiencies

2. Etiology and pathophysiology

a. SCID occurs as a result of x-linked recessive or autosomal recessive inheritence, as well as because of a spontaneous mutation

b. Characterized by absence of both humoral and cellular immunity

c. Maternal antibodies may protect the infant for a short period of time, but chronic infections become apparent around 3 months of age

d. Death usually occurs within the first 2 years of life

3. Assessment

NCLEX!

a. Initial infection often persistent thrush (oral candidiasis)

b. Followed by chronic infections

c. Organisms causing infection may include cytomegalovirus and *Pneumocystis carinii*

d. Failure to thrive also accompanies diagnosis

e. Leukocyte counts are usually reduced

4. Priority nursing diagnoses
   a. Risk for infection related to immunodeficiency
   b. Altered growth and development
   c. Altered nutrition: less than body requirements
   d. Risk for ineffective coping
5. Planning and implementation

NCLEX!

   a. Protecting the child from infection is of primary importance; careful handwashing is essential, as well as preventing contact with infected individuals
   b. Live plants and fresh flowers should be avoided as they harbor mold and bacteria
   c. While hospitalized, care should be taken in planning room assignment to reduce exposure to infection
   d. Bone marrow transplant offers the best hope for survival
6. Medication therapy
   a. Intravenous immune globulin (IVIG) (see Box 11-1)

Box 11-1

Nursing Considerations for the Administration of Intravenous Immune Globulin (IVIG)

Used in treatment of
- Immunodeficiency disease, such as severe combined immunodeficiency and acquired immunodeficiency syndrome (AIDS)
- Antibody deficiency associated with other conditions such as malignancy
- Kawasaki disease

Administration
- IVIG must be administered as stated in the package insert.
- Use separate tubing and do not mix with other medications.
- Start infusion slowly and increase to recommended rate after 30 minutes if no reaction occurs (see below).
- Monitor for hypersensitivity reaction (fever, increased pulse or respiration, decreased blood pressure, chest pain, shaking, chills).
- Schedule immunizations 14 days before or 3 months after IVIG infusion since immune response will be altered.

Possible adverse reactions
- Headache
- Fever
- Nausea, vomiting
- Arthralgia
- Anaphylaxis

Special types available
- RespiGam (helpful in respiratory syncytial virus)
- CytoGam (enriched with antibodies to cytomegalovirus)

Source: Ball, J. & Bindler, R. (1999). *Pediatric nursing: Caring for children* (2nd ed.). Stamford, CT: Appleton & Lange, p. 346.

NCLEX!

b. Immunizations should be administered 14 days prior to or 3 months after IVIG administration

c. Antibiotic therapy when indicated; monitor for overgrowth of nonsusceptible organisms

d. Maintain intact skin and mucous membranes

7. Client education

a. Teach the family ways to protect the child from infection

b. Provide emotional support and support group referrals

c. Genetic counseling provides the family with information about transmission

8. Evaluation: client remains free of infection; family demonstrates appropriate coping methods related to diagnosis and prognosis

V. Acquired Immunologic Health Problems

A. Allergies

1. Description

a. Hypersensitivity to a foreign protein

b. Antigen-antibody reaction causes release of histamine and other chemicals into the body; chemicals are responsible for allergic symptoms

c. Broad group of disorders; symptoms vary dependent on body cell that has been sensitized

2. Etiology and pathophysiology

a. First exposure to antigen causes the production of antibodies (usually IgE)

b. Subsequent exposure to same antigen causes an antigen-antibody reaction with cell damage causing release of histamine and other chemicals

c. Chemicals travel through bloodstream causing allergic symptoms

d. Most allergens are large molecular weight proteins

1) Common inhalant allergens include mold, pollen and house dust, pet dander

NCLEX!

2) Common food allergens include cow's milk, eggs, wheat, chocolate, citrus fruits

3) Drugs including oral and injectables

4) Animal serum/venom and insect stings

5) Contact allergens include plants, dyes, and chemicals

3. Assessment

a. Family history of allergies

b. History of reactions: allergy symptoms can be numerous

1) Respiratory system: allergic rhinitis, asthma, serous otitis media, allergic croup

2) Skin: eczema, atopic dermatitis, angioedema, urticaria
3) Gastrointestinal system: diarrhea, constipation, colic
4) Neurologic system: headache, tension-fatigue, convulsions
5) Genitourinary system: dysuria, enuresis
6) Miscellaneous: serum sickness and anaphylaxis

c. Elevated eosinophil counts

d. Allergy testing: Skin or RAST test

NCLEX!

1) Skin testing can involve a scratch or intradermal injection of small amounts of suspected allergens; the scratch test is often an initial diagnostic tool as it allows for testing a large number of allergens quickly with results in about 30 minutes; if the child is allergic to the allergen, a reddened wheal will form in 15 to 30 minutes; anaphylaxis is a rare but potential problem
2) The RAST test is a blood test looking for the specific IgE antibodies; used in individuals who have a history of a strong reaction, as this test allows no opportunity for anaphylaxis during testing; it is more expensive and felt to be less sensitive

4. Priority nursing diagnoses

a. Risk for injury

b. Altered tissue perfusion: cardiopulmonary

c. Impaired skin integrity

d. Diarrhea

e. Knowledge deficit

5. Planning and implementation

NCLEX!

a. Interventions are aimed at reducing exposure to allergen

1) Food: once food allergens are identified, all labels of prepared food should be carefully read to avoid allergens
2) Environment: create surface that's easily cleaned; focus in particular on child's bedroom; no carpet, bedroom curtains and bedding should be washable; avoid dust-collecting items in bedroom; avoid live plants and flowers; keep animals out of bedroom; no stuffed toys in bedroom
3) Inhalant: avoid cigarette smoking in child's presence and environment

b. Immunotherapy aims at increasing child's tolerance of allergen; also called hyposensitization or allergy shots, this therapy provides for the introduction of the allergen in small but increasing amounts by subcutaneous injections

1) Injections are given in controlled environment because of the risk of systemic reaction or anaphylaxis

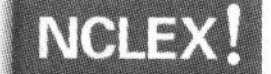

2) Child remains in controlled environment for 15 minutes post-injection to allow for monitoring of side effects
3) Emergency treatment must be readily available in case anaphylaxis occurs

6. Medication therapy

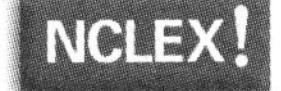

   a. Antihistamines are given prior to or early in the reactive phase; antihistamines compete with histamine on the receptor sites, therefore if given late in the reaction, will be ineffective

   b. Bronchodilators may be given for lower-respiratory symptoms

   c. Corticosteroids may be administered systemically or topically, depending upon symptoms

   d. Cromolyn sodium is a preventive medication for asthma; it is not useful during an acute attack

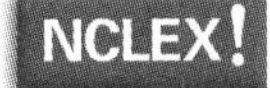

   e. Epinephrine is administered for anaphylaxis

7. Client education

   a. Parents and child should be taught to manage symptoms, control environmental exposure, and recognize medical emergencies

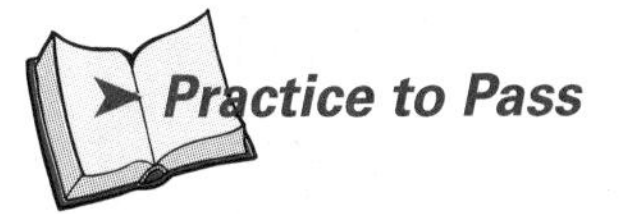

When a child develops an allergy, what kinds of life changes may need to be made?

   b. Obtain medic alert bracelets, especially for drug allergies

   c. Safe administration of medications

8. Evaluation: child and parents verbalize medication understanding, demonstrate their use correctly, and verbalize environmental control of allergens

VI. Infectious Immunologic Health Problems

A. TORCH

1. Description

NCLEX!

   a. **TORCH** is an acronym for a group of infections, which when acquired in utero, cause teratogenesis

      1) T is for toxoplasmosis: toxoplasmosis is an infectious disease by the organism *Toxoplasma gondii* and is usually contracted from cat feces and undercooked meats

      2) O is for other, which includes syphilis and hepatitis; congenital syphilis is caused by the spirochete *Treponema pallidum*

      3) R stands for rubella; also called German measles

      4) C refers to cytomegalovirus or CMV, a member of the herpes family

      5) H is for the herpes simplex virus

2. Etiology and pathophysiology

   a. Maternal exposure to organism allows fetal exposure through the placenta

   b. The earlier in the gestation that infection occurs, the greater the damage that may occur

   c. Mother may be asymptomatic during pregnancy and syndrome may not be recognized until after the baby is born

3. Assessment

   a. Assessment of the newborn is comprehensive, reviewing all systems

   b. Maternal history during pregnancy

c. Intrauterine growth retardation may be apparent at birth

NCLEX!

d. Symptoms including hydrocephalus, blindness, microcephaly, mental retardation, as well as failure to thrive, suggest TORCH infection; depending upon organism involved, the infant may also display jaundice, rash, deafness, cardiac defects

e. Serologic blood sampling for toxoplasmosis, rubella, CMV, and herpes; VDRL for syphlis and a hepatitis profile

4. Priority nursing diagnoses

   a. Altered nutrition: less than body requirements

   b. Risk for altered parent attachment

   c. Altered growth and development

5. Planning and implementation

NCLEX!

   a. The child should be isolated as virus may be shed for up to a year after birth; pregnant women are at increased risk

   b. Parents may grieve at the loss of the normal newborn; emotional support must be available

   c. Physical care supporting the infant's needs will be individualized

NCLEX!

   d. Nutritional support will be needed to support intake of food; the child may require a nasogastric or gastric tube or utilize a "premie" nipple to make sucking easier

6. Medication therapy

   a. Depends upon infectious organism

   b. For toxoplasmosis, an extended course of pyrimethamine (Daraprim) and sulfadiazine (generic) may be given; leucovorin may be added to reduce the bone marrow suppression

   c. Treatment for congenital syphlis is usually a 10 to 14 day course of penicillin

   d. Acyclovir (Zovirax) is used to treat infants with congenital herpes infection

7. Client education

   a. Parents are educated to meet the physical needs of their handicapped infant; nutrition support is of primary importance

   b. Infant stimulation to promote the physical development of the child; special instructions need to be given to assist the parents working with the blind or deaf child

   c. Instructions must be given about potential viral shedding; parents are instructed to avoid contact with pregnant women

8. Evaluation: parents verbalize and demonstrate appropriate child care measures including nutritional support; the parents express confidence in their ability to care for their child; the parents demonstrate safe medication administration

B. Sepsis

1. Description: **sepsis** is systemic bacterial infection spread through the bloodstream
2. Etiology and pathophysiology
   a. Neonates are at high risk because of the inability to localize an infectious organism; low birth weight is a risk factor for sepsis
   b. Immunocompromised children at high risk
   c. Children with skin defects/injuries or with invasive devices at high risk
   d. Organisms involved include *Escherichia coli,* pseudomonas, enterococcus, staphylococcus
3. Assessment
   a. Monitor clients for risk factors for sepsis

NCLEX!

   b. Hypothermia or hyperthermia
   c. Lethargy, poor feeding
   d. Jaundice or hepatosplenomegaly
   e. Respiratory distress
   f. Vomiting
   g. Hypoglycemia or hyperglycemia, metabolic acidosis
   h. CBC will indicate infection; blood culture will determine organism and sensitivities; spinal tap may be done to rule out meningitis
4. Priority nursing diagnoses
   a. Hypothermia
   b. Hyperthermia
   c. Ineffective infant feeding pattern
5. Planning and implementation

NCLEX!

   a. Maintain temperature within normal range with antipyretics as ordered, tepid sponge bath, appropriate clothing
   b. Monitor blood glucose; support nutrition; lethargy, hypoglycemia, and hyperthermia can all contribute to poor feeding
   c. Maintain antibiotic therapy on schedule, monitor for side effects
6. Medication therapy
   a. Antibiotic therapy based on culture and sensitivity
   b. Antipyretics such as acetaminophen (Tylenol) for elevated temperature
7. Client education
   a. Teach the parents how to monitor temperature and means of maintaining a neutral body temperature
   b. Instruct parents on the purpose of the antibiotics and potential side effects

8. Evaluation

a. Harmful sequelae of sepsis will be prevented

b. Parents are able to describe the purpose of the antibiotics and can list side effects for which the child is being monitored

C. Acquired immunodeficiency syndrome (AIDS)

1. Description: infection with retrovirus human immunodeficiency virus (HIV)

2. Etiology and pathophysiology

a. Virus transmitted through blood and body fluids of infected person

NCLEX!

b. Most common source of infection in children is perinatally, from an infected mother to her infant

1) Across the placenta

2) At the time of birth

3) Possibly through breast milk

c. Also could be contracted from transfusions with infected blood or blood products

d. Once in the body, the HIV enters the T lymphocytes, particularly the CD4 cell

e. The CD4 cell begins synthesis of the HIV DNA

f. Leads to death of CD4 cell

g. Infected child is susceptible to infection caused by deficiency in cell-mediated and humoral immunity

3. Assessment

a. Diagnostic tests for HIV start at birth; the child of the HIV-positive mother is followed up to 18 months before infection can be determined; tests are divided into early (birth, 3, and 6 months) and later (12, 15, and 18 months)

b. Early tests to detect the HIV antigen (p24 antigen), HIV (HIV culture and polymerase chain reaction [PCR])

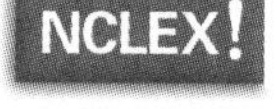

c. After maternal antibodies have disappeared, ELISA test (enzyme-linked immunosorbent assay)

d. CBC and CD4 levels

NCLEX!

e. Presenting symptoms include chronic diarrhea, failure to thrive, delayed development

NCLEX!

f. Frequent infections including candidiasis, *Streptococcus pneumoniae, Hemophilus influenzae, Staphylococcus aureus,* and herpes simplex

g. Opportunistic infections including *pneumocystis carinii*

4. Priority nursing diagnoses

a. Risk for infection related to immunosuppression secondary to HIV infection

b. Altered nutrition: less than body requirements

c. Ineffective family coping

5. Planning and implementation

NCLEX!

a. Focus on preventing infection

1) Normal health precautions including handwashing, avoiding contact with infected persons, maintaining nutritional status, good skin care, promoting a hygienic environment.

2) Immunizations on schedule; the child and all household contacts should avoid immunization with live virus vaccines

3) Following medical orders on prophylactic drugs

NCLEX!

b. Management of symptoms

1) Diarrhea management, monitoring hydration and nutrition status, maintaining skin integrity

2) Monitoring for infection including pneumonia, meningitis, otitis media and others

3) Support of family coping

a) Encourage participation in parent support groups

b) Demonstrate acceptance of child during everyday contact

c) Utilize communication skills to allow parents to verbalize feelings

6. Medication therapy

a. Prophylaxis treatment

1) Against HIV: zidovudine (AZT)

2) Against *pneumocystis carinii*: trimethoprim-sulfamethoxazole (Bactrim or Septra)

3) Against bacterial infections: intravenous immune globulin (IVIG)

NCLEX!

b. Infections: appropriate antimicrobial therapy; for antibiotic therapy, see Table 11-1

7. Client education

a. Information is presented on preventing the spread of HIV to other members of the household and those having contact with the child

b. Parents are taught to maintain a clean home environment and ways to reduce bacterial exposure

c. Information about nutritional support, diarrhea, and skin management as well as medication regimen is given

d. Developmental stimulation information is shared with the parents

e. Infection monitoring information is given to the parents

8. Evaluation: parents verbalize medication regimen, describe safety measures to prevent infection, identify symptoms of infection to be reported to physician, discuss their concerns about caring for this child, and join a support group

Table 11-1 Antibiotics

Classification and Examples	Mechanism	Common Side Effects	Nursing Responsibilities & Additional Comments
Penicillins 4 generations including natural penicillins (Penicillin G, Pen Vee K); Penicillinase resistant (Methicillin, Dynapen); Extended spectrum (Ampicillin, Amoxicillin); and Antipseudomonal (Ticar, Pipracil)	Inhibits cell wall synthesis; indicated for Gram-positive and Gram-negative infections	Allergic—rash, anaphylaxis; loss of normal flora—black furry tongue, diarrhea; hematologic—hemolytic anemia or leukopenia; electrolyte imbalances	First antibiotic; first cases of antibiotic resistance occurred when bacteria began forming penicillinase, which deactivates penicillin
Cephalosporins (Keflin, Ancef, Ceclor, Mandol)	Prevents production of enzymes which makes cell wall rigid; use for Gram-positive and Gram-negative infections	Allergy; may be neurotoxic and cause seizures in clients with preexisting renal disease	Use caution, many cephalosporins have similar names (keflex, keflin; cefoxitin sodium, ceftizoxime sodium) but are not the same drug or generation of cephalosporin
Aminoglycosides (Neomycin, Kanamycin, Gentamicin)	Gram-negative infections	Ototoxicity; nephrotoxicity	Not absorbed well through the GI tract, usually administered IM or IV; contraindicated with renal impairment or hearing disorders; peak and trough levels are usually ordered to monitor for toxicity; when concomitantly administered with penicillin, separate by time and use separate IV lines
Vancomycin (Vancocin)	Inhibits cell wall synthesis; used for Gram-positive infection, staphylococcus and *clostridium difficile*	Ototoxicity, nephrotoxicity, hypotension (red man syndrome)	Not given IM; give IV slowly to prevention hypotension; if hypotension occurs, stop drug and notify MD; after administration of antihistamine, may slowly restart drug
Macrolides (Erythromycin)	Bacteriostatic; use is similar to narrow-spectrum penicillin	Hepatotoxicity, ototoxicity, phlebitis	CDC has reported a possible link between erythromycin and pyloric stenosis; monitor infant for symptoms; inhibits metabolism of theophyllin—may lead to theophyllin toxicity
Quinolones (Cipro, Floxin)	Broad-spectrum; soft-tissue infections	Nausea, headache, dizziness, confusion	Contrindications include clients under 17; interferes with theophyllin and coumadin
Streptogramins (Synercid)	One of two new classes of antibiotics; bacteriostatic; effective against methicillin and vancomycin-resistant organisms	Thrombophlebitis, rash, arthralgia, elevated bilirubin levels	Incompatible with saline and heparin flush solutions—flush with D_5W; use with caution in clients with liver disease
Oxazolidinone (Zyvox)	New class of antibiotics; indicated for vancomycin- and methicillin-resistant organisms	Thrombocytopenia	Assess for signs of bleeding; monitor platelet count as ordered

D. Childhood communicable diseases

1. Description: a group of diseases common during childhood
2. Etiology and pathophysiology
    a. Variety of diseases spread from person to person
    b. Infectious organism often viral
    c. Mode of transmission describes how the organism moves from one individual to another
    d. **Incubation period** describes the time between exposure to the disease and disease outbreak; during this time, the child may be contagious
    e. **Period of communicability** is the time period when the organism can move from the host to another individual
3. Assessment
    a. Nurses in contact with children should be constantly alert to the appearance of symptoms associated with the childhood diseases and take measures to prevent the spread the infection to other children
    b. Client history will include record of vaccinations as well as history of exposure to children with communicable diseases
    c. Regardless of the reason the child is seeking treatment, all children should be assessed for symptoms of communicable diseases including rashes, temperature, and swollen glands
    d. The period of time between the initial symptoms and the presence of the full-blown disease is called the **prodromal period**
4. Priority nursing diagnoses
    a. Hyperthermia
    b. Risk for injury secondary to complications of childhood diseases
    c. Body image disturbance
    d. Risk for impaired skin integrity related to scratching secondary to itch
    e. Social isolation
5. Planning and implementation
    a. Immediate steps are taken to reduce exposure of other children to the possibly infected child
    b. Monitor temperature and use temperature control measures to reduce hyperthermia
        1) Tepid baths
        2) Limit clothing and bed coverings

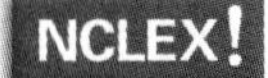

        3) Give NSAIDs as ordered; avoid aspirin as aspirin intake with a viral infection may contribute to the development of Reye syndrome
        4) Increase liquid intake

c. Provide skin care to prevent breakdown

1) If child is scratching, keep nails short, and use topical anti-itch medications

2) If skin is intact but dry, apply moisturizers

d. Bed rest is usually recommended during prodomal and/or febrile phases of the infectious diseases

1) Provide activities that allow quiet play

2) Activities that include socialization are preferred over solo activities

e. Monitor child for signs of complications of specific illness (see Table 11-2)

Table 11-2 Childhood Communicable Diseases

Disease Information	Clinical Manifestations	Clinical Management	Potential Complication
Rubeola: Red Measles *Causal agent:* Virus *Transmission:* Airborne *Incubation:* 10–20 days *Communicability:* Several days before rash appearance to 5 days after rash appearance *Immunity:* From vaccination or disease	*Prodromal:* Fever and lethargy, cough, and coryza; photophobia; koplik spots on buccal mucosa *Acute:* Red, flat rash (lasting about a week) begins behind ears, spreads to face, trunk and extremities	Manage temperature, keep room dim, vaporizer may improve respiratory secretions	Pneumonia: monitor lung sounds; otitis media: monitor ear pain; encephalitis: monitor for headache, vomiting, seizures
Rubella: German or 3-day measles *Causal agent:* Virus *Transmission:* Droplets *Incubation:* 2–3 weeks *Communicability:* 1 week before to 5 days after onset of rash *Immunity:* From vaccination or disease	*Prodromal:* Low-grade temperature, headache, sore throat and cough *Acute:* Flat red rash begins on face and spreads to rest of body; rash lasts 3 days	Nonaspirin antipyretics; encourage fluid; recommend to avoid contact with all pregnant women; nonimmune females should be immunized before reaching childbearing age	Usually benign childhood disease; greatest risk to fetus, especially in 1st trimester
Parotitis: Mumps *Causal agent:* Virus *Transmission:* Droplet or direct contact *Incubation:* 2 to 3 weeks *Communicability:* 1 week before parotid swelling until 1 week after swelling begins *Immunity:* From vaccination or disease	*Prodromal:* Fever, headache, earache that worsens with chewing *Acute:* Swelling of parotid glands	Nonaspirin antipyretics; fluids and soft liquids are easier to swallow; avoid sour foods	Orchitis: monitor for testicular swelling; encephalitis: monitor for headache and vomiting; deafness: monitor for signs of hearing loss
Varicella: Chickenpox *Causal agent:* Virus *Transmission:* Direct contact and airborne *Incubation:* 2–3 weeks *Communicability:* Day(s) before rash to 1 week after first lesions crust over *Immunity:* From vaccination or disease	*Prodromal:* Mild fever and malaise for 24 hours *Acute:* Rash that progresses from macule to vesicle to crusts; eruption lasts up to 5 days and lesions of all types will be present at one time	Acyclovir may be administered or IVIG may be administered to high-risk child; nonaspirin antipyretics, calamine lotion topically, oral antihistamines, oatmeal and Aveeno™ baths; keep nails short, discourage scratching	Encephalitis: Monitor for headaches and vomiting; Reye syndrome: monitor for vomiting and mental confusion—seek medical treatment immediately if seen

6. Medication therapy

   a. Antibiotic therapy usually not recommended unless secondary bacterial infection occurs

   b. Antipyretics, analgesics, and anti-inflammatory drugs may be ordered; aspirin is usually contraindicated in acute viral infections

7. Client education

   a. Instructions should be given regarding available vaccines to prevent the development of childhood contagious diseases

   b. Information should be given regarding isolation precautions for the illness

   c. Parents should be aware of symptoms that indicate the development of complications of the specific illness

8. Evaluation: client receives vaccinations on schedule; client develops no complications of childhood communicable disease; parents describe isolation precautions for their child with a communicable disease

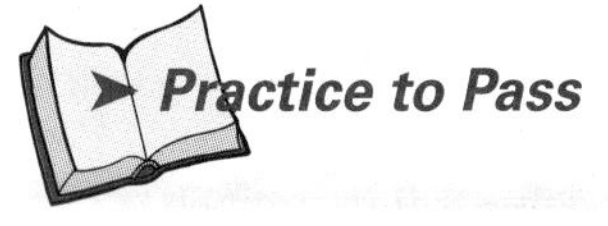

Discuss the four stages of a communicable disease.

Case Study

A 5-year-old child is admitted to the clinic with symptoms of elevated temperature, cough, and rhinitis. He also exhibits one small round red spot on his abdomen.

1. What diagnostic tests does the nurse prepare to do?
2. During the nursing assessment, what specific information does the nurse ask for?
3. What are three priority potential nursing diagnoses?
4. Discuss three nursing interventions appropriate for this child.
5. What criteria would guide the evaluation of this client?

For suggested responses, see pages 410–411.

Posttest

1 **The nurse has explained allergy-proofing the home to the mother of a child with dust allergies. Which statement by the mother indicates a clear understanding of appropriate allergy proofing?**

(1) "I'm going to replace the cotton curtains on the window with blinds."
(2) "The only toys allowed in his bedroom are his stuffed toys."
(3) "I should store his out-of-season clothes in his bedroom."
(4) "The mattress and box springs both need to be enclosed in a thick plastic cover."

2 **A child is in the clinic for a prick test. Because of the risk of anaphylaxis, the nurse has available for emergency treatment:**

(1) Epinephrine.
(2) Corticosteroids.
(3) Narcan.
(4) Cromolyn sodium.

3 A mother brings a 3-year-old child to the clinic for a well-child checkup. The child has not been to the clinic since 6 months of age. What is the priority of care for this child?

(1) Assess growth and development
(2) Begin dental care
(3) Update vaccinations
(4) Complete hearing screening

4 The mother of a 1-year-old child says that breast-feeding her infant is sufficient to provide immunity. She does not want to sign the permit for immunizations. What is the nurse's best response?

(1) Discuss active and passive immunity.
(2) Tell her immunizations are legally mandatory.
(3) Ask about the mother's diet.
(4) Allow her the right to refuse.

5 The nurse is caring for several children on a hospital unit where there has been a recent outbreak of diarrhea. None of these children were admitted for diarrhea, but the nurse is aware that they may be exposed. Of the children on the unit, the one most susceptible would be the:

(1) Toddler with SCID.
(2) Preschooler in traction for a fractured femur.
(3) School-age child with eczema.
(4) Teenager with frequent stools secondary to malabsorption syndrome.

6 A child is admitted to the hospital with an allergic reaction. The physician orders a CBC with differential. The nurse would expect to see an elevation in the level of:

(1) RBCs.
(2) Hemoglobin.
(3) Leukocytes.
(4) Eosinophils.

7 A child is being discharged from the nursery with a positive TORCH titer. Parents should be informed that:

(1) The child may shed the virus for a year.
(2) TORCH is a genetic disorder.
(3) No follow-up is necessary.
(4) Medication will not be needed for this condition.

8 An infant with AIDS will be attending daycare. The daycare workers are concerned about spreading the virus. The public health nurse is explaining to the workers the precautions they should take. These precautions include:

(1) Storing all of this infant's supplies separately from the other children.
(2) Wearing gloves when changing the child's diapers.
(3) Always wearing gloves and isolation gowns when handling the infant.
(4) Minimizing contact with the infant when he is febrile.

9 A mother overhears two nurses discussing a measles outbreak. The nurses are talking about the incubation period. The mother asks the nurses why it is important to know the incubation period for a childhood disease. The nurses' reply would be based on the knowledge that the incubation period:

(1) Describes a period when the child might be contagious.
(2) Determines the severity of the infection.
(3) Varies depending on the age of the child.
(4) Is a period of time when medications can prevent the development of symptoms.

10 An infant is admitted to the pediatric hospital straight from the birth hospital with numerous congenital defects and a diagnosis of rule out TORCH syndrome. The father tells the pediatric nurse that he and his wife had planned a beautiful birth experience and can't believe what's happened. An appropriate nursing diagnosis for this family would be:

(1) Risk for caregiver role strain.
(2) Situational low self-esteem.
(3) Risk for altered parent/infant attachment.
(4) Parental role conflict.

See pages 284–285 for Answers and Rationales.

Answers and Rationales

Pretest

1 **Answer: 3** ***Rationale:*** One of the most common side effects of gentamycin is nephrotoxicity. The nurse can monitor kidney function by monitoring intake and output.
Cognitive Level: Application
Nursing Process: Assessment; ***Test Plan:*** PHYS

2 **Answer: 3** ***Rationale:*** White blood cells are one component of the general nonspecific immune response. They among the first responders stimulated by a pathogenic organism. A white blood cell differential can often determine if the illness is of bacterial, viral, or allergic origin.
Cognitive Level: Application
Nursing Process: Planning; ***Test Plan:*** HPM

3 **Answer: 1** ***Rationale:*** Because of the itching, the child will be scratching. Intense scratching can break the skin, and the child might develop a bacterial infection secondary to the skin trauma. Altered nutrition, more than body requirements, does not clearly state the problem with the food allergies, nor does ineffective infant feeding behavior. There is no evidence of noncompliance.
Cognitive Level: Analysis
Nursing Process: Planning; ***Test Plan:*** HPM

4 **Answer: 4** ***Rationale:*** Oral polio virus vaccine contains a live virus, which could cause an infection in a child who is immune-depressed as a result of taking steroids.
Cognitive Level: Application
Nursing Process: Implementation; ***Test Plan:*** PHYS

5 **Answer: 2** ***Rationale:*** Care of the immunocompromised child focuses on preventing infection. The nursing interventions related to reaching this goal might include limiting contact with a large number of people, but that would not be the goal of the nursing care plan.
Cognitive Level: Application
Nursing Process: Planning; ***Test Plan:*** HPM

6 **Answer: 4** ***Rationale:*** Allergies are confirmed by RAST test. RAST is a radioallergosorbent test that detects IgE antibodies that are part of the allergic response. Urticaria is itching and is symptomatic of allergies and other diseases, and an increase in eosinophils is diagnostic of allergies.
Cognitive Level: Application
Nursing Process: Assessment; ***Test Plan:*** PHYS

7 **Answer: 3** ***Rationale:*** The acronym TORCH stands for toxoplasmosis, other (syphilis, hepatitis), rubella, cytomegalovirus, and herpes simplex virus. It is a study of common viruses that cause significant fetal damage.
Cognitive Level: Application
Nursing Process: Implementation; ***Test Plan:*** PHYS

8 **Answer: 1** ***Rationale:*** Neonates with sepsis may display either hypothermia or hyperthermia, but hypothermia is more common. The other symptoms are not associated with sepsis.
Cognitive Level: Analysis
Nursing Process: Assessment; ***Test Plan:*** PHYS

9 **Answer: 4** ***Rationale:*** Families need to know that casual contact cannot spread HIV. However, basic infection control practices must be maintained to prevent exposure through body fluids.
Cognitive Level: Analysis
Nursing Process: Planning; ***Test Plan:*** SECE

10 **Answer: 1** ***Rationale:*** The prodomal period refers to the period of time between the initial symptoms and the presence of the full-blown disease. The rash would not be apparent during this time. All the other statements are correct.
Cognitive Level: Analysis
Nursing Process: Evaluation; ***Test Plan:*** SECE

Posttest

1 **Answer: 4** ***Rationale:*** Cloth items hold in dust. Only essential items should be stored in the child's bedroom and those should be in drawers or closets. Stuffed animals retain dust and should be removed from the bedroom. Cotton curtains would be preferred over blinds because cotton curtains can be washed frequently. Both the mattress and the bed should be enclosed in special plastic covers to eliminate a source of dust.
Cognitive Level: Analysis
Nursing Process: Evaluation; ***Test Plan:*** HPM

2 **Answer: 1** ***Rationale:*** Prick tests determine allergens. Should the child have an allergy, epinephrine might be needed to counteract anaphylaxis.
Cognitive Level: Application
Nursing Process: Planning; ***Test Plan:*** SECE

3 **Answer: 3** ***Rationale:*** Every time a child enters the healthcare system, the immunization status should be checked. Some children have uncertain history of im-

munization because of parental noncompliance or special circumstances such as being refugees.
Cognitive Level: Application
Nursing Process: Planning; ***Test Plan:*** HPM

4 Answer: 1 ***Rationale:*** Infants receive passive immunity, which lasts 3 to 4 months through the placenta or breastmilk. Active immunity lasts long term and is acquired by exposure to disease or immunizations. Option 1 addreses the client's need for information.
Cognitive Level: Application
Nursing Process: Implementation; ***Test Plan:*** PSYC

5 Answer: 1 ***Rationale:*** The immunocompromised child would be the one at greatest risk for acquiring an infectious organism. The other children would be at less risk for acquiring the gastrointestinal infection.
Cognitive Level: Analysis
Nursing Process: Analysis; ***Test Plan:*** SECE

6 Answer: 4 ***Rationale:*** Eosinophils are the white blood cell associated with allergic reactions.
Cognitive Level: Analysis
Nursing Process: Analysis; ***Test Plan:*** PHYS

7 Answer: 1 ***Rationale:*** TORCH is an acronym for a set of microbes that includes toxoplasmosis, syphilis, hepatitis, rubella, cytomegalovirus, and herpes simplex. If an infant has one of the viruses, they could be shed for up to 1 year.
Cognitive Level: Analysis
Nursing Process: Implementation; ***Test Plan:*** SECE

8 Answer: 2 ***Rationale:*** The HIV virus is spread by blood and body fluids. Clean gloves should be worn when changing the diapers as it exposes the worker to body fluids. The other answers are incorrect.
Cognitive Level: Application
Nursing Process: Implementation; ***Test Plan:*** SECE

9 Answer: 1 ***Rationale:*** The incubation period is the time between exposure and outbreak of the disease. It is often a period when the child can be contagious without others being aware of the possible exposure.
Cognitive Level: Application
Nursing Process: Implementation; ***Test Plan:*** HPM

10 Answer: 3 ***Rationale:*** With the birth of a less-than-expected infant, the parents may have difficulty accepting the child. In addition, the prolonged hospitalization and separation from the parents inhibit bonding, which could lead to altered attachment.
Cognitive Level: Analysis
Nursing Process: Planning; ***Test Plan:*** PSYC

References

Ashwill, J. & Droske, S. (1997). *Nursing care of children: Principles and practice.* Philadelphia: W.B. Saunders Company, pp. 585–669.

Ball, J. & Bindler, R. (1999). *Pediatric nursing: Caring for children* (2nd ed.). Stamford, CT: Appleton & Lange, pp. 339–405, 915.

Bowden, V., Dickey, S., & Greenberg, C. (1998). *Children and their families: The continuum of care.* Philadelphia: W. B. Saunders Company, pp. 418–423, 1612–1683, 2077–2079.

Clinical Pharmacology 2000—Monograph. Dalfopristin; Quinupristin. *http://cp.gsm.com/apps/product/showmono.asp?cpnum=697&monotype=full&match=M.* 05/16/2000.

Ferris. R. & Kaplan, L. (2000). Treating vancomycin-resistant enterococcal infections, *Infusion, 6*(6), March/April: 11–17.

Hankins, J., Lonsway, R. A. W., Hedrick, C., & Perdue, M. B. (2001). *The Infusion Nurses Society: Infusion therapy in clinical practice* (2nd ed.). Philadelphia: W. B. Saunders Company, pp. 182–189.

Monahan, F. & Neighbors, M. (1998). *Medical-surgical nursing: Foundations for clinical practice* (2nd ed.). Philadelphia: W. B. Saunders, pp. 1429–1456.

CHAPTER 12

Cellular Health Problems

Leona M. Florek, MSN, RN

CHAPTER OUTLINE

OBJECTIVES

- Identify data essential to the assessment of alterations in cellular health in a child.
- Discuss the clinical manifestations and pathophysiology related to alterations in cellular health in a child.
- Discuss therapeutic management of a child with alterations in cellular health.
- Describe nursing management of a child with alterations in cellular health

[Media Link]

Use the CD-ROM enclosed with this text, or log onto the address given to access the free, interactive Companion Website created for this series. The CD-ROM and Companion Website accompanying this book offer additional practice opportunities and information—NCLEX Review, Case Studies, Glossary, In Depth with NCLEX, and more.

www.prenhall.com/hogan

Review at a Glance

anemia *a reduction in the number of circulating RBCs*

biopsy *the procedure for obtaining a representative tissue sample for microscopic examination*

chemotherapy *treatment of a disease with chemical agents that have specific toxicity on the disease process*

debulk *the process of surgically removing part of a neoplasm when complete excision is impossible*

infratentorial *below the tentorium cerebelli in the posterior one-third of the brain*

metastasis *a secondary growth in a distant location arising from a primary malignancy*

nadir *the lowest point, such as the blood count after chemotherapy*

neutropenia *abnormally small numbers of neutrophils in the blood*

palliation *treatment intended to relieve or reduce intensity without cure*

radiation therapy *the use of ionizing rays for therapeutic purposes in cancer therapy*

staging *the process of classifying tumors with respect to degree of differentiation, potential for responding to treatment and client prognosis*

supratentorial *above the tentorial notch in the anterior part of the brain*

thrombocytopenia *a reduction in the number of circulating platelets*

Pretest

1 An 18-month-old client is brought in for a well-child visit. The parent reports feeling a lump to the right of the "belly button" during bathing. Initial assessments should not include:

(1) Measuring weight and height.
(2) Further palpation of the area.
(3) Performing urine testing.
(4) Taking vital signs.

2 The parent of a child with neuroblastoma verbalizes regret at not coming in earlier for the client's complaints. An appropriate response is:

(1) This tumor may be diagnosed early because of obvious symptoms.
(2) This is a silent tumor, which is difficult to diagnose early.
(3) This is a very common brain tumor in children.
(4) This is the most common childhood cancer.

3 A 4-year-old is diagnosed with acute lymphocytic leukemia. Following teaching about the testing and therapy, the nurse evaluates the family's understanding of the problem. The statement by the family that indicates appropriate knowledge would be:

(1) "Tests will determine the extent of the tumor process and support the need for palliation."
(2) "Tests will help to determine if radiation or chemotherapy should be used in the treatment plan."
(3) "Tests will determine if surgery is needed."
(4) "Tests will determine the extent of the malignant process and stage the leukemia."

4 A school health nurse would suspect a brain tumor after noting the presence of which of the following symptoms that is compatible with this health problem?

(1) Ataxia and irritability
(2) Papilledema and positive red reflex
(3) Headache and vomiting
(4) Fever and seizures

5 An adolescent is being admitted for an amputation related to a bone tumor. Which age-related nursing diagnosis is most appropriate?

(1) Risk for disuse syndrome
(2) Body image disturbance
(3) Self-care deficit
(4) Activity intolerance

6 A child has been treated with chemotherapy for cancer. Neutropenia is an expected consequence. The nurse would teach the parents to do which of the following, anticipating that neutropenia may occur?

(1) Avoid contact sports.
(2) Avoid crowded spaces.
(3) Avoid spicy foods.
(4) Avoid all immunizations.

7 A child diagnosed with Ewing's sarcoma is being treated with chemotherapy. The results of a complete blood count (CBC) indicate severe thrombocytopenia. Nursing interventions related to this finding would include:

(1) Encouraging foods high in iron.
(2) Limiting physical contact with the child.
(3) Removing fresh flowers from the child's room.
(4) Clearing the floor of the child's room to prevent falls and bruises.

8 The parents of a child with neutropenia secondary to chemotherapy have been taught protective isolation behaviors. Nursing observations that indicate a need for further education is when the parents:

(1) Bring the child toys from home.
(2) Encourage friends to visit by phone rather than visit.
(3) Pull the child in a wagon around the nursing unit for entertainment.
(4) Wash their hands before entering the child's room but not upon exiting the room.

9 Following diagnosis of Wilms' tumor, the child undergoes removal of the affected kidney. In the postoperative period, priority nursing assessments should focus on:

(1) The incision.
(2) Lung sounds.
(3) Temperature.
(4) Kidney function.

10 A child will be undergoing chemotherapy. The nurse discusses the issue of hair loss with the child and family before chemotherapy begins. Later the family questions the nurse on why this information was given to the child at this time. The nurse's response will include the information that:

(1) Hair loss is a symptom of toxic blood levels of chemotherapy, so the child should be watching for this phenomenon.
(2) The presence or absence of hair is related to body image. Strategies for handling hair loss should precede the event.
(3) It is the nurse's legal responsibility to discuss this issue with the child.
(4) Hair loss can be prevented with appropriate nursing interventions.

See pages 306–307 for Answers and Rationales.

I. Introduction to Alterations in Cellular Health

A. Normal cell reproduction

1. The life of the cell is described as the cell cycle, beginning with its formation and ending with the division of the cell into two daughter cells

2. Different tissues have different lengths of cell cycles, varying from 16 hours to 400 hours; some cells, including neurons, never enter the cell cycle and thus never reproduce

B. Development of neoplasms

1. Any group of cells can develop abnormal growth and reproduction; this abnormal reproduction of cells is termed neoplasia; the immune system normally protects the body against the reproduction of these abnormal cells

2. Definitive causative agents for the development of neoplasms are unknown

   a. Numerous factors have been labeled as contributing to the development of a neoplasm, but the exact relationship between these factors and neoplasm development remains unknown

   b. Factors implicated in the development of neoplasms include genetics, radiation, exposure to power lines, the effect of cigarette smoking, viruses, and certain chemicals and drugs

3. Neoplasms can be either benign or malignant

   a. Benign neoplasms typically do not metastasize and do not tend to recur when surgically removed; they do not destroy tissue except secondarily by interfering with blood flow; benign tumors can be serious and even fatal if they interfere with vital functions

   b. Malignant neoplasms are those that tend to recur after removal and metastasize to distant tissues and organs; tissue is destroyed by invasion of these tumors and growth tends to be rapid

4. Treatment for neoplasms includes surgery, radiation, and chemotherapy, alone or in combination

   a. Cure of the tumor occurs when treatment removes all evidence of the tumor permanently

   b. **Palliation** (treatment intended to relieve or reduce intensity without cure) reduces the size of the tumor, thus decreasing symptoms and making the client more comfortable

II. Congenital Cellular Health Problems: Neuroblastoma

A. Description

1. Solid tumor outside the cranium originating in primitive neurocrest cells, which give rise to the adrenal medulla, paraganglia, and sympathetic nervous system of the cervical sympathetic chain and the thoracic chain

2. Is the most common tumor in children located outside the cranium

3. Usual age at onset is 22 months of age

4. Prognosis is based on client age and **staging** of the tumor (the process of classifying tumors with respect to degree of differentiation, potential for responding to treatment and patient prognosis); children under one year of age have a better prognosis

B. Etiology and pathophysiology

1. Cause is unknown although environmental factors, such as prenatal drug exposure, may be implicated

2. Oncogenes have been found to be present in neuroblastoma cells; the DNA sequence responsible for this is called *N-myc;* high *N-myc* levels are associated with rapid progression of disease and poorer prognosis

3. Tumor is often silent leading to late diagnosis and poor prognosis

C. Assessment

1. Symptoms are representative of location and stage of the disease

   a. A peritoneal tumor may present as an abdominal mass or may be evidenced by bowel and bladder dysfunction

   NCLEX!

   b. Typical signs include weight loss, abdominal fullness, irritability, fatigue, and fever

   c. Mediastinal tumors cause dyspnea and lead to neck and facial edema if the tumor is large

   d. Bone metastasis may lead to limp, fever, and malaise; ptosis and ecchymosis of the eyes can also occur

2. Computed tomography (CT) of the skull, neck, chest, abdomen, and bone are done to locate the tumor
3. Bone marrow aspiration helps to locate mass and determine **metastasis** (a secondary growth in a distant location arising from a primary malignancy)
4. Urine testing is done to detect the breakdown of products of adrenal catecholamines (epinephrine and norepinephrine), since some tumors secrete them; these breakdown products are vanillylmandelic acid (VMA) and homovanillic acid (HVA)

D. Priority nursing diagnoses

1. Knowledge deficit
2. Pain
3. Altered family processes

E. Planning and implementation

NCLEX!

1. Surgery is used for tumor removal following **biopsy** (the procedure for obtaining a representative tissue sample for microscopic examination)
2. **Radiation therapy** (the use of ionizing rays for therapeutic purposes in cancer therapy) is used in more advanced cases in addition to surgery and as palliation to reduce the symptoms of metastasis
3. **Chemotherapy**
   a. Is defined as treatment of a disease with chemical agents that have specific toxicity on the disease process
   b. Is a primary form of treatment for cancer; see Figure 12-1 for chemotherapy protocol

   NCLEX!

   c. Drug classifications, sample drugs, and side effects are identified in Table 12-1

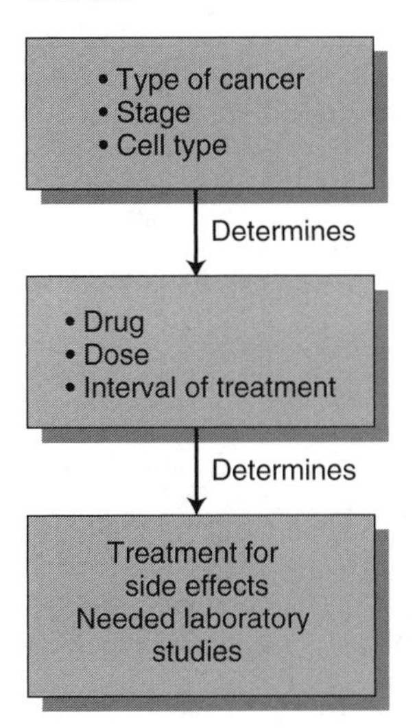

Figure 12-1

Chemotherapy protocol decision tree. *Source:* Ball, J. & Bindler, R. (1999). *Pediatric nursing: Caring for children* (2nd ed.). Stamford, CT: Appleton & Lange, p. 549.

Table 12-1

Classes of Chemotherapy, Commonly Used Examples, and Side Effects

Drug Classes with Selected Examples	Common Side Effects
I. Cell-cycle nonspecific drugs	
Alkylating Drugs	
Cyclophosphamide (Cytoxan); Mesna (Mesnex) is given with this to counteract hemorrhagic cystitis	Bone marrow depression (BMD), hemorrhagic cystitis, alopecia, and stomatitis
Antibiotics	
Doxorubicin (Adriamycin)	BMD, stomatitis, nausea, and vomiting
Hormones	
Prednisone (Meticorten)	Hyperglycemia, gastrointestinal upset, increased appetite, moon face, and increased risk for infection
II. Cell-cycle specific	
Antimetabolites	
6-Mercaptopurine (Purinethol)	BMD, stomatitis, nausea and vomiting, and anorexia
Cytarabine (Ara-C)	BMD, nausea and vomiting, and diarrhea
Methotrexate (Folex)	BMD, nausea and vomiting, and diarrhea (Note: leucovorin rescue—use of leucovorin, an analogue of folic acid—may be used to reduce normal cell kill due to methotrexate)
Plant Alkaloids	
Vincristine (Oncovin)	BMD, nausea and vomiting, fever, and neurologic toxicity (includes constipation)
Enzymes	
Aspiraginase (Elspar)	Allergic reaction, fever, nausea and vomiting, and anorexia
III. Miscellaneous	
Biologic Response Modifiers	
Interferon	Flu-like symptoms

d. Combination drug regimens allow for better cell kill with minimal toxicity and also decrease resistance of cancer cells

NCLEX!

e. Central venous access has facilitated safer drug administration of chemotherapeutic agents; it is important to check for blood return before, during, and after administration to prevent infiltration of vesicant drugs that will destroy the infiltrated tissue

4. If surgery is performed, monitor surgical site for hemorrhage and infection; use temperature as the most accurate measure of infection

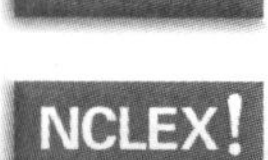

5. Monitor skin integrity at radiation site; see Table 12-2 for nursing care related to radiation therapy

6. Monitor mucous membrane integrity; use appropriate nursing interventions to prevent and treat mouth ulcers

7. Minimize exposure to infection

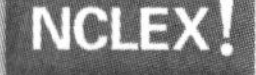

a. All visitors and staff should use good handwashing before contact

b. Private room may be indicated during the period of **nadir** (the lowest point, such as blood counts) after chemotherapy

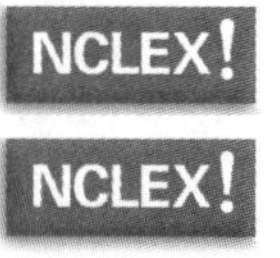

c. Monitor temperature

d. Avoid live attenuated immunizations

Table 12-2

Nursing Care of the Child Receiving Radiation Therapy

Nursing Diagnosis	Nursing Care
Risk for impaired skin integrity	Instruct the child to wear loose-fitting clothing. Use mild soap to wash and gently pat dry the area. Avoid lotions; may use water-soluble lubricant for dry desquamation. Use water-soluble lubricant or moist compresses for itching. Antihistamines may be ordered by the physician. Keep site protected from rubbing, scratching and sun exposure.
Risk for altered oral mucous membranes	Monitor oral mucosa at least daily. Offer oral hygiene after meals and snacks. Use soft toothbrush and mild toothpaste. Rinse mouth frequently; may use plain water or alcohol-free mouthwash. Child may suck on hard candy to stimulate saliva and remove bad taste. Physician may order medicated mouth rinse to reduce pain of mouth ulcers. Offer bland food and fluids, and avoid extremely hot or cold food and beverage temperatures.
Risk for infection	Restrict contact with infected healthcare workers, family and friends. Use good personal hygiene; keep nails short and clean. Remove sources of infectious organisms, including fresh flowers and vegetables; maintain clean environment.

8. Monitor bleeding

a. Take vital signs as ordered

b. Test all stools and body fluids for occult blood

NCLEX!

c. Avoid rectal temperatures, intramuscular injections, and hard tooth brushes

d. Avoid vigorous activities and contact sports

F. Child and family education

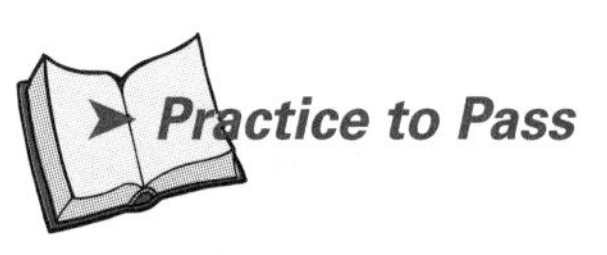

The parents of a 6-month-old with neuroblastoma are visiting their child in the hospital. They are tearful, protective, and insist on doing all personal care. How would you assess the family process?

1. Teach the family about the disease process as well as treatment modalities

2. Instruct the family about the blood dyscrasias and actions they can take to improve the child's condition

3. Give the family information about the need for good nutrition and management of nausea

G. Evaluation: the family displays appropriate coping mechanisms and actively participates in their child's care; the family describes the disease process and lists the side effects of the medications the child is receiving

III. Acquired Cellular Health Problems

A. Leukemia

1. Description

a. Cancer of the blood-forming tissues; a proliferation of immature, abnormal white blood cells (WBCs)

b. Most common malignancy of childhood

c. Peak age of development is four years; boys are affected more frequently than girls

d. Classification is based on type of WBC that becomes neoplastic and the immaturity of the neoplastic cell

1) Acute lymphocytic leukemia (ALL), which has a better prognosis

2) Acute non-lymphocytic leukemia (ANLL) or acute myelogenous leukemia (AML), which has the poorer prognosis

3) Chronic leukemias are rare in children

2. Etiology and pathophysiology

a. Although etiology is unknown, genetics is implicated by the increased incidence in identical twins; chromosomal factors are implicated by the increased risk in children with chromosomal abnormalities such as Down syndrome and Fanconi's syndrome

b. Unrestricted proliferation of immature WBCs occurs

c. Bone marrow infiltration crowds out stem cells that normally produce red blood cells and platelets; **anemia** (a reduction in the number of circulating red blood cells or RBCs) and **thrombocytopenia** (reduction in the number of circulating platelets) occur; the WBCs that are produced are immature and incapable of fighting infection

d. Spleen, liver, and lymph nodes become infiltrated and enlarged

e. Central nervous system (CNS) is at risk for infiltration

f. Clinical manifestations are directly related to area of involvement, such as bone pain from marrow proliferation

g. Prognosis is based on initial WBC count; prognosis is more favorable if initial WBC count is below 50,000/mm^3; children have a better prognosis if they are between the ages of 2 and 10 at the time of diagnosis; a better prognosis is given for ALL than for ANLL

h. Overall prognosis has improved; the majority of newly diagnosed children who receive multi-agent treatment will survive

3. Assessment

a. History, physical, and peripheral blood smear are performed

1) Peripheral blood count reveals anemia, thrombocytopenia, and **neutropenia** (abnormally small numbers of neutrophils in the blood)

2) Leukemic blasts (immature white blood cells) may be seen on the smear

NCLEX!

b. Bone marrow aspiration is the definitive test

1) Usually obtained from the iliac crest

2) Anemia, thrombocytopenia, and neutropenia

3) Normal marrow contains less than 5 percent blasts

4) Leukemic marrow has much higher percentage of blasts, often 60 to 100 percent

c. Other diagnostic tests may include spinal tap to determine if CNS involvement is occurring

NCLEX!

d. Physical assessments

1) Monitor temperature

2) Observe for evidence of new bleeding, such as bruises, bleeding gums, and blood in the stool

3) Observe level of consciousness; note and record irritability, vomiting, and lethargy which may be related to CNS infiltration

4. Priority nursing diagnoses

a. Risk for infection

b. Risk for injury

c. Activity intolerance

d. Anxiety

e. Risk for ineffective family coping

f. Pain

5. Planning and implementation

a. The aim of treatment is to induce a remission; combinations of chemotherapy are utilized to achieve this aim; remission refers to the absence of all signs of leukemia including less than 5 percent blasts in the bone marrow; once induction of remission is achieved, the child will be placed on maintenance therapy, which may last 2 to 3 years

b. Relapses occur when symptoms of leukemia return; reinduction places the child back into remission; relapse may occur at any time but the probability of it occurring decreases over time; bone marrow transplant may be utilized on children who have returned to remission after a relapse

c. Sanctuary therapy (CNS prophylaxis) is frequently administered during the initial period of treatment; the presence of leukemic cells in the CNS fluid leads to CNS involvement; most chemotherapy drugs do not cross the blood–brain barrier; failure to treat the leukemic cells in the CNS may allow for the return of the disease after remission appears to be achieved; CNS treatment can include radiation therapy to the brain and spinal cord or the administration of chemotherapy drugs into the CSF

NCLEX!

d. Nursing care is directed toward managing the symptoms of leukemia as well as preventing/treating side effects of the chemotherapy

NCLEX!

e. Supportive care for the anemia will include protection of the body from injury to prevent trauma to the RBCs present; the child will need rest periods to combat the fatigue associated with anemia; activity intolerance will require organization of nursing care to allow for adequate rest; adequate nutrient intake will be necessary for the production of new RBCs

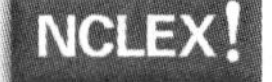

f. Platelet deficiency means the child will be prone to bleeding

1) Use a soft toothbrush or gauze over a finger for oral care to reduce bleeding of the gums

2) Avoid alcohol-containing mouthwashes to prevent drying of the oral mucous membranes
3) Keep the environment clear to avoid the risk of the child bumping into objects and sustaining falls that lead to bruises
4) Avoid rectal temperatures and test all stools for occult blood

NCLEX!

g. Although the white cell count may be high initially, the WBCs that are present are immature and unable to fight infections; ensure good handwashing by all who have contact with the child to protect the child from infection; prevent individuals with infections from coming in contact with the child; do not allow fresh flowers or fruits in the child's room because of the presence of mold and fungus on these items

h. Monitor vital signs, intake and output, weight and urine specific gravity

NCLEX!

i. Monitor for constipation

j. Inspect oral mucous membranes daily

NCLEX!

k. Monitor level of consciousness, degree of irritability, and overall behavior

l. Manage pain with medications and other alternative interventions

NCLEX!

m. See Table 12-3 for nursing interventions to treat side effects of chemotherapy

Table 12-3

Nursing Care of the Child Receiving Chemotherapy

Nursing Diagnosis	Nursing Care
Risk for infection	Perform careful handwashing. Avoid contact with infectious individuals. Avoid crowds. Eliminate fresh flowers and potted plants from the child's room. Cook all fruits and vegetables to reduce risk of introducing organisms into the environment. Protective isolation may be needed if white cell count drops significantly.
Risk for injury	Keep environment uncluttered to reduce bumping into objects and subsequent falls. Use soft toothbrush or gauze over finger to provide oral care. Avoid alcohol-containing mouthwash, which dries the mouth. Select toys that do not pose a risk of injury to the child.
Altered nutrition: less than body requirements	Provide antiemetics in anticipation of nausea. Allow parents to provide home-cooked foods if desired. Encourage foods of high nutrient value instead of non-nutritious snacks. Make meals pleasant; allow social meals. Keep environment aesthetically pleasant. Avoid visual reminders of vomiting, including keeping the emesis basin close but out of sight during meals.
Risk for altered oral mucous membranes	Rinse mouth frequently throughout the day with water. Avoid drying mouthwashes. Avoid foods that have high acidic content. Avoid spicy foods. Seek medical intervention for pain control for mouth ulcers.
Altered body image related to hair loss	Discuss possibility with child and family before it occurs. Plan with child for camouflage if desired; purchase wigs, hats, and scarves before hair loss occurs. Provide emotional support for hair loss. Avoid excessive hair combing/brushing.

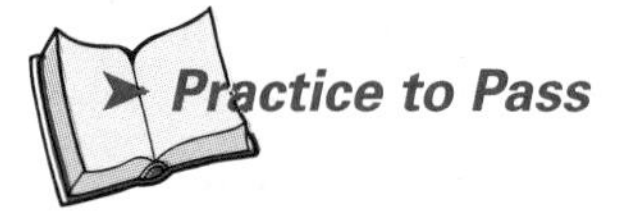

A 10-year-old with acute lymphocytic leukemia refuses all morning hygiene. What would you recommend to his parents when they seek your guidance on what to do?

6. Medication therapy

a. Combinations of chemotherapy drugs are used to enhance tumor cell death and reduce side effects; drugs are chosen that use different mechanisms to cause cell death; protocols often vary among institutions

b. The chemotherapy treatment can be divided into three phases

1) Induction, which is designed to achieve a remission

2) Intensification, which serves to maintain the remission

3) Maintenance, during which chemotherapy may be continued for 2 to 3 years; CNS prophylaxis may be used to eliminate the leukemic cells in the CNS

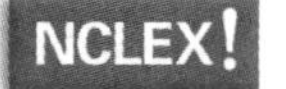

c. Induction: induces remission, lasts 4 to 6 weeks and uses prednisone (Meticorten), vincristine (Oncovin), asparaginase (Elspar), with or without doxorubicin (Daunomycin)

d. Intensification or consolidation: further decreases tumor burden and includes use of such drugs as asparaginase and methotrexate (Folex)

NCLEX!

e. CNS prophylaxis adds intrathecal chemotherapy consisting of methotrexate, cytarabine (Ara-C), and hydrocortisone (Cortef) during the other phases of treatment

f. Maintenance lasts 2½ to 3 years and includes oral 6-mercaptopurine (Purinethol) and weekly intramuscular methotrexate

g. Reinduction is used for relapses and adds drugs not previously used

h. Bone marrow transplants are not usually used for ALL until a second relapse occurs

7. Child and family education

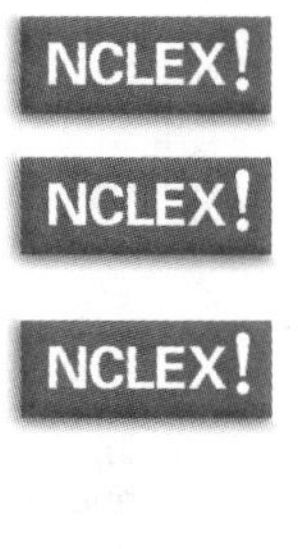

a. Explain the disease process and treatment modalities to the family

b. Provide the child and family with information that will assist them in reducing symptoms related to blood dyscrasias

c. Teach the family about the side effects of the chemotherapy and means of reducing the child's discomfort

d. Promote nutrition by providing information about nausea control

NCLEX!

e. Explain the need for good physical hygiene; explain means of protecting the child from infection

8. Evaluation: the child remains free of side effects of chemotherapy; blood values remain within normal limits; the family demonstrates appropriate coping mechanisms

B. Brain Tumors

1. Description

a. Most common solid tumor in children

b. Over half of brain tumors in children are **infratentorial** (below the tentorium cerebelli in the posterior third of the brain), primarily in the cerebellum and brainstem

c. The remaining are **supratentorial** (above the tentorial notch in the anterior part of the brain) and are mainly in the cerebrum (see Figure 12-2)

d. The terms benign and malignant are of little value since benign brain tumors can be fatal

2. Etiology and pathophysiology

a. Cause is unknown although radiation and environmental factors have been implicated

b. Supporting cells of brain, such as glias and astrocytes, frequently account for pediatric brain tumors

3. Assessment

a. Symptoms depend upon the location of the tumor and the age of the child

b. Since an infant's sutures are open, symptoms may be found late

NCLEX!

c. Increased intracranial pressure (ICP) occurs with brain tumors because of the presence of the tumor and obstructions in the flow of CSF; symptoms related to increased ICP include headache, especially on awakening, and vomiting unrelated to eating

d. Visual symptoms include diplopia and papilledema

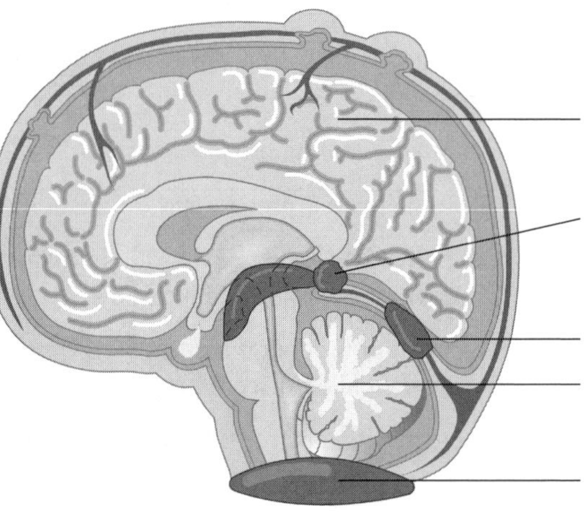

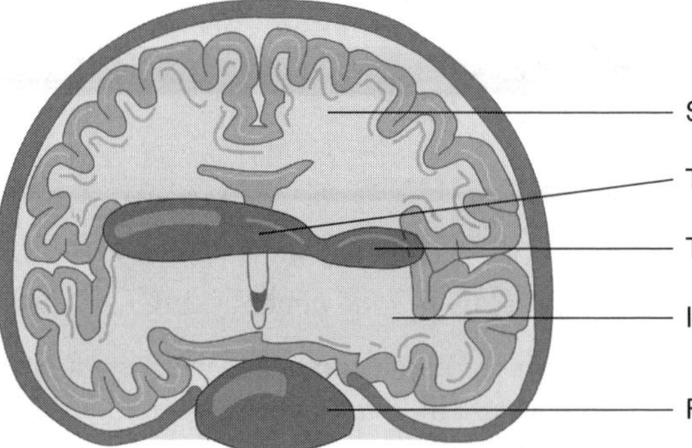

Figure 12-2

Sites of Pediatric Brain Tumors: Infratentorial tumors account for over half of all pediatric tumors.

Source: Ball, J. & Bindler, R. (1999). *Pediatric nursing: Caring for children* (2nd ed.). Stamford, CT: Appleton & Lange, p. 565.

e. Supratentorial tumors give rise to symptoms that include personality changes and seizures

f. Infratentorial tumor symptoms include ataxia, visual disturbances, delayed or precocious puberty, and growth failures

g. Diagnosis will be made based on results of MRI, CT scans, and radiographic studies with IV contrast; angiography is done when CT scans are positive; biopsy as a diagnostic procedure is done during surgery

4. Priority nursing diagnoses

a. Pain

b. Risk for altered nutrition

c. Impaired physical mobility

d. Anxiety

e. Risk for impaired family coping

5. Planning and implementation

a. Surgery is used for biopsy (diagnosis), to completely remove a tumor, or to **debulk** an unremovable tumor (surgically remove part of a neoplasm when complete excision is impossible); surgery may also be performed to restore the patency of the ventricles

b. Laser surgery can be used for more sensitive areas, where greater precision is needed

c. Radiation therapy may be used at the site postoperatively

d. Chemotherapy is commonly used, sometimes intrathecally

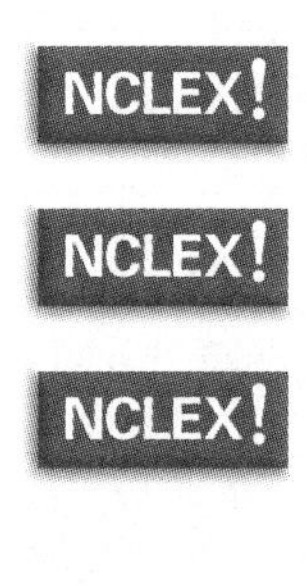

e. Complications such as hydrocephalus, seizures, sensorimotor deficits, and endocrine disorders may also need management

f. Maintain nutritional support; if the child vomits from increased ICP, provide hygiene and refeed; often the act of vomiting reduces the ICP

g. Monitor level of consciousness and observe for signs of increased ICP; monitor fluid status to prevent rises in ICP; observe for seizures and provide nursing care should they occur; protect the child from injury and have suction and oxygen available at the bedside

h. Monitor intake and output and measure urine specific gravity

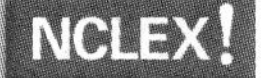

i. Postoperatively, position of the head may be critical

1) With an infratentorial incision, the head position is flat and on either side with neck slightly extended

2) With supratentorial incision, the head is elevated

3) The physician may order the degree of head elevation allowed, often 30 degrees

j. If a ventriculoperitoneal shunt has been placed to restore ventricle patency, nursing care will include maintaining the suture line and skin integrity over the shunt

k. Provide eye care because swelling of the eyes may occur postoperatively

NCLEX!

l. Monitor pain and provide relief; avoid medications that sedate the child, as it is difficult to determine level of consciousness when the child is sedated

m. Assess sensory-perceptual status and assist with loss of function

n. Assess surgical site for hemorrhage and infection

6. Child and family education

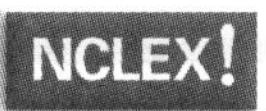

a. Reinforce information provided by the physician about the diagnosis and treatment; prepare the child and family for the surgical procedure, including the need to shave the head and to expect ecchymosis of the eyes, which is common following craniotomy

b. Teach the family activities that can reduce the child's pain preoperatively and postoperatively

c. Encourage the child and family to talk honestly about the diagnosis and their feelings

d. If diabetes insipidus occurs secondary to the brain tumor, teach the child and family about the medication to control the symptoms

7. Evaluation: the child's nutritional status is optimized; the child's pain is managed at an acceptable level; the family describes care of the ventriculoperitoneal shunt; the family safely and accurately describes the side effects of the child's medications

C. Wilms' tumor

1. Description

a. Intrarenal tumor that is also called a nephroblastoma

b. Common abdominal tumor during childhood

c. Most frequently occurs between 2 and 5 years of age

2. Etiology and pathophysiology

a. A small proportion of Wilms' tumors show a genetic basis with family members being at increased risk of development

b. The tumor may be unilateral or bilateral; bilateral tumors have poorer prognosis

c. The tumor is often encapsulated until relatively late

d. It metastasizes to the lungs and liver

e. Prognosis is based on stage of disease; over 75 percent of children have a 5-year survival rate

3. Assessment

a. Usually asymptomatic

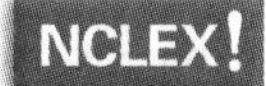

b. The most frequent admitting symptom is an abdominal mass; parent often finds the mass, which is located to one side of the midline of the abdomen

c. Pain and hematuria may be present in some children

d. Hypertension is present in approximately 25 percent of children because of increased renin production

e. Diagnosis is made by ultrasound of the abdomen and intravenous pyelogram (IVP)

f. CT scan and MRI of the lungs are done to detect metastasis

NCLEX!

g. Avoid palpating the abdomen preoperatively to reduce the risk of rupturing the capsule and causing tumor spillage; a sign is often placed over the child's bed with the instruction "No abdominal palpations"

4. Priority nursing diagnoses

a. Risk for altered urinary elimination

b. Pain

c. Alteration in cardiopulmonary tissue perfusion

d. Risk for impaired family coping

5. Planning and implementation

a. Unless bilateral tumors are present, surgery is performed to remove the affected kidney and look for metastasis

b. Radiation to the abdomen and chemotherapy can be used before and/or after surgery

NCLEX!

c. Postoperatively, monitor functioning of the remaining kidney

1) Measure intake and output

2) Monitor daily weight and urine specific gravity

3) Monitor fluid levels, intravenous infusions, and blood pressure

d. Complete pain assessment when measuring vital signs; provide pain relief with pharmaceuticals and nursing interventions; in addition to incisional pain, pain may result from the postoperative shift of internal organs to compensate for the loss of the kidney

NCLEX!

e. Assess bowel sounds, abdominal distention, and bowel movements

f. Monitor for infection, observing surgical wound and body temperature

6. Child and family education

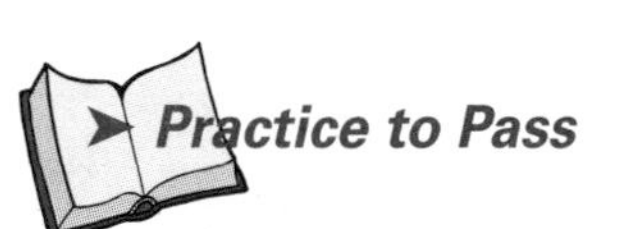

The parents of your client with Wilms' tumor are confused by your finding of hypertension. They state that the child is too young and maybe you could repeat the check. How would you explain this finding to them?

a. Explain to the family the need to avoid unnecessary palpation of the abdomen prior to surgical removal

b. Provide the parents with information they need to provide care to their child, including the nature of the disease, treatment options, and therapeutic and side effects of chemotherapy in use

c. Explain to the parents and child the need to protect the remaining kidney; teach signs and symptoms of urinary tract infections, and to avoid contact sports, during which injury to the kidney might occur

7. Evaluation: child and family describe disease process and treatment options; the child denies pain; the family members identify successful coping strategies; the child and family identify means of protecting the remaining kidney

D. Bone tumors

1. Osteogenic sarcoma

   a. Description: a tumor that arises from a bone cell, probably the osteoblast

   1) Most common bone cancer in children

   2) Most frequently affects the metaphysis of the long bones

   b. Etiology and pathophysiology

   1) Osteogenic sarcoma usually occurs in adolescent boys; tumor growth is detected at time of rapid bone growth

   2) Most frequently affects the distal portion of femur; also affects humerus, tibia, pelvis, jaw, and phalanges

   3) It is a malignant tumor that frequently metastasizes to the lungs; metastasis may be present at the time of diagnosis

   4) Etiology is unknown except for increased incidence noted in children who have had retinoblastoma; an abnormal gene may also be implicated, as osteogenic sarcoma has been found in several members of the same family

   c. Assessment

NCLEX!

   1) Pain and swelling are initial symptoms

   2) X-rays following traumatic injury may be first indication of disease

   3) Followup assessments will include CT or MRI imaging to detect areas of metastasis

   d. Priority nursing diagnoses

   1) Pain

   2) Anxiety, ineffective individual or family coping

   3) Risk for injury, impaired physical mobility, self-care deficit

   4) Altered health maintenance

   5) Risk for body image disturbance

   6) Anticipatory grieving

   e. Planning and implementation

   1) Treatment may include radical resection or amputation

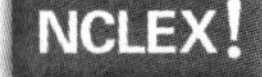

   2) Selected clients may have limb-salvaging procedures with prosthetic replacement

   3) Thoracotomy may be performed for metastasis to the lung

   4) Chemotherapy may be administered pre- and postoperatively

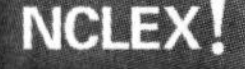

   5) Emotional support of the child is important both pre- and postoperatively, as the child and family deal with a life-threatening disease where the treatment involves body image as well as mobility issues

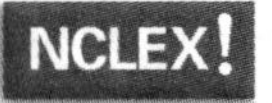

   6) Employ a straightforward approach when amputation is indicated; allow for verbal expression of feelings

7) Postoperative care includes sterile stump care and special bandaging as ordered

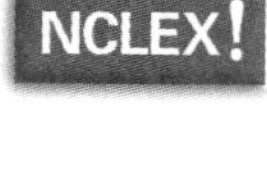

8) Elevate stump for 24 hours, if prescribed, but avoid prolonged elevation
9) Maintain body alignment
10) Perform range of motion to joints above amputation

NCLEX!

11) Assist with early ambulation; assist with temporary prosthesis use
12) Teach appropriate use of assistive devices

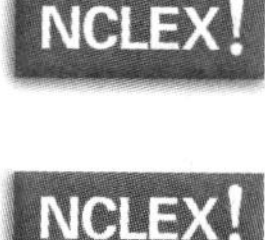

13) Encourage early interaction with peers

f. Child and family education

1) Teach the child and family about the disease process and treatment options
2) Teach the child and family stump care
3) Demonstrate safe use of prosthesis; teach the child to monitor the condition of the stump
4) Discuss with the child and family phantom limb pain and its management

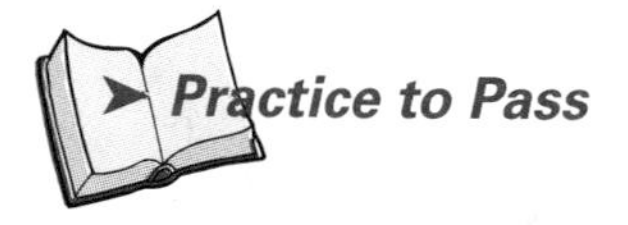

Practice to Pass

The parents of a 5-year-old have been told their child's tumor has not responded to treatment and the child is terminally ill. The child is later heard to be asking what happens when someone dies. The family asks the nurse how they should respond to the child's questions. What would you tell the parents?

g. Evaluation: child demonstrates appropriate stump care; child ambulates safely with prosthesis and ambulation assistive devices; child and family demonstrate appropriate coping strategies; child demonstrates positive body image by making positive comments about himself; child maintains relationships with peers

2. Ewing's sarcoma

a. Description

1) Ewing's sarcoma is a malignant, small round cell tumor
2) Usually involves the diaphysial (shaft) portion of the long bones; commonly found in the femur, pelvis, tibia, fibula, ribs, scapula, humerus, and clavicle

b. Etiology and pathophysiology

1) Tumor arises in the marrow spaces of the bone
2) Tends to occur in individuals between the ages of 4 and 25
3) It is a highly malignant tumor that metastasizes to the lung

NCLEX!

c. Assessment

1) Pain
2) Soft tissue mass
3) Secondary symptoms of anorexia, malaise, fever, fatigue, and weight loss
4) Diagnosed with X-rays of affected area
5) Radionuclide bone scans and CT scans of the chest are uses to assess for metastasis

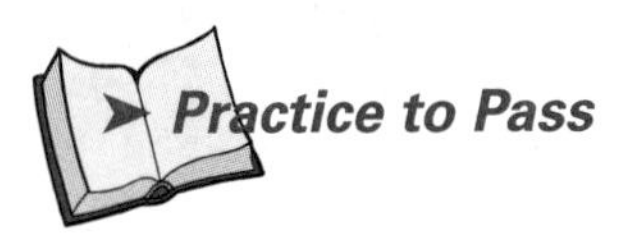

A pediatric patient has been diagnosed with a brain tumor and after years of treatment, death is near. The mother has reached the stage of bereavement where she is calm and accepting. The father expresses anger at the doctors and nurses for their failure to save his child. How would you support this family?

d. Priority nursing diagnoses

1) Pain
2) Anxiety, ineffective individual or family coping
3) Risk for injury, impaired physical mobility, self-care deficit
4) Altered health maintenance
5) Risk for body image disturbance
6) Anticipatory grieving

e. Planning and implementation

1) Amputation usually not recommended
2) Treatment includes extensive radiation along with chemotherapy
3) Emotional support of the child is important, as the radiation therapy can affect the appearance and mobility of the extremity
4) Encourage mobility of the extremity as tolerated
5) Refer to Tables 12-1, 12-2, and 12-3 for information on chemotherapy and radiation therapy
6) Allow open communication with the child and family relative to the disease and its prognosis

f. Child and family education

1) Discuss with the child and the family the disease process and treatment options
2) Teach skin care related to radiation therapy

g. Evaluation: the child and family demonstrate adequate coping behaviors; the child's skin remains intact; the child maintains mobility of the extremity

Case Study

A 6-year-old is being admitted to your pediatric unit for the first round of chemotherapy in treating newly diagnosed acute lymphocytic leukemia (ALL). You are assigned this admission and are to prepare the child and family for insertion of a central venous access device and the subsequent chemotherapy.

❶ What physical assessments would you make of the child?

❷ What emotional assessments are relevant to the situation?

❸ What priorities of care should be addressed?

❹ What education would the child and family need?

❺ How would you respond when the parents ask if they will be able to go to Disney World, as planned, in 2 weeks?

For suggested responses, see page 411.

Posttest

1 A school-age child is being admitted for surgical removal of a brain tumor. Expected nursing assessments during the preoperative period would include:

(1) Bulging fontanels.
(2) Vomiting.
(3) Drainage from the ear or nose.
(4) Elevated blood glucose levels.

2 A child is receiving chemotherapy to induce remission in acute leukemia. When considering common side effects of chemotherapy, an appropriate nursing diagnosis early in the course of therapy would include:

(1) Sleep pattern disturbance.
(2) Altered mucous membranes.
(3) Risk for infection.
(4) Risk for impaired tissue perfusion: peripheral.

3 A client is to begin radiation therapy after the removal of Wilms' tumor. The parent statement that indicates a lack of understanding of related skin care would be:

(1) "We will use loose-fitting clothes on our child."
(2) "We will protect our child from sun exposure."
(3) "We will keep the area moist with Vaseline."
(4) "We will prevent our child from scratching the site."

4 An adolescent on consolidation chemotherapy for acute lymphocytic leukemia (ALL) asks the nurse to come quickly to evaluate "blood in my urine." The nurse would do which of the following as the most important action?

(1) Explain this is normal for these drugs.
(2) Measure intake and output.
(3) Force fluids to improve the hematuria.
(4) Recognize that this is untoward and report the event.

5 A client is being admitted for mild neutropenia and a severe oral monilial infection. The nurse should assign the child to which room?

(1) A semi-private room with a medical patient
(2) A semi-private room with a surgical patient
(3) A private room without further precautions
(4) A private room with protective isolation

6 You are assigned to the postoperative care of a client with a below-the-knee amputation for osteogenic sarcoma. Nursing care of the child would include:

(1) Maintaining bedrest until able to use permanent prosthesis.
(2) Keeping stump elevated continuously until prosthesis applied.
(3) Applying a dressing to the stump that allows continuous visualization of the distal stump.
(4) Encouraging early visits from friends.

7 The nursing diagnosis for a child undergoing chemotherapy for leukemia is Altered nutrition: less than body requirements related to nausea and anorexia. An appropriate goal for this client would be:

(1) Administer antiemetics PRN.
(2) The child's caloric intake will be within normal range.
(3) The child does not complain of nausea.
(4) Intake and output are approximately equal.

8 A child is to receive chemotherapy intravenously with a vesicant drug. The nurse can ensure safe administration of this drug by:

(1) Administering the drug using a positive pressure infusion pump.
(2) Checking for blood return before, during and after administration of the drug.
(3) Maintaining the infusion site below the level of the heart.
(4) Delivering the infusion as rapidly as possible.

9 **A child with leukemia has developed pancytopenia. Measures designed to reduce stomatitis in this child while receiving chemotherapy would include:**

(1) Alcohol-based mouthwash to reduce oral organisms.
(2) Brushing the teeth twice a day with a firm-bristled toothbrush.
(3) Increasing intake of citrus juices, such as orange juice, that contain vitamin C.
(4) Rinsing the mouth several times a day with plain water.

10 **During rounds, the interdisciplinary team is discussing a child with leukemia who has just been diagnosed as terminally ill. The nurses describe the mother's behavior as angry, claiming the nurses are not providing care for her child. The team leader will focus on the probable cause of the mother's anger, which is:**

(1) Poor care on the part of the nurses.
(2) Lack of attention for the mother's needs.
(3) Overwhelming guilt for having caused the leukemia.
(4) A stage of bereavement over the anticipated loss of the child.

See pages 307–308 for Answers and Rationales.

Answers and Rationales

Pretest

1 **Answer: 2** ***Rationale:*** This is the usual presentation of Wilms' tumor (nephroblastoma), and palpating the area may cause the tumor to spread. Since Wilm's tumor is a cancer of the kidney, it important to assess growth and development, kidney function, and blood pressure, which may be elevated because of increased renin production.
Cognitive Level: Application
Nursing Process: Assessment; ***Test Plan:*** PHYS

2 **Answer: 2** ***Rationale:*** This tumor occurs in 1 in 10,000 live births. It arises out of embryonic neural crest cells and, therefore, is usually found in the adrenals or retroperitoneal sympathetic chain. Symptoms are vague and depend on location.
Cognitive Level: Application
Nursing Process: Implementation; ***Test Plan:*** PSYC

3 **Answer: 4** ***Rationale:*** Acute lymphocytic leukemia is staged at diagnosis to determine treatment. The goal is remission, which is usually accomplished using chemotherapy. Radiation therapy to the central nervous system is rarely used because of untoward side effects.
Cognitive Level: Application
Nursing Process: Evaluation; ***Test Plan:*** PHYS

4 **Answer: 3** ***Rationale:*** The most common reported symptoms of brain tumors in children are headache, especially upon awakening, and vomiting that is unrelated to eating. Both are related to increased intracranial pressure. Irritability and ataxia may also be present; however, presenting symptoms are often vague. Fever is not a symptom of a brain tumor. Papilledema may be noted, but red reflex is not indicative of brain tumors.
Cognitive Level: Application
Nursing Process: Assessment; ***Test Plan:*** PHYS

5 **Answer: 2** ***Rationale:*** Bone tumors usually occur in otherwise healthy children. Given the interruption of normalcy and the developmental tasks of the adolescent, body image disturbance can occur when a limb is lost.
Cognitive Level: Analysis
Nursing Process: Analysis; ***Test Plan:*** PSYC

6 **Answer: 2** ***Rationale:*** Neutropenia is a reduced white blood cell count, which increases the risk for infection. Only live vaccines are contraindicated in children who are immunocompromised. Contact sports would be a problem with thrombocytopenia, and spicy foods would increase discomfort if an alteration in mucous membranes occurred.
Cognitive Level: Application
Nursing Process: Implementation; ***Test Plan:*** SECE

7 **Answer: 4** ***Rationale:*** Thrombocytopenia refers to a decrease in platelets. Preventing falls and bruises would be appropriate for an individual with platelet deficiencies. Fresh flowers may contain molds and fungus that can lead to infection and would be a concern for a child with neutropenia. Providing foods high in iron would be appropriate to restore red blood cells. Limiting contact with the child could affect his

or her body image and self-esteem. Contact is acceptable as long as the individual is not infectious.
Cognitive Level: Analysis
Nursing Process: Implementation; ***Test Plan:*** PHYS

8 **Answer: 3** ***Rationale:*** Healthy children are often a source of infectious organisms. Children in hospitals may carry a number of infectious organisms. Hospitalized neutropenic children should be protected from exposure to other children whenever possible. Toys from home would not carry a high risk. Hand washing before contact with the child is the important intervention. Limiting physical contact with peers would decrease exposure to infectious organisms. Telephone contacts allow for the peer support the child needs.
Cognitive Level: Analysis
Nursing Process: Evaluation; ***Test Plan:*** PHYS

9 **Answer: 4** ***Rationale:*** All of these assessments look at possible postoperative complications. Since the child is left with only one kidney, failure of that kidney caused by inadequate blood flow, infection, or any other cause could be fatal.
Cognitive Level: Analysis
Nursing Process: Planning; ***Test Plan:*** PHYS

10 **Answer: 2** ***Rationale:*** Preparation helps individuals handle stressful situations. If the child had not been prepared for hair loss, it could be more anxiety-provoking for the child. Hair loss cannot be prevented.
Cognitive Level: Analysis
Nursing Process: Planning; ***Test Plan:*** PSYC

Posttest

1 **Answer: 2** ***Rationale:*** Vomiting is a symptom of increased intracranial pressure. Bulging fontanels would not be present in a school-age child. Drainage from the ear or nose might indicate a basilar skull fracture, not a brain tumor. Some brain tumors display the symptom of diabetes insipidus, not diabetes mellitus, thus the symptom would be dilute urine rather than elevated blood glucose.
Cognitive Level: Application
Nursing Process: Analysis; ***Test Plan:*** PHYS

2 **Answer: 2** ***Rationale:*** Nausea and vomiting, anorexia, mouth sores, constipation, and pain are early and common side effects of chemotherapy. Bone marrow suppression reaches its peak 7 to 10 days after induction. Sleep pattern disturbance may be related but is not directly caused by chemotherapy.
Cognitive Level: Analysis
Nursing Process: Planning; ***Test Plan:*** PHYS

3 **Answer: 3** ***Rationale:*** Self-care during external radiation therapy includes loose-fitting clothes, gentle washing with mild soap, avoiding sun exposure, and avoiding scratching and other irritation. Any lubricant must be water-soluble.
Cognitive Level: Analysis
Nursing Process: Evaluation; ***Test Plan:*** PHYS

4 **Answer: 4** ***Rationale:*** This is an untoward effect of the commonly used cancer medication cyclophosphamide (Cytoxan) and should be reported. Fluids are usually forced prior to administration and the bladder is emptied frequently to prevent hematuria. Measuring intake and output should be done routinely on all clients and is not specific to managing this complication.
Cognitive Level: Analysis
Nursing Process: Implementation; ***Test Plan:*** PHYS

5 **Answer: 3** ***Rationale:*** A private room assignment is indicated for children with chemotherapy-related neutropenia. Careful handwashing is also an essential element to reduce the risk of infection.
Cognitive Level: Application
Nursing Process: Implementation; ***Test Plan:*** SECE

6 **Answer: 4** ***Rationale:*** Nursing care must be supportive of body image adjustment. The child would be encouraged to sit in a chair and ambulate on crutches while waiting for the permanent prosthesis. The stump dressing is a continuous ace bandage, which supports the stump shape in preparation for the prosthesis.
Cognitive Level: Application
Nursing Process: Implementation; ***Test Plan:*** PSYC

7 **Answer: 2** ***Rationale:*** The client's goal is stated in terms of behaviors of the child that demonstrate the problem is solved. Option 1 is a nursing action, not a goal. Absence of nausea does not guarantee adequate intake. Equal intake and output does not indicate adequate nutrition.
Cognitive Level: Application
Nursing Process: Planning; ***Test Plan:*** PHYS

8 **Answer: 2** ***Rationale:*** By checking for blood return throughout the administration, the nurse can stop the infusion at any time a blood return does not occur. A positive pressure infusion pump, maintaining the infusion site below the level of the heart, or rapid drug delivery does not guarantee the infusion will not extravasate.
Cognitive Level: Application
Nursing Process: Implementation; ***Test Plan:*** PHYS

9 Answer: 4 ***Rationale:*** Studies have shown that simply rinsing the mouth with water decreases the onset of stomatitis in clients receiving chemotherapy. Alcohol-based mouthwash would be avoided as it is drying to the oral mucous membranes. A stiff toothbrush may cause the gums to bleed. Should oral lesions be present, acidic foods and liquids will increase discomfort.
Cognitive Level: Application
Nursing Process: Implementation; ***Test Plan:*** PHYS

10 Answer: 4 ***Rationale:*** The stages of grief and bereavement include denial, anger, bargaining, depression, and acceptance. The anger expressed may often be displaced and directed towards persons who have a role in the loss. Nursing and other healthcare personnel must be aware of this in order to help the family cope with the impending loss.
Cognitive Level: Analysis
Nursing Process: Planning; ***Test Plan:*** PSYC

References

Ball, J. & Bindler, R. (1999). *Pediatric nursing: Caring for children* (2nd ed.). Stamford, CT: Appleton & Lange, pp. 60–88, 367–404, 541–580, 983.

Bowden, V. R., Dickey, S. B., & Greenberg, C. S. (1998). *Children and their families: The continuum of care.* Philadelphia: W. B. Saunders, pp. 618–619.

Clark, M. (1999). *Nursing in the community: Dimensions of community health nursing* (3rd ed.). Stamford, CT: Appleton & Lange, pp. 454–484, 738–741.

Gorski, L. (2000). *Best practices in home infusion therapy.* Gaithersburg, MD: Aspen Publishers, Inc., pp. 10:8, 11:17.

Lehne, R. A. (1998). *Pharmacology for nursing care* (3rd ed.). Philadelphia: W. B. Saunders, pp. 1007–1041.

Monahan, F. D. & Neighbors, M. (1998). *Medical-surgical nursing: Foundations for clinical practice* (2nd ed.). Philadelphia: W. B. Saunders, pp. 1518–1523, 1536–1538.

Wong, D. L. & Hess, C. S. (2000). *Wong and Whaley's clinical manual of pediatric nursing* (5th ed.). St. Louis: Mosby, Inc., pp. 183–208, 444–445, 486–502, 533.

Wong, D. L., Hockenberry-Eaton, M., Wilson, D., Winkelstein, M. L., Ahmann, E., & DiVito-Thomas, P. A. (1999). *Whaley and Wong's nursing care of infants and children.* St. Louis: Mosby, Inc., pp. 7–12, 594–606, 690–691, 720–730, 914, 1709–1751.

CHAPTER 13

Gastrointestinal Health Problems

Gina M. Orta, MS, RN
Jennifer Jeames Coleman, MSN, RN

CHAPTER OUTLINE

OBJECTIVES

- Identify data essential to the assessment of alterations in health of the gastrointestinal system of a child.
- Discuss the clinical manifestations and pathophysiology of alterations in health of the gastrointestinal system of a child.
- Discuss therapeutic management of a child with alterations in health of the gastrointestinal system.
- Describe nursing management of a child with alterations in health of the gastrointestinal system.

[Media Link]

Use the CD-ROM enclosed with this text, or log onto the address given to access the free, interactive Companion Website created for this series. The CD-ROM and Companion Website accompanying this book offer additional practice opportunities and information—NCLEX Review, Case Studies, Glossary, In Depth with NCLEX, and more.

www.prenhall.com/hogan

Review at a Glance

acholic *free of bile*

anicteric *without jaundice*

cachexia *a state of ill health, malnutrition, and wasting*

dehiscence *bursting open or separation*

fecalith *solidified feces*

hematemesis *vomiting of blood*

icteric *with jaundice*

McBurney's point *point of tenderness in acute appendicitis, situated between the umbilicus and the right anterosuperior iliac spine*

omentum *a double fold of peritoneum attached to the stomach which connects to certain abdominal viscera*

peristalsis *a progressive, wavelike muscular movement that occurs involuntarily*

reflux *a return or backward flow*

steatorrhea *increased fat in the stools*

Pretest

1 **An 18-month-old child with a history of cleft lip and palate has been admitted for palate surgery. The nurse teaches the parents not to use a toothbrush immediately after surgery because:**

(1) The toothbrush would be frightening to the child.
(2) The child no longer has deciduous teeth.
(3) The suture line could be interrupted.
(4) The child will be NPO.

2 **The nurse instructs the parents about the postoperative feeding schedule following their infant's pyloromyotomy. The nurse evaluates that the parents understand the instructions when they state they may begin feedings:**

(1) 6 hours postoperatively.
(2) 8 hours postoperatively.
(3) 10 hours postoperatively.
(4) 12 hours postoperatively.

3 **Shortly after the delivery of an infant with an omphalocele, the nurse would initially:**

(1) Weigh the infant.
(2) Insert an orogastric tube.
(3) Call the blood bank for 2 units of blood.
(4) Cover the sac with moistened sterile gauze.

4 **While gathering admission data on a 16-month-old child, the nurse notes all the following abnormal findings. Which finding is related to a diagnosis of Hirschsprung's disease?**

(1) Projectile vomiting lacking bile
(2) Decreased urine output
(3) Weighs less than expected for height and weight
(4) Intermittent sharp pain

5 **A 6-week-old infant is brought into the pediatrician's office with a history of frequent vomiting after feedings and failure to gain weight. The diagnosis of gastroesophageal reflux is made and discharge instructions are begun. While planning discharge teaching on feeding techniques with the parents, the nurse should include instructions to:**

(1) Dilute the formula.
(2) Delay burping to prevent vomiting.
(3) Change from milk-based formula to soy-based formula.
(4) Position the infant at a 30- to 45-degree angle after feedings.

6 **A 14-year-old boy is brought into the Emergency Department with a diagnosis of rule out appendicitis. He is complaining of right lower quadrant pain. The nurse's most appropriate action to assist in managing his pain would be to:**

(1) Insert a rectal tube.
(2) Apply an ice bag.
(3) Apply a heating pad.
(4) Administer an intravenous antispasmodic agent.

7 **The nurse has completed discharge teaching on the dietary regimen of a child with celiac disease. The nurse recognizes that client education has been successful when the mother states that the child must comply with the gluten-free diet:**

(1) Throughout life.
(2) Until the child has achieved all major developmental milestones.
(3) Only until all symptoms are resolved.
(4) Until the child has reached adolescence.

8 **An appropriate nursing assessment of an infant suspected of having necrotizing enterocolitis would be:**

(1) pH evaluation of the stomach.
(2) Neurological status every 2 hours.
(3) Rectal temperature every 2 hours.
(4) Abdominal girth every 4 hours.

9 **The nurse is developing a teaching plan for the parents of an infant diagnosed with hepatitis A. Which of the following instructions would be included to reduce the risk for transmission of this disease?**

(1) Disinfect all clothing and eating utensils on a daily basis.
(2) Tell family members to wash their hands frequently.
(3) Spray the yard to eliminate infected insects.
(4) Vacuum the carpets and upholstery to rid the house of the infectious host.

10 **Which of the following signs would the nurse recognize as an indication of moderate dehydration in a preschooler?**

(1) Sunken fontanel
(2) Diaphoresis
(3) Dry mucous membranes
(4) Decreased urine specific gravity

See pages 345–346 for Answers and Rationales.

I. Overview of the Anatomy and Physiology of the Gastrointestinal System

A. Development

1. The gastrointestinal (GI) system begins to develop during the third week of gestation

2. The primitive gut is initially formed and then divides into the foregut, midgut, and hindgut; the structures continue to develop in an intricate fashion to become the digestive tract and accessory organs

B. Structure: the GI tract extends from the mouth to the anus; it includes organs of digestion and accessory organs such as the liver, gallbladder, and pancreas

1. The mouth serves as the entryway into the GI tract; the tongue senses the taste and texture of food; the submandibular, parotoid, and sublingual glands secrete saliva

2. The esophagus transports food from the mouth to the stomach by **peristalsis** (waves of gut movement); the upper esophageal sphincter prevents air from being swallowed while breathing; the lower esophageal sphincter prevents the reflux of gastric contents into the lower esophagus

3. The stomach is a food reservoir that receives partially processed food and drink funneled from the mouth and esophagus and gradually releases it into the small intestine

4. The small intestine's primary function is the absorption of nutrients (carbohydrates, fats, proteins, minerals, and vitamins) into the systemic circulation; after appropriate absorption of nutrients, the small intestine is left with the initial fecal liquid

5. The large intestines receive this fecal material from the small intestine; the water is removed from the stool, which is stored for a short period of time

6. The rectum receives the fecal material and defecation ensues

C. Gastrointestinal functions: the primary functions of the GI tract are the digestion and absorption of nutrients and water, secretion of various substances, and elimination of waste products

1. Digestion

   a. The mouth serves as the principal site for initial preparation of food for the body to use

   b. Two basic activities are involved in the digestive process

      1) Muscular activity, which produces GI movement; three types of muscles contribute to the motility and are controlled by the central nervous system

         a) Circular muscles churn and mix the food particles

         b) Longitudinal muscles propel the food bolus

         c) Sphincter muscles control the passage of food from one segment to the next segment

      2) Enzymatic activity, which results from stimulating the GI tract and aids in food breakdown and the utilization process; the enzymatic and chemical process of digestion involves many types of GI secretions; there are enzymes for degradation of nutrients, hormones to stimulate or inhibit GI secretions, hydrochloric acid to produce the pH necessary for enzyme activity, mucus for lubrication and protection of the GI tract, and water and electrolytes to transport nutrients for digestion and absorption

2. Absorption of nutrients primarily occurs in the small intestine

   a. The large intestine completes the process of absorption and functions primarily to absorb sodium and additional water

   b. Several mechanisms of absorption include passive diffusion, carrier-mediated diffusion, active energy-driven transport, and engulfment

II. Assessment of the Gastrointestinal System

A. Medical history

1. Assess for the presence of pain (location, type, duration, quality, aggravating or alleviating factors)
2. Identify normal bowel habits (frequency, consistency, color, associated pain, medications, or enemas)
3. Obtain data regarding constipation and diarrhea (client's definition, frequency, and treatment)
4. Assess for changes in appetite
5. Identify thirst level (increased or decreased desire for liquids)
6. Identify food intolerances (which foods, symptoms, and treatment)
7. Assess for belching, vomiting, heartburn, flatulence (when, frequency, quality, treatments)

8. Identify feeding routine (what, when, amount, toleration)

9. Past medical history related to GI system (illnesses, surgeries, accidents or injuries, family history)

B. Physical assessment

1. Assess weight and height

2. Determine hydration status (skin turgor, mucous membranes, peripheral pulses, and tears)

3. Inspect the abdomen (contour, visible peristalsis, rash, lesions, asymmetry, masses, enlarged organs, or pulsations)

4. Auscultate bowel sounds (normal is 5 to 20/minute)

5. Palpate (light and deep)

6. Assess for rebound tenderness

7. Assess rectal patency

C. Common diagnostic studies related to GI function

1. Serum chemistry study, liver profile, lipid profile, erythrocyte sedimentation rate (ESR), C-reactive protein (CRP), thyroid function

2. Stool examination for ova and parasites, blood, white blood cells, pH, Clinitest for reducing substances, stool culture

3. Fecal fat collection for 72 hours to rule out fat malabsorption

4. Bowel studies: upper GI series, barium enema, biopsy, rectosigmoidoscopy

5. Abdominal radiographs

6. Abdominal and pelvic ultrasound

III. Congenital Gastrointestinal Health Problems

A. Cleft lip and cleft palate

1. Description

   a. Cleft lip is a congenital anomaly involving one or more clefts in the upper lip; the degree of cleft varies from a small notch to a complete separation (see Figure 13-1)

   b. Cleft palate is a congenital anomaly consisting of a cleft ranging from soft palate involvement alone to a defect including the hard palate and portions of the maxilla in severe cases

2. Etiology and pathophysiology

   a. Causes include hereditary, environmental, and teratogenic factors

   b. Cleft lip occurs in approximately 1 in every 1,000 births; it is more common in boys than girls

   c. Cleft palate occurs in 1 in 2,500 births; the incidence in girls is double that in boys

Figure 13-1

A. Unilateral cleft lip, B. Bilateral cleft lip.

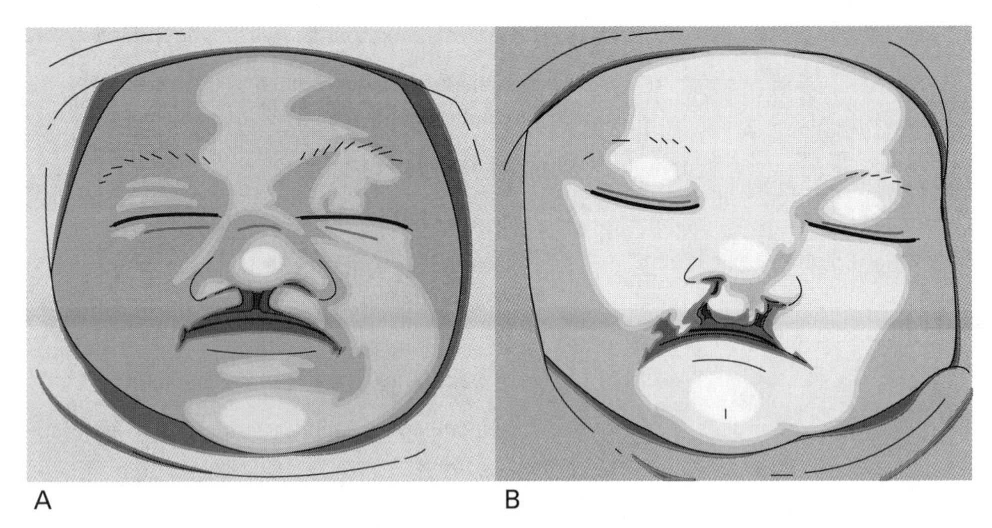

d. These defects occur during embryonic development; cleft lip results from failure of fusion of lateral and medial tissues forming the upper lip occurring around 7 weeks gestation; cleft palate is a failure of fusion of tissues forming the palate which occurs around 9 weeks gestation

3. Assessment
   a. These defects are readily apparent at birth
      1) Cleft lip involves a notched upper lip border, nasal distortion, and may include unilateral or bilateral involvement
      2) Cleft palate is a visible or palpable gap in uvula, soft palate, hard palate, and/or incisive foramen with exposed nasal cavities and associated nasal distortion
   b. Careful physical assessment should be performed to rule out other midline birth defects
4. Priority nursing diagnoses: Ineffective airway clearance; Altered family processes; Risk for infection; Risk for injury; Knowledge deficit; Altered nutrition: less than body requirements; Pain
5. Planning and implementation

NCLEX!

   a. Depending on the severity of the defect and the general health of the child, surgical correction of cleft lip typically is done at 1 to 2 months; cleft palate is generally repaired between the age 6 and 18 months; cleft palate may be corrected through several operations performed in stages
   b. Early correction of cleft palate enables development of more normal speech patterns; delayed closure of large defects may require the use of orthodontic devices
   c. Preoperative nursing care
      1) Assess respiratory status continuously during feedings
      2) Feed infant in upright position
      3) Feed the infant slowly and burp frequently

NCLEX!

4) Use ESSR (Enlarged nipple, Stimulate suck by rubbing nipple on lower lip, Swallow, Rest after each swallow to allow for complete swallowing)
5) Use alternate feeding devices such as elongated nipple (lamb's nipple) or breast shield
6) Assess degree of cleft and ability to suck

NCLEX!

7) Provide postoperative feeding instructions
8) Encourage parents to verbalize fears, concerns, negative emotions
9) Facilitate grief responses of shock, denial, anger, and mourning
10) Encourage touching, holding, cuddling, and bonding
11) Provide parents with pictures of other children before and after surgical repair
12) Discuss infant's positive characteristics
13) Refer to community resources and parent support groups

d. Postoperative care

1) Monitor the child for respiratory distress during the postoperative period; monitor lung sounds, encourage deep breathing without placing stress on suture line
2) No oral temperatures
3) Advance feedings as tolerated

NCLEX!

4) No straws, pacifiers, spoons, or fingers in or around the mouth for 7 to 10 days
5) For cleft lip, resume preoperative feeding techniques

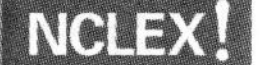

6) For cleft palate, liquids can be taken from a cup; no straws are allowed; soft foods can be taken off the side of the spoon; the child is not allowed to feed himself or herself to reduce risk of injury
7) Clean lip from suture line out after feedings and PRN
8) Apply antibacterial ointment as ordered
9) Use elbow restraints to keep infant from putting fingers in mouth or touching the surgical site

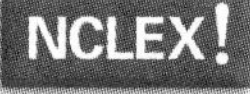

10) No tooth brushing for 1 to 2 weeks
11) Place infant in side lying position on unaffected side to avoid excessive contact with the bed linens

NCLEX!

12) Monitor site for redness, swelling, excess bleeding, purulent drainage, or fever
13) Assess pain using appropriate tools
14) Provide comfort measures to decrease stress, such as crying, on suture line; encourage rocking, cuddling, and holding
15) Provide analgesics and sedatives on a scheduled basis
16) Provide age-appropriate activities for diversion

6. Child and family education

a. Teach precautions to prevent aspiration of formula and provide emergency phone numbers in case of emergency

b. Provide instruction on CPR

c. Teach parents safety and care issues regarding the use of restraints

1) Do not apply restraints too tightly

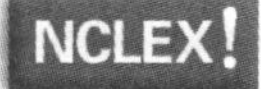

2) Remove at least every 2 hours and play games to encourage flexion

3) Remove only one restraint at a time

d. Stress importance of follow-up care and referral appointments

e. Make appropriate and early referrals for speech and language disabilities

f. Encourage early speech attempts and arrange for speech therapy

g. Encourage good dental hygiene and orthodontic follow-up

7. Evaluation

a. Infant maintains a patent airway

b. Infant completes a feeding within 30 minutes and follows appropriate growth curve

c. Parents verbalize and demonstrate an understanding of alternate feeding techniques

d. Parent and infant demonstrate bonding behaviors

e. Parents assume responsibility for the infant's home care and follow-up care

f. Surgical site heals without infection

g. Pain control is achieved as evidenced by the infant's engagement in age-appropriate activities, lack of irritability, and ability to sleep undisturbed

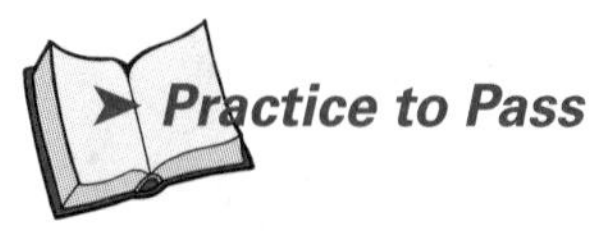

What feeding techniques would you discuss with the parents of a newborn with cleft lip and cleft palate?

B. Pyloric stenosis

1. Description: pyloric stenosis results when the circular areas of muscle surrounding the pylorus hypertrophy and block gastric emptying

2. Etiology and pathophysiology

a. The exact cause remains unknown, however, heredity is thought to play an important role

b. Incidence is 1 in 500 live births; firstborn children and offspring of affected children are at highest risk; males are affected five times more often than females and full-term infants more than premature infants; there is also a higher incidence in white infants

c. The pylorus narrows because of progressive hypertrophy and hyperplasia of the circular pyloric muscle

d. This leads to obstruction of the pyloric sphincter, with subsequent gastric distention, dilatation, and hypertrophy (see Figure 13-2)

e. Pyloromyotomy, which is the creation of an incision along the anterior pylorus to split the muscle, is commonly performed to relieve the obstruction

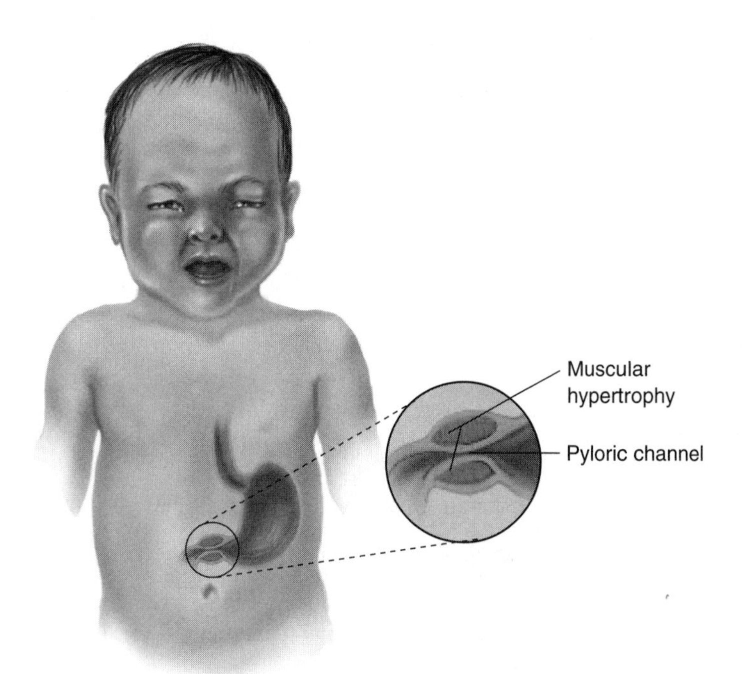

Figure 13-2

Pyloric stenosis.
Source: Ball, J. & Bindler, R. (1999). *Pediatric nursing: Caring for children* (2nd ed.). Stamford, CT: Appleton & Lange, p. 607.

3. Assessment

NCLEX!

NCLEX!

   a. Previously healthy infant with progressive, projectile, non-bilious vomiting
   b. Movable, palpable, firm, olive-shaped mass in right upper quadrant (RUQ)
   c. Visible, deep, peristaltic waves from left upper quadrant (LUQ) to RUQ immediately before vomiting
   d. Irritability, hunger, and crying
   e. Sunken fontanels, poor skin turgor, dry mucous membranes, and decreased urine output, constipation, jaundice, metabolic alkalosis
   f. Ultrasonography and upper GI series may reveal delayed gastric emptying and an elongated pyloric canal
   g. Laboratory findings may include an increased pH and bicarbonate level, indicating metabolic alkalosis; the serum chloride, sodium, and potassium levels may be decreased; an increased hematocrit and hemoglobin may also be present, indicating hemoconcentration
4. Priority nursing diagnoses: Risk for aspiration; Ineffective breathing pattern; Risk for fluid volume deficit; Altered nutrition: less than body requirements; Risk for altered parenting
5. Planning and implementation
   a. Assess skin turgor, mucous membranes, and fontanels at least every shift, monitor urine specific gravity, weigh daily

NCLEX!

   b. Maintain NPO status prior to surgery, monitor I & O hourly, administer IV fluids and electrolytes as ordered
   c. Maintain NG tube patency and monitor NG output

d. Keep infant warm and quiet

NCLEX!

e. Small frequent feedings of clear liquids should be initiated within 4 to 6 hours after surgery; follow strict diet regimen of gradual advancement of feedings until normal formula feedings have been resumed

f. Continue IV hydration until age- or weight-appropriate amounts of formula are tolerated

NCLEX!

g. Assess incision for redness, swelling, and drainage; immediately report signs of infection to the physician

h. Monitor vital signs at least every 4 hours

i. Encourage parental involvement and rooming-in

6. Child and family education

a. Explain what pyloric stenosis is and how it is treated

b. Explain all equipment such as the NG tube and IV

c. Discharge instructions for the parents include instructions to report any vomiting, abdominal tenderness, fever, incisional redness, or drainage to the physician

d. Provide verbal and written feeding instructions if the child has not returned to full-strength formula feedings prior to discharge

e. Inform the parents of the importance of follow-up care with the physician

7. Evaluation

a. Infant exhibits signs of adequate hydration

b. Infant consumes age- and weight-appropriate amounts of formula and regains weight

c. Incision is clean, dry, intact, and well-approximated

d. Infant is free of signs and symptoms of infection

e. Parents actively participate in infant's care and verbalize understanding of condition, surgical treatment, and home care

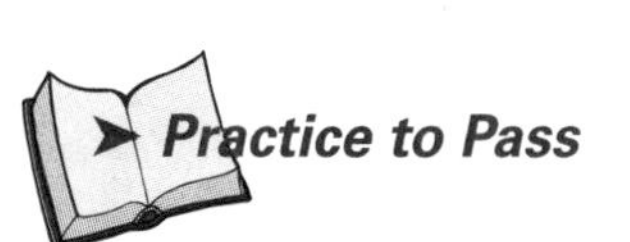

You have just admitted a child to the nursing unit. The child is scheduled for a pyloromyotomy. What information would you include in your preoperative teaching?

C. Omphalocele and gastroschisis

1. Description

a. Omphaloceles are congenital malformations in which intraabdominal contents herniate through the umbilical cord

b. Gastroschisis occurs when the bowel herniates through a defect in the abdominal wall, usually to the right of the umbilical cord, and through the rectus muscle; there is no membrane covering the exposed bowel

2. Etiology and pathophysiology

a. Omphalocele

1) An omphalocele results from failure of the abdominal contents to return to the abdomen when the abdominal wall begins to close by the tenth week of gestation

2) Viscera is outside of abdominal cavity but inside translucent sac covered with peritoneum and amniotic membrane

3) Omphalocele is often associated with other congenital anomalies such as cardiac defects, genitourinary anomalies, chromosomal defects, craniofacial abnormalities, and diaphragmatic abnormalities

4) Incidence is 1 in 3,000 to 10,000 births

b. Gastroschisis

1) Controversy exists regarding the etiology of gastroschisis; some suggest that at some point a tear occurs at the base of the umbilical cord, allowing the intestine to herniate

2) Viscera outside of abdominal cavity and not covered with peritoneal sac

3) Gastroschisis is rarely associated with other major congenital anomalies, but jejunoileal atresia, ischemic enteritis, and malrotation may occur as a result of the defect itself

4) Gastroschisis occurs in about 1 to 3 in 10,000 births

3. Assessment

a. Obvious protrusion of abdominal contents present at time of delivery

b. The size of the sac varies depending on the extent of the protrusion

NCLEX!

c. Rupture of the sac results in evisceration of the abdominal contents

d. Defect may be noted on prenatal ultrasound

4. Priority nursing diagnoses: Ineffective thermoregulation; Risk for infection; Risk for fluid volume deficit; Ineffective family coping

5. Planning and implementation

a. Assess body temperature continuously using skin probe; place infant in warmer immediately after birth

NCLEX!

b. Use sterile technique in dealing with defect

NCLEX!

c. Immediately cover with warm, moist, sterile gauze, and wrap with plastic to keep moisture in and preserve heat

d. Minimize movement of infant and handling of intestines

e. Assess respiratory status continuously during immediate newborn period by placing on cardiac and apnea monitor with pulse oximetry

f. Monitor for circulatory compromise by monitoring temperature, pulses, capillary refill, skin color, and heart rate and respiratory rate

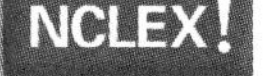

g. Assess mucous membranes for moisture and skin for elastic turgor; monitor I & O, weigh daily, assess fontanels, monitor electrolytes, and maintain IV and administer fluids and TPN as ordered

h. Maintain NG tube for decompression

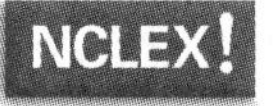

i. Monitor for signs of ileus by auscultating of bowel sounds, measuring abdominal girth, assessing bowel movements and maintaining an NPO status

j. Assess parents' coping mechanisms

k. Encourage parents to verbalize feelings of loss of "perfect" child and guilt that may accompany congenital anomaly

l. Encourage parental participation in infant's care

6. Child and family education

a. Provide written and verbal information on growth and developmental needs

b. Teach parents appropriate techniques for developmental stimulation

c. Provide information regarding support groups and other community resources

d. Teach parents the signs of bowel obstruction

7. Evaluation

a. Infant maintains appropriate body temperature

b. Infant is free from infection

c. Infant maintains effective breathing pattern as evidenced by absence of respiratory distress or circulatory compromise

d. Infant maintains adequate hydration and nutrition status

e. Parents verbalize their feelings and actively participate in infant's care

D. Diaphragmatic hernia

1. Description: congenital diaphragmatic hernia (CDH) results when abdominal contents protrude into the thoracic cavity through an opening in the diaphragm

2. Etiology and pathophysiology

a. CDH occurs when there is failure of the transverse septum and the pleuroperitoneal folds to completely develop and form the diaphragm

b. Intestines and other abdominal structures enter the thoracic cavity

c. Lung growth may cease; after birth, respiration becomes further compromised by pulmonary hypoplasia and compression of the lung including the airways and blood vessels

3. Assessment

a. Clinical findings depend on the severity of the defect

b. Fetal ultrasound shows abdominal organs in chest

c. Postnatal diagnosis is confirmed by chest x-ray examination

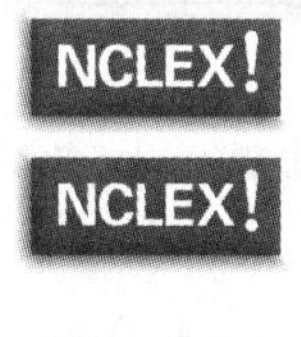

d. Diminished or absent breath sounds on affected side

e. Bowel sounds may be heard over chest

f. Cardiac sounds may be heard on right side of chest

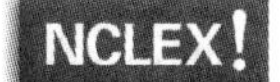

g. Dyspnea, cyanosis, nasal flaring, tachypnea, retractions

h. Sunken abdomen, barrel-shaped chest

4. Priority nursing diagnoses: Ineffective breathing pattern; Impaired gas exchange; Risk for fluid volume deficit; Pain; Risk for infection

5. Planning and implementation

   a. Preoperative nursing care

      NCLEX! 1) Assess vital signs frequently with ongoing respiratory assessment

      NCLEX! 2) Elevate head of bed and position on affected side

      3) Maintain patency of NG tube to decompress the stomach

      4) Monitor IV fluids

      NCLEX! 5) Maintain mechanical ventilation, extracorporeal membrane oxygenator (ECMO), chest tubes

      6) Provide minimal stimulation

   b. Postoperative care focuses on promoting lung function

      NCLEX! 1) Monitor for signs of infection and respiratory distress

      NCLEX! 2) Continue to support respirations by positioning in semi-Fowler's position on affected side; organize care to decrease exertion

      3) Promote nutrition when feedings resumed

      4) Support family through crisis

6. Child and family education

   a. Instruct parents on wound care, prevention of infection, and feeding techniques

   b. Provide written and verbal information on growth and developmental needs

   c. Provide information regarding long-term problems and necessity of regular follow-up visits

7. Evaluation

   a. Infant establishes effective breathing pattern

   b. Infant maintains adequate hydration status

   c. Infant is free from pain

   d. Infant is free from infection

   e. Parents actively participate in infant's care and verbalize an understanding of condition, surgical treatment, and home care

E. Biliary atresia

1. Description: biliary atresia is a progressive inflammatory process that causes both intrahepatic and extrahepatic bile duct fibrosis

2. Etiology and pathophysiology

   a. The cause of biliary atresia is unknown; because the problem originates during the prenatal period, viruses, toxins, and chemicals are believed to be a few of the suspected causes

b. Obstruction of the extrahepatic bile ducts causes obstruction of the normal flow of bile out of the liver and into the gallbladder and small intestine

c. Bile plugs form and cause bile accumulation in the liver

d. Inflammation, edema, and irreversible hepatic injury occur

e. The liver becomes fibrotic, and cirrhosis and portal hypertension develop, leading to liver failure

f. Because of the lack of bile in the intestines, fat and fat-soluble vitamins cannot be absorbed; this leads to malnutrition, deficiencies of fat-soluble vitamins, and growth failure

g. Without treatment this disease is fatal

h. Treatment involves surgery (Kasai procedure) to temporarily correct the obstruction and supportive care

i. Liver transplantation is eventually necessary

3. Assessment

a. Healthy appearing infant at birth

b. Jaundice occurs within 2 weeks to 2 months

c. **Acholic** stools: puttylike, clay-colored stools

d. Increased bilirubin levels

e. Abdominal distention

f. Hepatomegaly

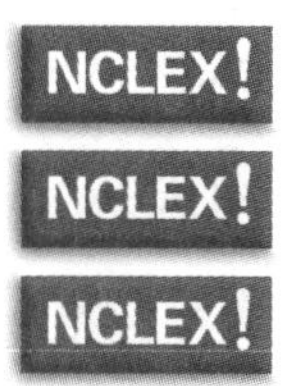

g. Increased bruising of the skin, prolonged bleeding time

h. Intense itching

i. Tea-colored urine

j. Ultrasound and liver biopsy are also used in the confirmation process

4. Priority nursing diagnoses: Altered nutrition: less than body requirements; Anticipatory grieving; Altered family processes

5. Planning and implementation

a. Weigh daily

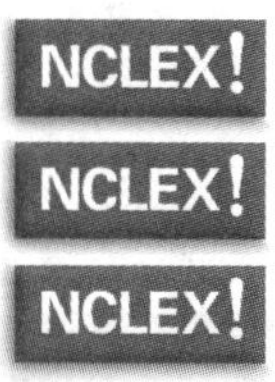

b. Administer TPN or intralipids as ordered

c. Administer fat-soluble vitamins A, D, E, and K as ordered

d. Monitor stool pattern

e. Establish an open, caring relationship with family

f. Refer parents to support groups

6. Child and family education

a. Instruct the parents in meticulous skin care

b. Provide verbal and written information regarding nutritional needs

c. Provide instructions on home medication regimen and allow time for return demonstration

d. Inform parents of the signs and symptoms for which to call the physician

NCLEX!

e. If a transplant is performed, post-transplant medications should be discussed in depth including their administration and side effects

7. Evaluation

a. Infant's weight is maintained; the skin remains intact

b. Parents understand treatment plan and discharge instructions

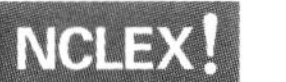

c. If a liver transplant has been performed, the parents identify signs of rejection

F. Hirschsprung's disease

1. Description

a. Hirschsprung's disease is a congenital anomaly resulting from an absence of ganglion cells in the colon

b. This disease is also known as megacolon and congenital aganglionosis

2. Etiology and pathophysiology

a. Hirschsprung's disease is believed to be a familial, congenital defect

b. The rate of occurrence is about 1 in 500 live births and is about 4 times more common in males than in females; there is a higher incidence in children with Down Syndrome and genitourinary abnormalities

c. The rectosigmoid region is most commonly affected

d. Absence of autonomic parasympathetic ganglion cells in one portion of the colon results in lack of innervation in that portion

e. Peristalsis cannot occur without proper innervation; this lack of peristalsis causes accumulation of intestinal contents and distention of the bowel proximal to the defect

3. Assessment

a. Clinical manifestations vary according to the child's age at the time of diagnosis

1) Newborns

a) Failure to pass meconium stools

b) Reluctant to ingest fluids

c) Abdominal distention

NCLEX!

d) Bile-stained emesis

2) Infants

NCLEX!

a) Failure to thrive

b) Constipation

c) Abdominal distention

d) Vomiting

e) Episodic diarrhea

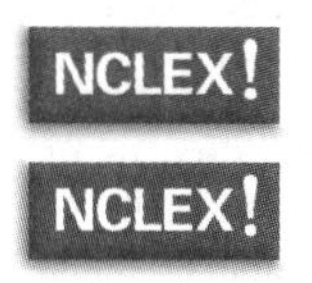

3) Toddlers and older children
   a) Chronic constipation
   b) Foul-smelling stools
   c) Abdominal distention
   d) Visible peristalsis
   e) Palpable fecal mass
   f) Malnourishment
   g) Signs of anemia and hypoproteinemia

b. Rectal examination typically reveals an absence of stool

c. Laboratory studies and diagnostic tests commonly reveal an enlarged portion of the colon and a rectal biopsy will confirm the absence of ganglion cells

4. Priority nursing diagnoses: Constipation; Risk for fluid volume deficit; Impaired skin integrity; Risk for infection; Altered nutrition: less than body requirements; Body image disturbance

5. Planning and implementation

a. Medical treatment involves removing the aganglionic bowel; a temporary colostomy is created soon after diagnosis; this colostomy will be closed and the bowel reanastomosed at a later time, usually around the age of two years

NCLEX!

b. Preoperatively, assess bowel function and characteristics of stool; measure abdominal circumference; monitor the child for vomiting and respiratory distress

c. Monitor urine specific gravity; monitor electrolytes; assess hydration status

d. Prepare child for surgery and temporary placement of colostomy

e. Administer antibiotics as ordered

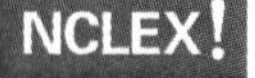

f. Monitor vital signs; measure abdominal girth; assess surgical site for redness, swelling, drainage after surgery

g. Assess stoma for color, bleeding, breakdown of surrounding skin

h. Assess anal area after pull-through for patency of any appliance that may be in place, presence of stool, redness, drainage

NCLEX!

i. Provide meticulous skin care, use appropriately sized stoma supplies

j. Notify the physician of any fever, unusual drainage, redness, or odor

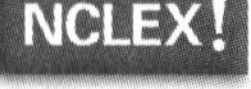

k. Keep child NPO until bowel sounds return or flatus is passed, maintain NG tube, administer IV fluids as ordered, daily weights, begin with clear liquids and progress as tolerated

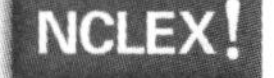

l. Assess pain using age-appropriate scales, provide comfort measures and involve parents, provide pain medications on regular basis as ordered, notify physician if pain is not managed

m. Involve child in quiet age-appropriate activities for diversion

n. Assess parents' level of understanding of condition, home care, and treatment, encourage parents to share feelings, anxieties, and concerns about rectal irrigations and ostomy care, explain surgical repair and recovery process

o. Refer to support groups and make appropriate referrals

6. Child and family education

a. Encourage preschool and early school-age children to draw pictures, use dolls, and play to express concerns about bodily appearance, irrigations, and colostomy

b. Provide parents with instructions about how to complete rectal irrigations and allow time for return demonstration

c. Teach ostomy care in the immediate postoperative period and encourage parents to participate and learn while in the hospital, encourage the child to assume care as soon as appropriate

NCLEX!

d. Teach parents how to assess for distention and obstruction and the importance of reporting these findings to the physician

NCLEX!

e. Teach ostomy care and provide for return demonstration by parents and child

7. Evaluation

a. Child remains free of fluid and electrolyte imbalances

b. Child experiences no breakdown of skin surrounding the colostomy

c. Child exhibits no signs or symptoms of infection

d. Child demonstrates adequate nutrition for age and age-appropriate hydration status

e. Child receives effective pain control and resumes age-appropriate play

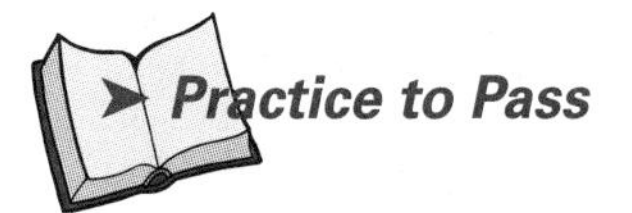

What information would you consider when planning your preoperative teaching with the parents of a child with Hirschsprung's disease?

f. Child and parents verbalize and demonstrate an understanding of condition, rectal irrigations, colostomy care, and routine postoperative home care

g. Child and parents verbalize feelings about condition and altered body image and use effective coping mechanisms

IV. Acquired Gastrointestinal Health Problems

A. Gastroesophageal reflux

1. Description: gastroesophageal reflux (GER) is a regurgitation of gastric contents into the esophagus; this is a result of relaxation or incompetence of the lower esophageal (cardiac) sphincter

2. Etiology and pathophysiology

a. The exact cause of GER is unknown, but is believed to be a result of delayed maturation of lower esophageal neuromuscular function or impaired local hormonal control mechanisms

b. Repeated **reflux** (backward flow) of gastric contents can damage delicate esophageal mucosa

c. GER is typically self-limiting, usually resolving by 1 year of age; in more severe cases, the child may require surgery, such as Nissen fundoplication, in which the gastric fundus is wrapped around the distal esophagus

d. There is a higher rate of occurrence in children with neurologic impairments like cerebral palsy, Down Syndrome, and head injuries

e. GER is the most common esophageal problem in infancy; some reflux may normally occur in infants, children, and even adults; however, GER is pathologic when it is severe or when complications arise

f. Pathologic GER occurs in approximately 3 percent of all newborns, with a higher incidence in premature infants; boys are affected three times as often as girls, and almost all infants with GER are symptomatic by 6 weeks of age

3. Assessment

NCLEX!

a. Frequent vomiting, possibly with **hematemesis** (bloody vomitus), hiccuping

NCLEX!

b. Weight loss, failure to thrive

c. Aspiration and recurrent respiratory infections, recurrent otitis media

d. Near-miss sudden infant death syndrome and cyanotic episodes

e. Esophagitis and bleeding caused by repeated irritation of esophageal lining with gastric acid

NCLEX!

f. Heartburn, abdominal pain, irritability, melena

g. Laboratory studies and diagnostic findings indicate absence of gastric or duodenal obstruction on barium swallow and upper GI radiograph

h. Low resting lower esophageal sphincter pressure on esophageal manometry

i. Endoscopy and pH probe studies

j. Anemia secondary to blood loss

4. Priority nursing diagnoses: Risk for aspiration; Fluid volume deficit; Altered nutrition: less than body requirements; Risk for infection; Impaired home maintenance management

5. Planning and implementation

a. Medical treatment depends on severity of condition

NCLEX!

1) Mild: change feeding habits; keep the child upright; rice cereal may be added to the formula to thicken the feedings; fatty foods and citrus juices are avoided

2) Severe: surgical treatment may be required in the form of a Nissen fundoplication; a gastrostomy tube may be utilized for 6 weeks after surgery

b. Assess breath sounds and respiratory status particularly before and after feedings

NCLEX!

c. Position infant upright to reduce respiratory complications, place on cardiac and respiratory monitor, keep suctioning equipment at the bedside; the best post-feeding position is prone with the head elevated; the parents are taught to avoid placing the infant in an infant seat as this increases intrabdominal pressure

d. Administer GER medications as ordered, which may include drugs that promote gastric emptying or pyloric sphincter relaxation, or antacids to neutralize the acidity of refluxed contents (Table 13-1)

NCLEX!

e. Assess hydration status, monitor I & O, administer IV fluids as ordered, weigh daily

f. Assess the amount, frequency, and characteristics of emesis, assess the relation of vomiting to the time of feedings and the infant's activity level

g. Provide frequent, small feedings

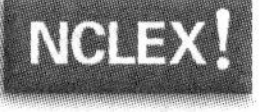

h. If taking solids, offer solids first and then liquids, improve nutritional status through feeding techniques such as thickening formula with cereal, enlarging nipple openings, and burping the infant frequently

NCLEX!

i. Assess for dumping syndrome 30 minutes after feeding if postoperative for Nissen fundoplication

j. Assess parents' ability to provide home care

k. Assess parents' coping mechanisms

l. Encourage parental participation in child's care and offer positive reinforcement

NCLEX!

6. Medications: see Table 13-1 for drugs commonly used to treat gastroesophageal reflux

7. Child and family education

a. Explain proper feeding techniques, such as thickening the formula, crosscutting the nipples and upright positioning of infant

b. Provide information about medication administration

c. Inform parents of problems that may arise and when to notify the physician

8. Evaluation

a. Infant gains weight and tolerates diet

b. Infant maintains balanced fluid and electrolyte status

c. Infant exhibits clear breath sounds and is free from respiratory distress

d. Parents verbalize and demonstrate proper feeding techniques

e. Parents comply with follow-up care

Table 13-1

Medications Used to Treat Gastroesophageal Reflux

Drug	Action
Antacids (aluminum hydroxide, aluminum carbonate)	Neutralize refluxed material and decrease resultant discomfort
Histamine blockers Ranitidine (Rantac) Cimetidine (Tagamet)	Decrease gastric acid production
Metoclopramide (Reglan)	Increase esophageal motility and tone
Cisapride (Propulsid)	Increase esophageal motility and tone
Acetaminophen (Tylenol)	Control pain

Source: Ball, J. & Bindler, R. (1999). *Pediatric nursing: Caring for children* (2nd ed.). Stamford, CT: Appleton & Lange, p. 610.

B. Appendicitis

1. Description: appendicitis is the inflammation and infection of the vermiform appendix, a small lymphoid, tubular blind sac at the end of the cecum

2. Etiology and pathophysiology

   a. The exact cause of appendicitis is poorly understood, but it is a result of an obstruction of the lumen of the appendix by hardened fecal material (**fecalith**), foreign bodies, microorganisms, or parasites

   b. The obstruction of the lumen causes an accumulation of normal mucous secretions causing the appendix to become distended; this distention causes capillary and venous engorgement and increased intraluminal pressure

   c. The process of ischemia can lead to necrosis and perforation of the intestinal wall; if this occurs the bacteria from the bowel contaminates the peritoneum and may lead to peritonitis and sepsis

   d. Appendicitis is the most common reason for abdominal surgery in childhood; frequency increases with age with the peak incidence between ages 15 and 30 years old

   e. Appendicitis occurs equally in males and females

3. Assessment

   NCLEX!

   a. Generalized abdominal pain progressively worsening and localizing in the right lower quadrant at **McBurney's point** (Figure 13-3)

   b. Nausea and vomiting, fever, and chills

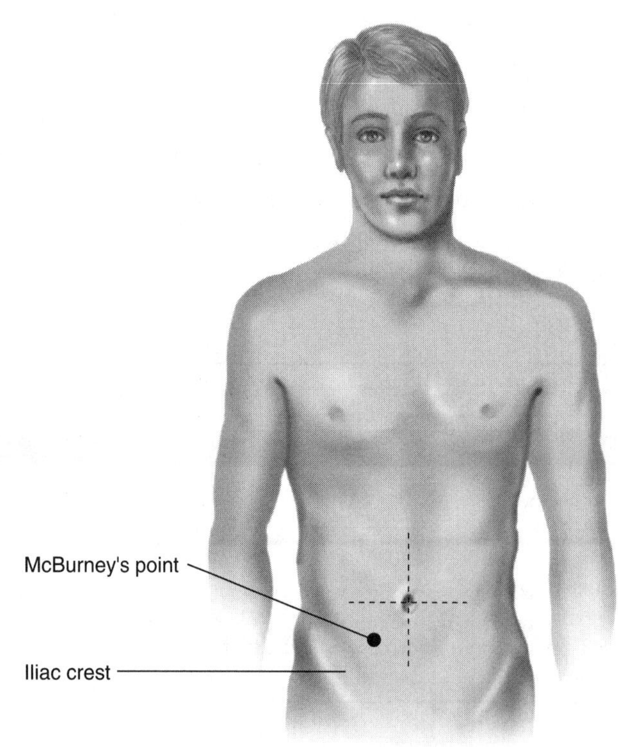

Figure 13-3

McBurney's point in appendicitis.
Source: Ball, J. & Bindler, R. (1999). *Pediatric nursing: Caring for children* (2nd ed.). Stamford, CT: Appleton & Lange, p. 618.

   c. Anorexia, diarrhea, or acute constipation
   d. Elevated WBC count: 15,000 to 20,000 cells/mm^3
   e. Ultrasound indicating an enlarged incompressible appendix

4. Priority nursing diagnoses: Risk for infection, Pain, Anxiety, Risk for fluid volume deficit, Altered nutrition: less than body requirements
5. Planning and implementation
   a. Surgical removal (appendectomy) is done as soon as diagnosis made
   b. Preoperative nursing care
      1) Prepare the child for an appendectomy; explain the procedure and postoperative care to child and family
      2) Keep the child NPO before surgery and prevent dehydration by administering IV fluids as ordered

NCLEX!

      3) Place the child in semi-Fowler's or right-side lying position to help localize and prevent the spread of any infection; this position is used both preoperatively and postoperatively
      4) Assess bowel activity by evaluating for abdominal distention, auscultating bowel sounds, and observing elimination patterns

NCLEX!

      5) Do nothing to stimulate peristalsis, which would hasten perforation; avoid laxatives, enemas, or heat applications
      6) Apply cold packs to the child's abdomen to help relieve discomfort

NCLEX!

      7) Sudden relief of pain usually indicates a ruptured appendix
   c. Postoperative nursing care

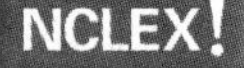

      1) Monitor vital signs, assess for abdominal distention and inspect the surgical wound for signs of infection
      2) Encourage ambulation within 6 to 8 hours after surgery, if not contraindicated
      3) Encourage the child to turn, cough, and breathe deeply
      4) Monitor intake and output and ensure that spontaneous voiding occurs
      5) Assess for pain and administer analgesics as ordered

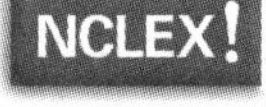

      6) If appendix ruptures, postoperative recovery is slowed; child will probably have a NG tube to decompress the stomach, and a penrose drain; antibiotics may be administered
6. Child and family education
   a. Explain to child and family diagnostic procedures, cause of appendicitis, surgical treatment and anticipated postoperative care
   b. Provide instruction on assessing the surgical incision for signs and symptoms of infection
   c. Provide information on other problems that should be reported to the physician, such as, fever, increased discomfort, and incision **dehiscence** (separation)

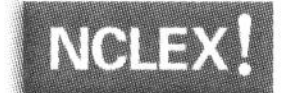

d. Instruct parents to have child avoid lifting, stretching, and strenuous activities until all follow-up care is completed

e. Provide information on fluids and nutrition during the recovery process and the advancement of the diet; include signs and symptoms to notify the physician for, such as, vomiting, abdominal distention, and increased pain

7. Evaluation

a. The child expresses, through verbal and nonverbal behaviors, that pain is being controlled

b. The child is free from fever and infection

c. The child remains hydrated

d. The child demonstrates early ambulation

e. Family and the child verbalize feelings and understanding of condition and treatment

Practice to Pass

A 12-year-old just arrived at the Emergency Department. The admitting diagnosis is rule out appendicitis. What signs and symptoms would you anticipate this child has?

C. Umbilical hernia

1. Description

a. A hernia is a protrusion of the bowel through an abnormal opening in the abdominal wall

b. An umbilical hernia is a soft, skin-covered protrusion of intestine and **omentum** (double fold of peritoneum) through a weakness in the abdominal wall around the umbilicus

2. Etiology and pathophysiology

a. In an umbilical hernia, incomplete closure of the umbilical ring results in protrusion of portions of the omentum and intestine through the opening

b. The defect usually closes spontaneously by age 3 or 4 years; surgical correction is necessary if closure does not occur or if incarceration of herniated bowel occurs

c. This defect is most common in low birthweight infants or black infants and commonly occurs in children with Down Syndrome, hypothyroidism, and Hurler syndrome

3. Assessment

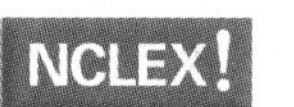

a. Clinical manifestations of umbilical hernias typically include a soft swelling or protrusion around the umbilicus, usually reducible with the finger

b. An incarcerated hernia is one that cannot be reduced and increases the risk of ischemia of the bowel

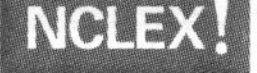

c. An incarcerated hernia produces such symptoms as irritability, tenderness at the site, anorexia, abdominal distention, and difficult defecation

4. Priority nursing diagnoses: Altered family processes; Risk for fluid volume deficit; Risk for injury; Pain

5. Planning and implementation

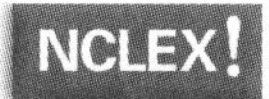

a. Most umbilical hernias disappear spontaneously by 1 year of age

b. No surgical repair is needed unless it causes symptoms, persists past 5 years of age, becomes strangulated, or continues to grow

c. Binding is not effective in reducing or minimizing the protrusion

d. Monitor for changes in size of hernia

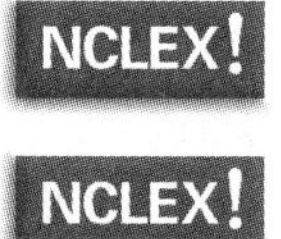

e. Assess for increased bowel sounds and irreducible mass, which may indicate strangulation

f. Postoperatively, assess for wound infection, maintain hydration, assess and manage pain, allow for self-expression

6. Child and family education

NCLEX!

a. Teach parents the signs of strangulation, such as vomiting, pain, and an irreducible mass at the umbilicus

b. Instruct parents to avoid ineffective and potentially harmful home remedies such as “belly binders”

c. Teach parents the signs and symptoms of wound infection

d. Inform the parents of any precautions and restrictions, such as, tub bathing, or strenuous activity if surgery was performed

7. Evaluation

a. Parents identify care of the child with an umbilical hernia

b. Parents avoid use of belly binders or coins as reduction devices

c. Infant has an unremarkable postoperative period, including proper wound healing, effective pain management, and appropriate hydration status

D. Celiac disease

1. Description

a. A genetic GI malabsorption condition also known as gluten-sensitive enteropathy

b. Celiac disease is a chronic inability to tolerate foods containing gluten

c. This disease results from the inability to fully digest the gliadin and glutenin or protein components of certain grains like wheat, barley, rye, and oats

NCLEX!

d. This deficiency in digestion requires lifelong dietary modifications

2. Etiology and pathophysiology

a. The exact cause is unknown, but it is believed there is an inherited predisposition with an influence by environmental factors and an immunologic abnormality

b. Incidence of celiac disease ranges from 1 in 3,000 to 5,000 live births; this disease is more common in white and European children and is rarely reported in Asians or blacks

c. When exposed to gluten, changes occur in the intestinal mucosa; the intestinal mucosa becomes damaged; the villi will eventually atrophy which reduces the absorptive surface of the small intestine and affects absorption of ingested nutrients; chronic diarrhea results

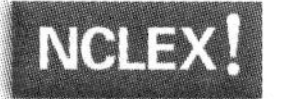

d. Acute episodes characterized by a general flare-up of symptoms occur and are precipitated by infections, prolonged fasting, ingestion of gluten, or exposure to anticholinergic drugs; these episodes are called celiac crises and can lead to electrolyte imbalance, rapid dehydration, and severe acidosis

3. Assessment

   a. Symptoms typically appear within 3 to 6 months after introduction of gluten (usually in the form of grains) into the child's diet

   b. Frequent bulky, greasy, malodorous stools with frothy appearance due to fat in stool (**steatorrhea**)

   c. Abdominal distention, vomiting, and anorexia

   d. Growth retardation with lack of fat deposits and muscle wasting

   e. Anemia, irritability, edema

   f. In a celiac crisis, severe diarrhea and dehydration ensue; electrolyte imbalances and metabolic acidosis can create life-threatening disease

   g. For unknown reasons, some children do not exhibit symptoms until after age 5 years with growth retardation and delayed sexual maturation as the predominant manifestations

   h. Laboratory studies and diagnostic tests

      1) Flat mucosal surface, absence or atrophy of villi, and deep crypts visible on biopsy of small intestine

      2) Steatorrhea on analysis of 72-hour quantitative fecal fat study

      3) Presence of serum antigliadin antibody (AGA) and reticulin antibody levels are elevated

4. Priority nursing diagnoses: Altered nutrition: less than body requirements; Fluid volume deficit; Altered growth and development; Knowledge deficit; Risk for injury

5. Planning and implementation

   a. Nursing care focuses on supporting the child and parents in maintaining a gluten-free diet (see Table 13-2)

   b. Assess child's growth and evaluate using a standard growth chart

   c. Administer fluids for hydration

   d. Monitor I & O, assess skin turgor, mucous membranes, and urine specific gravity

   e. Encourage participation in age-appropriate activities

Table 13-2

Suggestions for a Gluten-Free Diet

Unrestricted Food Items	Restricted Food Items
Beef, pork, poultry, fish	Breaded items using wheat, oats, rye or barley
Eggs	Any food made from wheat, rye, oats, or barley (bread, rolls, cookies, cakes, crackers, cereal, spaghetti, macaroni)
Milk, cream, cheese	Beer and ale, Ovaltine, instant tea mix, commercially prepared ice cream, malted milk, prepared puddings
Vegetables	Canned baked beans, commercially seasoned vegetable mixes or vegetables with sauce
Fruit	Salad dressings and mayonnaise, ketchup, gravy
Rice, corn, gluten-free wheat flour, puffed rice, corn flakes, corn meal	

f. Inform parents of organizations such as the American Celiac Society, the Celiac Sprue Association/United States of America, and the Gluten Intolerance Group

6. Child and family education

a. Provide written and verbal instructions on gluten-free diet

NCLEX!

b. Instruct parents to read labels of processed foods, because most contain gluten as a filler

c. Provide instructions about the urgency of seeking medical care in the event of celiac crisis

NCLEX!

d. Teach the importance of lifelong compliance with dietary modifications and follow-up medical care

7. Evaluation

a. Child has soft, formed stools without diarrhea

b. Child resumes normal growth pattern and participates in age-appropriate activities

c. Parents verbalize an understanding of the disease process, dietary modifications, and the prevention of celiac crisis

d. Parents will contact one of the suggested organizations for further information and support

E. Necrotizing enterocolitis

1. Description

a. Necrotizing enterocolitis (NEC) is an inflammatory disease of the intestinal tract that occurs primarily in premature infants

b. NEC is characterized by varying degrees of mucosal or transmural necrosis of the intestine

c. The usual onset is in the first 2 weeks of life but can be later in very low birthweight infants

2. Etiology and pathophysiology

a. NEC can be caused by several factors, such as intestinal ischemia, bacterial or viral infection, and immaturity of the gut; the disease occurs most often in the terminal ileum and colon

b. The onset of pathology appears to begin when the blood flow to the bowel leads to bowel wall ischemia; this ischemia allows bacteria to enter the bowel wall and colonize

c. Damage to the bowel can lead to perforation, which leads to the necessity of bowel resection

3. Assessment

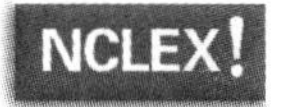

a. History may include prematurity, small for gestational age, maternal hemorrhage, preeclampsia, cocaine exposure in utero, exchange transfusions, umbilical catheters, or asphyxia

b. Typically, suspected NEC (stage I) consists of nonspecific clinical findings that simply represent physiologic instability and may resemble other common conditions in premature infants; these findings include:

1) Temperature instability

2) Lethargy

3) Recurrent apnea and bradycardia

4) Hypoglycemia

5) Poor peripheral perfusion

6) Increased pregavage gastric residuals

7) Feeding intolerance, vomiting, abdominal distention

8) Guaiac positive stools

NCLEX!

c. NEC (stage II) consists of nonspecific signs and symptoms plus the following:

1) Severe abdominal distention

2) Abdominal tenderness

3) Grossly bloody stools

4) Palpable bowel loops

5) Edema of the abdominal wall

6) Bowel sounds may be absent

NCLEX!

d. NEC (stage III) occurs when the infant becomes acutely ill; signs and symptoms include:

1) Deterioration of vital signs

2) Evidence of septic shock

3) Edema and erythema of abdominal wall

4) Right lower quadrant mass

5) Acidosis (metabolic and/or respiratory)

6) Disseminated intravascular coagulation

e. Diagnostic testing includes an abdominal x-ray revealing free peritoneal gas, dilated bowel loops, bowel distention, and bowel thickening

4. Priority nursing diagnoses: Altered nutrition: less than body requirements; Risk for infection; Risk for injury; Risk for fluid volume deficit; Ineffective breathing pattern; Risk for altered parenting

5. Planning and implementation

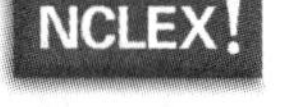

a. Nursing care focuses on early detection to minimize bowel necrosis

b. Measure abdominal girth frequently

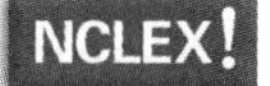

c. Observe toleration of feedings

d. Monitor cardiac and respiratory status

e. Assess and maintain optimal hydration status

f. Promote and maintain adequate body temperature

g. Administer antibiotics as ordered

h. Encourage family interaction and promote the attachment process

i. Provide developmentally appropriate activities

6. Child and family education

a. Encourage parents to ventilate concerns about outcomes of surgery

b. Instruct parents on the signs of intestinal obstruction, strictures, poor tolerance of feedings, and impaired healing processes

c. Instruct parents about care of ostomy and intravenous central line

7. Evaluation

a. Infant regains normal gastrointestinal function

b. Infant's growth improves as evidenced on the growth chart

c. Parents verbalize an understanding of home care and follow-up needs

F. Failure to thrive

1. Description

a. Failure to thrive (FTT) is a term used to describe a child whose weight falls below the 5th percentile on a standardized growth chart; growth measurements in addition to a persistent deviation from an established growth curve is generally a cause for concern

b. There are two basic types of FTT: organic and non-organic

2. Etiology and pathophysiology: the type of FTT is determined by the causes involved

a. Organic FTT is the result of a physical cause; cystic fibrosis is the leading cause of organic FTT; other physical causes include celiac disease, congenital heart defects, chronic renal failure, gastroesophageal reflux, malabsorption syndrome, or endocrine dysfunction

b. Non-organic FTT is caused by psychosocial factors and is suspected in the absence of history, physical, or laboratory findings of any organic disease; lack of bonding to the primary caregiver is the most common non-organic cause, however, other factors that can play a role are poverty, health beliefs, inadequate nutritional knowledge, family stress, feeding resistance, or insufficient breast milk

3. Assessment

a. Physical findings

1) Weight below the 5th percentile

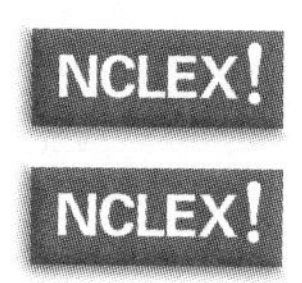

2) Sudden or rapid deceleration in growth curve

3) Delay in developmental milestones

4) Decreased muscle mass

5) Abdominal distention

6) Muscular hypotonia

7) Generalized weakness and **cachexia** (malnutrition accompanied by wasting)

b. Behavioral indicators

1) Avoidance of eye contact or physical touch

2) Intense watchfulness

3) Sleep distrubances

NCLEX!

4) Disturbed manner, such as apathy, extreme irritability, extreme compliance

NCLEX!

5) Repetitive rocking, head banging, intense sucking, intense chewing of fingers or hands, or head rolling

c. Diagnostic tests

1) Developmental screening

2) Tuberculin skin test

3) Bone scan, chest x-ray, ECG, intravenous pyelogram, upper and lower gastrointestinal series

4) Urinalysis, complete blood count, sweat chloride test, stool tests, T4 test

5) Bowel and muscle biopsies

4. Priority nursing diagnoses: Altered nutrition: less than body requirements; Altered growth and development; Altered family processes; Altered parenting

5. Planning and implementation

a. Document child's eating patterns

b. Document parent-child interaction

c. Encourage parents to discuss positive and negative feelings of care, procedures, and interaction with the child

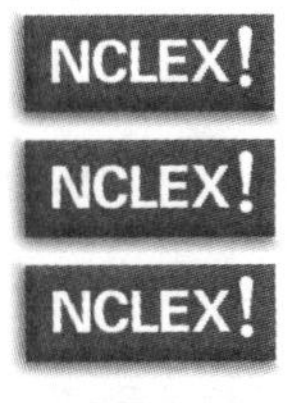

d. Feed on demand or increase intake as tolerated

e. Offer high-protein, high-calorie snacks

f. Offer frequent, small portions of a wide variety of foods

g. Monitor I & O, daily weights

h. Provide consistency in nursing care

6. Child and family education

a. Reinforce information about normal growth and development

b. Provide written and verbal information on ways to make mealtimes less of a control issue

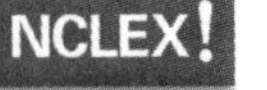

c. Provide information on effective feeding practices

7. Evaluation
    a. Infant gains weight and eats foods that are offered
    b. Parents participate in feeding the infant, and demonstrate appropriate interactions with the infant during meals

V. Infectious Gastrointestinal Health Problems

A. Hepatitis

1. Description: hepatitis is an inflammation of the liver; it ranges greatly in severity and can be caused by several different viruses, toxins, or disease states
2. Etiology and pathophysiology
    a. Hepatitis viruses cause local necrosis of the parenchymal cells of the liver; the inflammatory response leads to swelling and blockage of the liver's drainage system
    b. Hepatitis occurs in varying levels of severity from asymptomatic or mild cases, in which the liver cells regenerate completely in 2 to 3 months, to more severe forms, in which hepatic necrosis and death may occur in 1 to 2 weeks
    c. There are five major hepatitis viruses

NCLEX!

1) Hepatitis A is transmitted via the GI tract (oral–fecal route); hepatitis A is highly contagious and easily spread throughout households and day-care centers

NCLEX!

2) Hepatitis B is bloodborne; hepatitis B is transmitted through the exchange of blood or body fluids; hepatitis A and B are the most common forms
3) Hepatitis C, also called post-transfusion hepatitis, is spread by blood and body fluids; it is the most common cause of chronic hepatitis
4) Hepatitis D, Delta-agent hepatitis, is transmitted by the percutaneous route and occurs only in people infected with hepatitis B
5) Hepatitis E is transmitted enterically

3. Assessment
    a. Children less than 5 years of age diagnosed with hepatitis A are usually asymptomatic or have mild, nonspecific symptoms
    b. Individuals with hepatitis B can be asymptomatic or have acute fulminating hepatitis, which can be fatal
    c. If symptomatic, symptoms usually occur in two stages: anicteric and icteric

NCLEX!

1) **Anicteric** (absence of jaundice), lasting 5 to 7 days
    a) Anorexia, nausea, and vomiting
    b) Right upper quadrant (RUQ) abdominal or epigastric pain
    c) Fever, malaise, fatigue, depression, irritability
    d) Hepatosplenomegaly

NCLEX!

2) **Icteric** (presence of jaundice), lasting up to 4 weeks

a) Jaundice, urticaria

b) Dark urine and light-colored stools

c) Child temporarily feels better as jaundice appears

d. Acute fulminating hepatitis: bleeding problems, hepatic encephalopathy, ascites, acute liver failure, death; this complication is seen infrequently but quickly leads to liver decompensation that can lead to death within a week

e. Other assessment findings

1) A positive history of exposure to jaundiced children

2) A confirmed outbreak in daycare center

3) Percutaneous exposure to blood or body fluid

4) Elevated liver function tests (SGOT, SGPT), bilirubin levels, sedimentation rate

5) Antigen identification markers (IgM anti-HAV and IgM anti-HBV)

6) Positive liver biopsy

NCLEX!

4. Priority nursing diagnoses: Risk for altered health maintenance; Altered nutrition: less than body requirements; Risk for injury; Body image disturbance; Activity intolerance

5. Planning and implementation

a. In uncomplicated cases, treatment is usually supportive; hospitalization is rarely indicated; in fulminating hepatitis, intensive care may be needed to provide homeostasis, nutritional, and hydration support, as well as neurologic assessment to increase the chances of survival

NCLEX!

b. With cases of hepatitis A, controlling the spread of infection is a major nursing focus; this is accomplished through disinfection of contaminated diaper-changing surfaces, use of universal precautions, and reporting to the local public health department; exposed individuals should receive immune globulin as soon as possible

NCLEX!

c. With cases of hepatitis B, prevention is the major health focus; hepatitis B vaccines are begun during the neonatal period and are recommended for all infants as part of their well-child care

6. Child and family education

a. Teach parents how to maintain adequate nutrition

NCLEX!

b. Teach parents how to prevent the spread of infection

c. Advise parents to call for signs and symptoms of fulminant hepatitis

7. Evaluation

a. The child maintains a pre-illness weight, is free of vomiting and abdominal pain, and stools will remain normal

b. Family members remain free from infection

c. The child does not experience fulminant hepatitis

d. Family verbalizes an understanding of disease process, use of universal precautions, and complies with immunization recommendations

B. Vomiting and diarrhea

1. Description

a. Vomiting is the forceful ejection of gastric contents through the mouth

1) Vomiting in children is common and is usually self-limiting

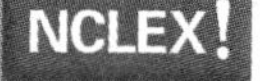

2) Vomiting requires no specific treatment unless complications occur (including dehydration and electrolyte imbalances, malnutrition, and aspiration)

b. Diarrhea is defined as frequent, watery, loose stools and is actually a symptom rather than a disease

1) Diarrhea accompanies many childhood disorders, including respiratory infections and gastrointestinal disorders, and it can be an adverse effect of certain medical management modalities such as antibiotic therapy

2) Diarrhea can be acute or chronic, inflammatory or non-inflammatory, or viral or bacterial in nature

3) Diarrhea can lead to a state of dehydration, electrolyte imbalance, hypovolemic shock, and even death in pediatric clients

2. Etiology and pathophysiology

a. Vomiting is a well-defined, complex, coordinated process that is under the control of the central nervous system; the act of vomiting involves both voluntary and involuntary muscles; a certain position is assumed, the glottis is closed, the diaphragm and abdominal muscles contract, and the cardiac sphincter relaxes while anti-peristaltic waves occur

b. Vomiting can be an associated symptom of an acute infectious disease, increased intracranial pressure, toxic ingestion, food intolerance and allergy, mechanical obstruction of the GI tract, metabolic disorder, or a psychogenic problem

c. The child's age, pattern of vomiting, and duration of symptoms help to determine the etiology

d. The color and consistency of the emesis vary according to the etiology

1) Green bilious vomiting suggests bowel obstruction

2) Curdled stomach contents, mucus, or fatty foods that are vomited several hours after ingestion suggest poor gastric emptying

3) Vomitus having the appearance and consistency of coffee grounds (due to blood being mixed with stomach contents) is associated with GI bleeding disorders

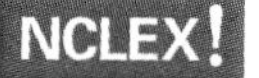

e. Associated symptoms also help to identify the etiology

1) Fever and diarrhea accompanying vomiting suggest an infection

2) Constipation associated with vomiting suggests an obstruction

3) Localized abdominal pain and vomiting often occur with appendicitis, pancreatitis, or peptic ulcer disease

4) A change in level of consciousness or a headache associated with vomiting indicates a central nervous system or metabolic disorder

5) Forceful vomiting (projectile) is associated with pyloric stenosis

f. Diarrhea

1) Increased intestinal motility and rapid emptying results in impaired absorption of nutrients and excessive excretion of water and electrolytes

2) The electrolytes most affected are sodium and potassium; sodium is necessary for fluid and acid–base balance; potassium is a neurotransmitter necessary for muscle contractility

3) Diarrhea can have many different causes (Table 13-3)

4) Diarrhea is the leading cause of death and a major cause of morbidity in children throughout the world; children in daycare centers and those living in substandard housing environments lacking proper sanitation are at an increased risk

g. Fluid and electrolyte imbalance

1) Body fluids are contained in the extracellular and intracellular compartments and contain electrolytes, which perform varying functions in the body; the normal exchange of fluids between compartments occurs across the cell membrane; young children have more fluid outside the cell, interactions with the environment can significantly compromise the composition of that fluid

2) The ratio of water and solute determines fluid and electrolyte balance; the primary electrolytes are sodium, potassium, chloride and calcium

3) Extracellular sodium is responsible for the degree of concentration of body fluids and whether cells swell or shrink; decreased sodium (hyponatremia) in children can occur with increased intake of water, dilute formula, or physiological causes

4) Intracellular potassium is responsible for muscle function; imbalances cause flaccid skeletal muscles, gastrointestinal cramping and cardiac arrhythmias (see Table 13-4)

Table 13-3

Common Causes of Diarrhea in Children

Causative Factor	Effect on Bowel Function
Colon disease	Trauma to intestinal wall
Stress	Increased motility
Food Intolerance	Increased motility, increased mucus secretion in colon
Food Sensitivity	Decreased digestion of food
Intestinal Infection	Inflammation of mucosa, increased mucus secretion in colon
Medication	Irritation and superinfection
Surgical Procedure	Reduced size of colon, decreased absorption surface

Table 13-4 **Summary of Clinical Assessment of Electrolyte Imbalances**

Assessment Category	Specific Assessments	Changes with Electrolyte Imbalances
Skeletal muscle function	Muscle strength	Weakness, flaccid paralysis—hyperkalemia; hypokalemia
Neuromuscular excitability	Deep tendon reflexes	Depressed—hypercalcemia; hypermagnesemia
		Hyperactive—hypocalcemia; hypomagnesemia
	Chvostek's sign (not infants)	Positive—hypocalcemia; hypomagnesemia
	Trousseau's sign	Positive—hypocalcemia; hypomagnesemia
	Paresthesias	Digital or perioral—hypocalcemia
	Muscle cramping or twitching	Present—hypocalcemia; hypomagnesemia
Gastrointestinal tract function	Bowel sounds	Decreased or absent—hypokalemia
	Elimination pattern	Constipation—hypokalemia; hypercalcemia
		Diarrhea—hyperkalemia
Cardiac rhythm	Arrhythmia	Irregular—hyperkalemia; hypokalemia; hypercalcemia; hypocalcemia; hypermagnesemia; hypomagnesemia
	Electrocardiogram	Abnormal—hyperkalemia; hypokalemia; hypercalcemia; hypocalcemia; hypermagnesemia; hypomagnesemia
Cerebral function	Level of consciousness	Decreased—hyponatremia; hypernatremia

Source: Ball, J. & Bindler, R. (1999). *Pediatric nursing: Caring for children* (2nd ed.). Stamford, CT: Appleton & Lange, p. 325.

h. Acid–base imbalance

1) The degree of acidity or alkalinity of body fluids determines proper functioning of the cells of the body; the body maintains proper balance by constantly producing acids and buffers, regulating concentrations via the kidneys and respiratory system

2) Acidosis is determined by the number of hydrogen ions in fluid; increased hydrogen ions indicate acidosis; the lungs attempt to compensate by increasing rate and depth of respirations to remove carbon dioxide; the kidneys increase secretion of hydrogen ions, thereby raising serum pH

3) Alkalosis refers to the buffer bicarbonate; increased levels of bicarbonate cause alkalosis, respiratory rate decreases and the kidneys conserve hydrogen ions and excrete bicarbonate

3. Assessment

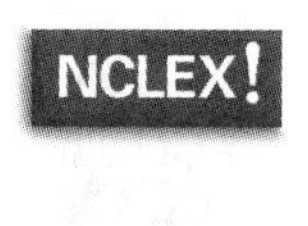

a. Assessment of the child's hydration status is highest priority (see Table 13-5)

b. Assess amount, color, consistency, and time of stools and vomitus

NCLEX!

c. Assess daily weights; daily weights are the best indication of fluid balance

d. Assess I & O and child's activity level

e. Assess for abdominal cramping, fever, and other related symptoms

f. Laboratory and diagnostic tests

1) Stool examination to rule out bacteria, ova, parasites, or rotaviruses

2) Stool examination for pH, leukocytes, glucose, and presence of blood

3) Electrolytes, BUN, creatinine, and glucose

4) X-rays, ultrasound, or endoscopy

Table 13-5 Severity of Clinical Dehydration

	Mild	Moderate	Severe
Percent of body weight lost	Up to 5%	6%–9%	10% or more
Level of consciousness	Alert, restless, thirsty	Restless or lethargic (infants and very young children); alert, thirsty, rest less (older children and adolescents)	Lethargic to comatose (infants and young children); often conscious apprehensive (older children and adolescents)
Blood pressure	Normal	Normal or low; postural hypotension (older children and adolescents)	Low to undetectable
Pulse	Normal	Rapid	Rapid, weak to nonpalpable
Skin turgor	Normal	Poor	Very poor
Mucous membranes	Moist	Dry	Parched
Urine	May appear normal	Decreased output (<1 mL/kg/hr); dark color	Very decreased or absent output
Thirst	Slightly increased	Moderately increased	Greatly increased unless lethargic
Fontanel	Normal	Sunken	Sunken
Extremities	Warm; normal capillary refill	Delayed capillary refill (>2 sec)	Cool, discolored; delayed capillary refill (>3–4 sec)

Source: Ball, J. & Bindler, R. (1999). *Pediatric nursing: Caring for children* (2nd ed.). Stamford, CT: Appleton & Lange, p. 294.

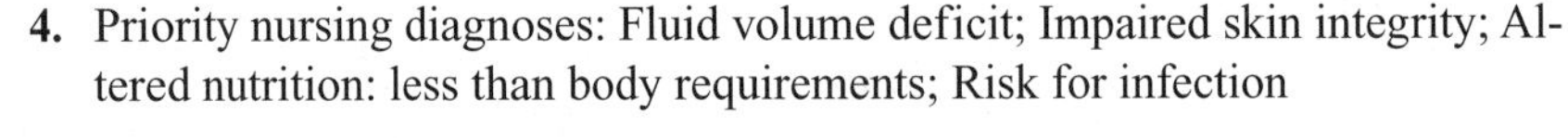

4. Priority nursing diagnoses: Fluid volume deficit; Impaired skin integrity; Altered nutrition: less than body requirements; Risk for infection
5. Planning and implementation
    a. Priority nursing interventions are focused on assessing signs and symptoms of dehydration

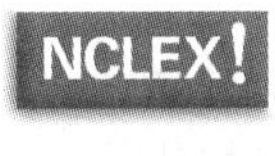

    b. Weigh child on admission and daily using the same scale at the same time of day

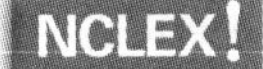

    c. Monitor and document I & O hourly, weigh each diaper after voiding and bowel movements, monitor urine specific gravity
    d. Monitor vital signs, avoiding rectal temperatures
    e. Child is usually NPO to allow bowel rest; administer I.V. fluids as ordered

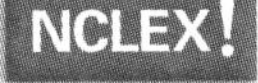

    f. Begin oral rehydration with frequent, small feedings; oral rehydration fluids include commercial preparations such as Pedialyte; frequent small amounts of liquids should be offered—1 to 3 teaspoons of fluid every 10 to 15 minutes; infants progress from clear liquids to a bland, milk-free diet; bananas, rice cereal, applesauce, and toast diets (BRAT) may still be prescribed for the child recovering from diarrhea; as vomiting/diarrhea improves, the child may resume regular diet
    g. Administer antidiarrheals, antibiotics, antiprotozoals as ordered
    h. Monitor lab tests (electrolytes, hematocrit, pH, serum albumin)
    i. Implement measures to reduce fever if needed
    j. Cleanse diaper area with mild soap and water after each stool, avoid the use of baby wipes

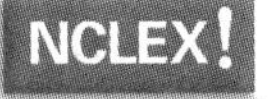

    k. Practice universal precautions

6. Child and family education

a. Provide information on causes of vomiting and diarrhea

b. Provide instructions on oral rehydration therapy

c. Demonstrate skin care to the family

d. Instruct parent what signs and symptoms require medical attention

7. Evaluation

a. Child is well hydrated as evidenced by moist mucous membranes, elastic skin turgor, urine specific gravity of 1.005–1.020, 1–2 mL/kg/hr of urine output

b. Child is free of frequent, loose stools as evidenced by soft, formed stools of less than four per 24-hour period

c. Child is free from vomiting

d. Child tolerates a regular diet

e. Child maintains skin integrity

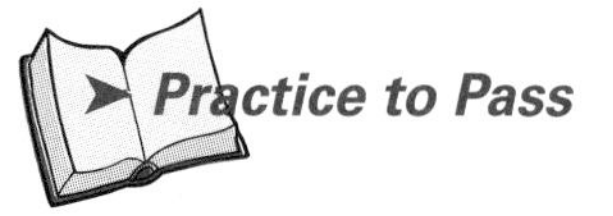

A mother brings her 4-month-old son to the pediatrician's office with a history of vomiting and diarrhea. What are your immediate assessments?

Case Study

A 4-year-old has been admitted for rule out appendicitis. She has just arrived in your nursing unit. The child is crying stating her stomach hurts. No surgery has been scheduled, but close observation is warranted. The child and her parents are very anxious.

1. What questions will you ask her and/or her parents?
2. What general nursing orders do you expect for this client during her observation phase?
3. What can you do to help relieve this child's pain?
4. How can you decrease the parent's anxiety? The child's anxiety?
5. What postoperative nursing orders do you expect depending on whether there is rupture or no rupture?

For suggested responses, see page 411.

Posttest

1 **The best rationale to give parents who are questioning the use of elbow restraints with their child who has had cleft palate repair is:**

(1) "This device is frequently used postoperatively to protect the IV site in small children."
(2) "The restraints will help us maintain proper body alignment."
(3) "Elbow restraints are used postoperatively to keep their hands away from the surgical site."
(4) "The restraints help us remember that the child is NPO after surgery."

2 **The nurse is caring for an infant vomiting secondary to pyloric stenosis. The mother questions why the vomitus of this child appears different from that of her other children when they have the flu. The nurse would explain that the emesis of an infant with pyloric stenosis does not contain bile because:**

(1) The GI system is still immature in newborns and infants.
(2) The obstruction is above the bile duct.
(3) The emesis is from passive regurgitation.
(4) The bile duct is obstructed.

3 **The nurse is teaching the parents of a child with celiac disease about the dietary restrictions. The nurse would explain that the most appropriate diet for their child is:**

(1) Gluten-free.
(2) Salt-free.
(3) Fat-free.
(4) High-calorie, low-fat.

4 **A high school experiences an outbreak of hepatitis B. In teaching the high school students about hepatitis B, the nurse would explain:**

(1) Hepatitis B cannot exist in carrier state.
(2) Hepatitis B is primarily transmitted through the fecal–oral route.
(3) Immunity to all types of hepatitis will occur after this current attack.
(4) Hepatitis B can be prevented by receiving the HBV vaccine.

5 **A 4-year-old child is admitted to the unit with moderate dehydration. Which of the following symptoms led the physicians to the diagnosis of moderate dehydration in this child?**

(1) Elevated heart rate and sunken fontanel
(2) Increased thirst and urine specific gravity of 1.038
(3) Weight gain and decreased skin turgor
(4) Oliguria and urine specific gravity of 1.010

6 **While performing a newborn assessment, the nurse notices the infant is having difficulty breathing. Nasal flaring, cyanosis, and retractions are observed and there are no breath sounds on the left side. The apical pulse is auscultated on the right side of the chest. The nurse would notify the physician immediately because he or she suspects:**

(1) Diaphragmatic hernia.
(2) Pyloric stenosis.
(3) Cleft palate.
(4) Omphalocele.

7 **The nurse has taught dietary restrictions to the 7-year-old child with celiac disease. After teaching, the child is allowed to choose a correct menu. The nurse would know that teaching was effective when the child chooses:**

(1) Beef and barley soup, rice cakes, and celery.
(2) Ham and cheese sandwich with lettuce and tomato on rye toast.
(3) Beef patty on a hamburger bun and french fries.
(4) Baked chicken, green beans, and a slice of cornbread.

8 **An infant returns from initial surgery for Hirschsprung's disease. Because of the type of surgery the child had, the nurse would exclude from the routine postoperative plan-of-care instructions to:**

(1) Maintain the child NPO until bowel sounds return.
(2) Monitor rectal temperature every 4 hours.
(3) Reunite the parents with the child as soon as possible.
(4) Assess the surgical site every 2 hours.

9 **A 3-month-old infant has gastroesophageal reflux (GER) but is thriving without other complications. The mother wants to know if there is anything she can do differently to decrease the reflux. Which of the following interventions should the nurse suggest to minimize reflux?**

(1) Discontinue breast-feeding immediately.
(2) Decrease frequency of feedings as much as possible.
(3) Place the baby in prone position with the head elevated.
(4) Place the infant in a car seat after feeding.

10 **A 10-year-old boy has been admitted with a diagnosis of "rule out appendicitis." While the nurse was conducting a routine assessment, the boy stated, "It doesn't hurt anymore." The nurse suspects that:**

(1) The boy is afraid of going to surgery.
(2) The boy is having difficulty expressing his pain adequately.
(3) The appendix has ruptured.
(4) This is a method the boy uses to receive attention.

See page 346 for Answers and Rationales.

Answers and Rationales

Pretest

1 **Answer: 3** ***Rationale:*** During the immediate postoperative period, protecting the operative site is a priority in the nursing care of this child. A toothbrush should be a familiar object to an 18-month-old child. Deciduous (primary) teeth are still present at this age and are replaced by permanent (secondary) teeth around 6 years of age. Oral care will be performed according to the physician's orders but usually consists of cleansing the area with sterile water.
Cognitive Level: Application
Nursing Process: Implementation; ***Test Plan:*** PHYS

2 **Answer: 1** ***Rationale:*** Clear liquids are usually prescribed 4 to 6 hours after surgery.
Cognitive Level: Application
Nursing Process: Evaluation; ***Test Plan:*** PHYS

3 **Answer: 4** ***Rationale:*** Omphaloceles are congenital malformations in which abdominal contents protrude through the umbilical cord. The protrusion is covered by a translucent sac; immediately after birth, the sac requires priority attention. The sac is covered with sterile gauze soaked in normal saline solution to prevent drying and injury.
Cognitive Level: Application
Nursing Process: Implementation; ***Test Plan:*** PHYS

4 **Answer: 3** ***Rationale:*** Infants with Hirschsprung's disease usually display failure to thrive, with poor weight gain and delayed growth. Projectile vomiting is usually associated with pyloric stenosis. Decreased urine output and intermittent sharp pain are nonspecific symptoms that can be associated with many different diseases and disorders.
Cognitive Level: Analysis
Nursing Process: Analysis; ***Test Plan:*** PHYS

5 **Answer: 4** ***Rationale:*** Small, frequent feedings followed by placing the infant at a 30- to 45-degree angle has been shown to be beneficial in treating gastroesophageal reflux. Diluting the formula would not be recommended because the infant needs the calories from the full-strength formula. It may be recommended to thicken the formula with rice cereal. It is recommended to burp frequently; to delay burping would only increase the occurrences of reflux. Gastroesophageal reflux is not related to milk intolerance so changing the formula would not help the child.
Cognitive Level: Application
Nursing Process: Planning; ***Test Plan:*** HPM

6 **Answer: 2** ***Rationale:*** An ice bag may help relieve his pain. A rectal tube is contraindicated because it stimulates bowel motility, which would increase the pain. A heating pad is contraindicated because it increases the flow of blood to the appendix and may lead to rupture. An antispasmodic agent would not be beneficial for the pain associated with appendicitis. Antispasmodic agents are typically used to inhibit smooth muscle contractions.
Cognitive Level: Application
Nursing Process: Implementation; ***Test Plan:*** PHYS

7 **Answer: 1** ***Rationale:*** Discharge planning focuses on educating the parents in maintaining a gluten-free diet for the child. Dietary modifications are lifelong and should not be discontinued when the child is symptom-free. Symptoms will return if dietary restrictions are not maintained.
Cognitive Level: Application
Nursing Process: Evaluation; ***Test Plan:*** HPM

8 **Answer: 4** ***Rationale:*** Measuring the abdominal girth frequently aids in early detection of necrotizing enterocolitis, which, in turn, minimizes loss of bowel. Assessment of stomach pH is not done. Frequent assessment of the neurologic status is not specific to this disease. Rectal temperatures are contraindicated because of the increased risk of perforation.
Cognitive Level: Analysis
Nursing Process: Assessment; ***Test Plan:*** PHYS

9 **Answer: 2** ***Rationale:*** Hepatitis A is highly contagious and is transmitted primarily through the fecal–oral route. The virus is transmitted by direct person-to-person contact or through ingestion of contaminated food or water, especially shellfish growing in contaminated water. The remaining answers are related to other infectious diseases.
Cognitive Level: Application
Nursing Process: Implementation; ***Test Plan:*** SECE

10 **Answer: 3** ***Rationale:*** Mucous membranes typically appear dry when moderate dehydration is observed. Other typical findings associated with moderate dehydration include restlessness with periods of irritability (especially infants and young children), rapid pulse, poor skin turgor, delayed capillary refill, and decreased urine output. Both anterior and posterior fontanels are closed in a preschool-aged child. The skin is usually dry with decreased elasticity, not diaphoretic. Urine specific gravity increases with decreased urine output associated with dehydration.
Cognitive Level: Application
Nursing Process: Assessment; ***Test Plan:*** HPM

Posttest

1 **Answer: 3** ***Rationale:*** Elbow restraints are used to keep hands away from the mouth after cleft palate surgery. This precaution will be maintained at home until the palate is healed, usually 4 to 6 weeks.
Cognitive Level: Application
Nursing Process: Implementation; ***Test Plan:*** PHYS

2 **Answer: 2** ***Rationale:*** In pyloric stenosis, bile is unable to enter the stomach from the duodenum because the pylorus muscle is hypertrophied, which causes the obstruction.
Cognitive Level: Application
Nursing Process: Analysis; ***Test Plan:*** PHYS

3 **Answer: 1** ***Rationale:*** Most children who remain on a gluten-free diet are healthy and free of symptoms and complications.
Cognitive Level: Application
Nursing Process: Implementation; ***Test Plan:*** PHYS

4 **Answer: 4** ***Rationale:*** HBV vaccine provides active immunity and current recommendations include immunizations for all newborns, as well as several high-risk groups. Hepatitis B is spread by blood and body fluids, including through sexual contact.
Cognitive Level: Application
Nursing Process: Implementation; ***Test Plan:*** HPM

5 **Answer: 2** ***Rationale:*** The nurse would expect an increased desire to drink fluids and a higher specific gravity caused by the concentration of urine. Although the heart rate would be elevated, the fontanels are closed on a 4-year-old. The degree of dehydration is based on the percent of weight loss so a weight gain would not be likely. Diminished urine output is an expected normal finding in dehydration, however the urine specific gravity would also be affected.
Cognitive Level: Analysis
Nursing Process: Analysis; ***Test Plan:*** PHYS

6 **Answer: 1** ***Rationale:*** Clinical findings will vary in infants born with congenital diaphragmatic hernias but the first indications are of respiratory distress. Further assessment will reveal bowel sounds auscultated over the chest, cardiac sounds on the right of the chest, and a sunken abdomen with a barrel-shaped chest.
Cognitive Level: Analysis
Nursing Process: Analysis; ***Test Plan:*** HPM

7 **Answer: 4** ***Rationale:*** Celiac disease is characterized by an intolerance for gluten. Gluten is found in wheat, barley, rye, and oats. This includes bread, cake, doughnuts, cookies, and crackers, as well as processed foods that contain gluten as a filler.
Cognitive Level: Analysis
Nursing Process: Evaluation; ***Test Plan:*** HPM

8 **Answer: 2** ***Rationale:*** The corrective surgery for Hirschsprung's disease requires pulling the end of the normal bowel through the muscular sleeve of the rectum. With this type of procedure, rectal temperatures and any invasive procedure would be avoided to allow proper healing to occur.
Cognitive Level: Analysis
Nursing Process: Planning; ***Test Plan:*** PHYS

9 **Answer: 3** ***Rationale:*** Infants with GER should be given small, frequent feedings. After a feeding the infant should be placed in a prone position with the head of the bed elevated. A harness can be used to help maintain this position. Infant seats should be avoided because of the increased intrabdominal pressure this position creates.
Cognitive Level: Application
Nursing Process: Implementation; ***Test Plan:*** HPM

10 **Answer: 3** ***Rationale:*** Signs and symptoms of a ruptured appendix include fever, sudden relief from abdominal pain, guarding, abdominal distention, rapid shallow breathing, pallor, chills, and irritability.
Cognitive Level: Application
Nursing Process: Analysis; ***Test Plan:*** PHYS

References

Ashwill, J. & Droske, S. (1997). *Nursing care of children: Principles and practice.* Philadelphia: W. B. Saunders, pp. 558–560, 679–766, 1295–1300.

Ball, J. & Bindler, R. (1999). *Pediatric nursing: Caring for children* (2nd ed.). Stamford, CT: Appleton & Lange, pp. 293–301, 593–650, 972–973.

Bowden, V. R., Dickey, S. B., & Greenberg, C. S. (1998). *Children and their families: The continuum of care.* Philadelphia: W. B. Saunders, pp. 1028–1109.

Jarvis, C. (2000). *Physical examination and health assessment* (2nd ed.). Philadelphia: W. B. Saunders, pp. 605–608, 626–629.

Monahan, F. D., & Neighbors, M. (1998). *Medical-surgical nursing: Foundations for clinical practice* (2nd ed.). Philadelphia: W. B. Saunders, pp. 947–1199.

Olds, S., London, M., & Ladewig, P. (2000*). Maternal newborn nursing: A family and community-based approach* (6th ed.). Upper Saddle River, NJ: Prentice Hall, Inc., pp. 845–847.

Wilson, B., Shannon, M., & Stang, C. (2000). *Nurses drug guide 2000.* Stamford, CT: Appleton & Lange, pp. 136–137, 442–443, 589–590.

Wong, D., Hockenberry-Eaton, M., Wilson, D., Winkelstein, M., Ahmann, E., & DiVito-Thomas, P. (1999). *Whaley and Wong's nursing care of infants and children* (6th ed.). St. Louis: Mosby, Inc., pp. 451–452, 514–536, 643–647, 1316–1328, 1533–1577.

CHAPTER 14

Hematologic Health Problems

Gwendolyn T. Martin, MS, RN, CNS, CPN

CHAPTER OUTLINE

OBJECTIVES

- Identify data essential to the assessment of the hematologic system in a child.
- Discuss the clinical manifestations and pathophysiology related to alterations in health of the hematologic system of a child.
- Discuss therapeutic management of a child with alterations in the health of the hematologic system.
- Describe nursing management of a child with alterations in health of the hematologic system.

[Media Link]

Use the CD-ROM enclosed with this text, or log onto the address given to access the free, interactive Companion Website created for this series. The CD-ROM and Companion Website accompanying this book offer additional practice opportunities and information—NCLEX Review, Case Studies, Glossary, In Depth with NCLEX, and more.

www.prenhall.com/hogan

Review at a Glance

anemia *a decrease in the number of red blood cells, the amount of hemoglobin, and the volume of packed red cells to less-than-normal levels*

ecchymosis *the initial black or blue mark resulting from the release of blood into the tissue; this may occur because of injury or the spontaneous leaking of blood from the vessels*

erythrocytes *red blood cells*

erythropoiesis *red blood cell formation*

hemarthrosis *bleeding into the joint spaces of bones*

hematopoiesis *the production of blood cells*

hemochromatosis *the presence of excessive iron stores in the body*

hemoglobinopathy *a group of disorders associated with abnormal forms of hemoglobin*

hemolysis *the destruction of red blood cells*

leukocytes *white blood cells*

petechiae *pinpoint hemorrhages that cause tiny red or purple spots on the skin or mucous membranes*

thrombocytes *platelets*

x-linked recessive trait *also called sex-linked recessive trait; a form of inheritance where the mother passes the defective gene to her sons; the defective gene is carried on the X chromosome; the mother does not have the disease but is a carrier of the disease; affected fathers do not pass the gene to their sons, but their daughters will be carriers of the disorder*

Pretest

1 The nurse has completed some child and family education for a child diagnosed with thalassemia. The medical plan of treatment includes blood transfusions when the anemia reaches a severe point. Which statement by the parents indicates a need for further education?

(1) "Because of the anemia, my child will need extra rest periods."
(2) "My child inherited this disorder from both of us."
(3) "We should be alert to periods when our child seems paler than usual."
(4) "My child needs an iron supplement."

2 The nursing assistant is setting up a hospital room preparing to admit a child with disseminated intravascular coagulopathy. Which item would the nurse remove from the set-up?

(1) Rectal thermometer
(2) Bedpan
(3) Intravenous therapy start kit
(4) Sphygmometer

3 At a hemophilia camp, several children with injuries arrive at the clinic at the same time. When prioritizing care for the children, the child who requires the most immediate care from the nurse is the child with:

(1) A swollen knee.
(2) Abrasions on both arms.
(3) A slight head injury.
(4) A puncture wound in the foot.

4 A 14-year-old boy with sickle cell anemia is admitted with severe pain in his abdomen and legs. He asks why the doctor ordered oxygen when he is not having any problems breathing. The nurse would reply that the main therapeutic benefit of oxygen is to:

(1) Prevent further sickling.
(2) Prevent respiratory complications.
(3) Increase the oxygen-carrying capacity of red blood cells (RBCs).
(4) Decrease the potential for infection during the crisis.

5 You are administering a liquid iron preparation to a 3-year-old with iron deficiency anemia. It will be most appropriate to:

(1) Mix the medication in his milk and give it to him at lunch.
(2) Give the medication after lunch with a sweet dessert to disguise the taste.
(3) Give the medication to him in a small cup and allow him to sip it through a straw.
(4) Allow him to decide whether to take the medicine with breakfast or dinner.

6 **The nurse is admitting a child newly diagnosed with disseminated intravascular coagulopathy (DIC). Although the physician has explained the plan of care to the family, they continue to ask about each nursing activity. The nurse notes that the family seems unable to comprehend the answers. The nurse would:**

(1) Notify the doctor because the family seems to have a comprehension problem.
(2) Ask the doctor to write down the information for the family.
(3) Recognize that the family is under stress and continue to answer their questions.
(4) Determine if they are an English-as-a-second-language (ESL) family.

7 **You are administering factor VIII to a child with hemophilia. You should observe for which potential complication during the infusion?**

(1) Fluid overload
(2) Transfusion reaction
(3) Emboli formation
(4) Contracting AIDS

8 **As you make a plan of care for a child experiencing a sickle cell crisis, you should base your actions on the knowledge that the pain of a vaso-occlusive crisis is caused primarily by:**

(1) Obstruction of small blood vessels.
(2) Sequestration of blood.
(3) Hepatosplenomegaly.
(4) Increased RBC destruction.

9 **Which of the following statements should be included when teaching the parents of a 7-month-old infant about preventing anemia?**

(1) Anemia for the duration of infancy is unusual as infants use fetal iron stores until 18 months of age.
(2) Cow's milk is an excellent source of iron, and infants should be changed from formula to milk as soon as possible after 6 months of age.
(3) Milk is a poor source of iron, and infants should be given solid foods high in iron such as cereals, vegetables, and meats.
(4) Anemia can easily occur during infancy and all infants should receive iron supplements.

10 **What precautions should the nurse take when discontinuing an IV for a child with alterations in platelet function?**

(1) Restrict movement of the arm for 12 hours.
(2) Obtain a culture of the tip of the IV catheter.
(3) Place steri-strips over site and have child hold the arm above heart level for 15 minutes.
(4) Apply direct pressure to the site for at least 5 minutes.

See pages 373–374 for Answers and Rationales.

I. Overview of the Anatomy and Physiology of the Hematologic System

A. Hematologic function

1. The hematologic system facilitates the regulation of all other body systems directly or indirectly via blood and lymph circulating through every tissue and organ

2. The hematologic system is responsible for supplying and transporting oxygen to the other cells of the body

   a. It transports food, wastes, and hormonal messengers

   b. It functions as a part of the immune system to protect against and fight infection

   c. It also helps prevent hemorrhage when there is injury

B. Hematologic system

1. Blood forming organs

   a. Early production of blood cells (**hematopoiesis**) in the fetus occurs in the liver until 5 months gestation

   b. After birth, the liver is the primary site for production of most of the blood clotting factors and prothrombin; proper liver function is necessary for two sources of vitamin K to exist; vitamin K is produced by bacteria in the bowel, as well as being absorbed from the food digested; vitamin K is essential to the development of clotting factors VII, IX, X, and prothrombin; clotting factors, predominantly those that are activated by vitamin K, are lower in infants; many physicians recommend a preventative dose of vitamin K at the time of birth

   c. The spleen helps balance blood cell production and destruction by destroying aged or imperfect red blood cells (RBCs) and stores platelets

   d. Bone marrow, the major hematopoietic organ, takes over production at 5 months gestation; at birth, hematopoiesis occurs in almost every bone; however only the flat bones, such as hips, pelvic and shoulder girdles, ribs, sternum, and vertebrae maintain their hematopoietic activity throughout life

2. Blood is composed of cellular elements and plasma

   a. Cellular elements; see Table 14-1 for normal pediatric blood values

      1) RBCs or **erythrocytes** are formed through the process of **erythropoiesis** and make up the largest component of blood cells

         a) Hemoglobin (Hbg) is a component of RBCs and transports oxygen from the lungs to the tissues as well as carrying carbon dioxide back to the lungs

         b) The RBC count, hemoglobin (Hgb) and hematocrit (Hct) levels are high in infants

         c) These values will stabilize in childhood

         d) However, adolescent males demonstrate increased Hgb compared to the lowered value of adolescent females

Table 14-1

Normal Blood Values in Children

	Newborn	1 Year	5 Years	8–12 Years
Red blood cells (RBCs) (millions/μL)	5.9 (4.1–7.5)	4.6 (4.1–5.1)	4.7 (4.2–5.2)	5 (4.5–5.4)
Hemoglobin (Hgb) (g/dL)	19 (14–24)	12 (11–15)	13.5 (12.5–15)	14 (13–15.5)
White blood cells (WBCs) (per μL)	17,000 8–38	10,000 5–15	8000 5–13	8000 5–12
Platelets (per μL)	200,000	260,000	260,000	260,000
Hematocrit (Hct) (%)	54	36	38	40

Adapted from Merenstein, G. B., Kaplan, D. W., & Rosenberg, A. A. (1997). *Handbook of Pediatrics* (18th ed.). Stamford, CT: Appleton & Lange, pp. 986–989. © now held by McGraw-Hill.

2) White blood cells (WBCs) or **leukocytes** are formed primarily in the bone marrow; production also takes place in the lymph tissue

    a) Leukocytes provide immunity and help protect against the consequences of infection and injury

    b) Leukocytes are divided into five types, each having a specific purpose imperative to inflammation or immunity (Table 14-2)

    c) Alterations in the levels of the five different leukocytes can be seen in a differential blood count and may be indicative of a specific disease or condition

3) Platelets (**thrombocytes**) are cell fragments that work to stop blood flow from an injury by adhering to the walls of blood vessels and forming platelet plugs

    a) Platelets are produced in the bone marrow and then are stored in the spleen; from the spleen, they are released as needed by the body

    b) On average, 20 percent of platelets are stored in the spleen, and 80 percent are circulating; newborns will have lower levels of platelets

b. The liquid component of blood is plasma; plasma contains three plasma proteins

1) Albumin prevents plasma from leaking into the tissue through increasing the osmotic pressure of the blood

2) Fibrinogen molecules accumulate to form essential structures for the blood clotting process

3) Globulins are the main components of antibodies and protect the body against infection; globulins also transport other substances

c. Lymphatic fluid is similar to blood plasma but contains less protein; it does not produce cells, but rather has a necessary role in regulating blood cells; it is the extra interstitial fluid that is returned to systemic circulation by components of the auxiliary venous system referred to as lymph vessels or lymphatics; this balances the systemic circulation

II. Diagnostic Tests of the Hematologic System

A. History

NCLEX!

1. Assess for a history of easy or frequent bruising as well as frequent or heavy nosebleeds

NCLEX!

2. Assess for history of recurrent or chronic infections

Table 14-2

White Blood Cells and Their Functions

Type	Function
Neutrophils	Phagocytosis
Eosinophils	Allergic reactions
Basophils	Inflammatory reactions
Monocytes (macrophages)	Phagocytosis, antigen processing
Lymphocytes	Humoral immunity (B cell), cellular immunity (T cell)

Source: Ball, J. & Bindler, R. (1999). *Pediatric nursing: Caring for children* (2nd ed.). Stamford, CT: Appleton & Lange, p. 518.

3. Assess for medication use that might impair hematologic function, including those that cause bone marrow suppression, **hemolysis** (the destruction of blood cells), or those that disrupt platelet function
4. Remember to question family closely as to over-the-counter medications that client or family might not associate with impaired hematologic function
5. Asses for dietary patterns that might contribute to anemia or altered blood cell function
6. Assess for family housing, occupations, or hobbies that might indicate exposure to chemicals or agents that affect hematologic function
7. Assess for past medical history related to hematologic dysfunction: illnesses, surgeries, or injuries
8. Assess for family history of illnesses related to hematologic dysfunction

B. Physical assessment

1. Assess skin for the presence of pallor or jaundice; assess the mucous membranes and nailbeds for pallor or cyanosis
2. Assess skin turgor and pruritus as dry skin and itching may be indicators of a hematologic dysfunction

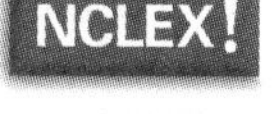

3. Assess skin for **petechiae,** the red or purple pinpoint hemorrhages; assess also for **ecchymosis** or bruising caused by the release of blood into the tissues
4. Assess for spontaneous bleeding or bruising; assess for bleeding or bruising disproportionate to the causative trauma
5. Assess the gums for active bleeding; as appropriate, also assess for excessive menstrual flow
6. If indicated, assess for bleeding from invasive medical interventions such as peripheral IV sites, central lines, nasogastric tubes, endotracheal tubes, or indwelling urinary catheters
7. Assess heart for increased rate or audible murmur
8. Assess for swollen or tender lymph nodes; assess for increased liver or spleen size at the costal margins

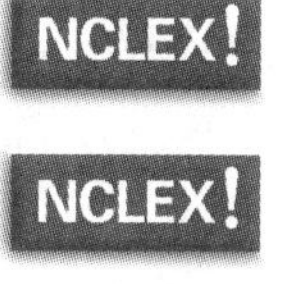

9. Assess for level of activity, fatigue, needing more rest than usual, decreasing endurance during routine activities, or dyspnea upon exertion
10. Assess for frequent infections, fevers, or weight loss

C. Common diagnostic studies

1. Complete blood count (CBC) with differential
   - **a.** Complete blood counts evaluate red blood cell counts, white blood cell counts, platelet counts, including hemoglobin and hematocrit; CBCs also evaluate the shape of the red blood cells
     - 1) The hemoglobin level is an evaluation of the amount of hemoglobin per 100 mL of blood
     - 2) The hematocrit is a comparison of the amount of RBCs in a volume of whole blood; thus the hematocrit is the percentages of solids to liquids;

changes in the amount of solids or the amount of liquids will affect the results; a low hematocrit can indicate a decreased amount of RBCs or an increase in the liquid volume of blood

b. The differential is an evaluation of the types of WBCs present; by evaluating the percentages of each type of WBC present in whole blood, the physician can determine the cause of the alteration in the white cell count

1) Bands: immature WBCs; an increase in the bands often indicates a response to a pathologic process

NCLEX!

2) Neutrophils are elevated in inflammatory process, infectious diseases, stress and in leukemia; an increase in bands and neutrophils are often called a shift to the left (based on typical order of lab reports) and indicate an acute infectious process

3) Eosinophils are elevated in allergic diseases

4) Basophils are associated with chronic conditions

5) Monoctyes are also associated with chronic infections and with infections

6) Lymphocytes respond to specific microorganisms and foreign proteins

2. Direct and indirect Coombs' tests evaluate the presence of antibodies associated with the RBCs

a. Direct Coombs' test evaluates the amount of antibodies coating the red cells

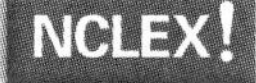

b. An indirect Coombs' test evaluates the presence of unattached, circulating antibodies

NCLEX!

3. Prothrombin time (PT) and partial thromboplastin time (PTT) evaluate the clotting sequence, looking primarily at the factor function

4. Bleeding time differentiates hemostasis disorders from coagulation defects

5. Platelet agglutination/aggregation evaluates platelet clumping ability

6. Hemoglobin electrophoresis differentiates the types of hemoglobin present and notes abnormal forms of hemoglobins

7. Serum ferritin measures the iron stores in the body

NCLEX!

8. Bone marrow aspiration and biopsy involves the removal of a small amount of bone marrow to evaluate the production of blood cells; the iliac crest is the site of choice for pediatric bone marrow aspirations

III. Congenital Hematologic Health Problems

A. Hemophilia

1. Description

a. A group of disorders characterized by a deficiency in a specific clotting factor

b. The disease is a chronic inherited bleeding disorder

c. Hemophilia is without cure and is a lifelong condition

2. Etiology and pathophysiology

a. There are three forms of hemophilia: the two most common types are inherited as an **X-linked recessive trait** expressed almost exclusively as carrier females and affected males; when a female inherits the hemophilia trait from her father, she has a 50 percent chance of transmitting it to her son

1) Hemophilia A (classic hemophilia) is the result of a factor VIII deficiency; it accounts for approximately 80 percent of the hemophilia cases; hemophilia A is the result of approximately 1 in 5,000 male births

2) Hemophilia B (Christmas Disease) is the result of a deficiency of factor IX; hemophilia B accounts for 15 percent of hemophilia cases

b. Up to one-third of all hemophiliacs have no family member who is affected by a clotting disorder; these cases are caused by a new mutation

c. Bleeding tendencies may be mild, moderate, or severe; symptoms may not become evident until after 6 months of age; at that time, the child's increasing mobility results in more accidents; there may be bleeding from falls as well as the eruption of teeth

d. Bleeding into the joint spaces (**hemarthrosis**) is one of the symptoms most commonly seen; this leads to impaired range of motion and pain, tenderness, and swelling

e. Significant deep tissue and intramuscular hemorrhages may occur; obstruction of the airway may result from bleeding into tissues of the mouth, neck, or chest; critical bleeding may be seen in the retroperitoneal or intracranial areas

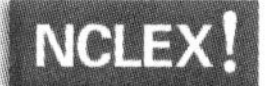

f. Extensive bleeding may be seen after circumcision, tooth extractions, lesser injuries, and minor surgical procedures; there may also be nosebleeds and hematuria

3. Assessment

a. Diagnosed by history, presenting symptoms, and laboratory data

NCLEX!

b. Presenting laboratory data will include prolonged activated PTT and decreased factor VIII or IX levels; PT, thrombin time, fibrinogen, and platelet count are normal

c. Genetic testing can be used to identify carriers; carriers and affected individuals can also be identified prior to birth via amniocentesis or chorionic villi sampling

d. Obtain medical history, with close attention to episodes of bleeding as well as a history of familial bleeding disorders

e. Assess for active bleeding, joint swelling, pain, or deformities

f. Assess for hematuria or flank pain

g. Complete a neurological assessment to rule out peripheral neuropathies secondary to intracranial bleeding

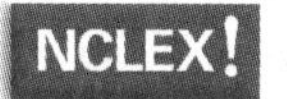

h. Factor contamination is reduced by careful screening of donors as well as lab techniques; hemophiliacs who have received some of the more impure forms in the past could be at risk for developing AIDS

4. Priority nursing diagnoses
   a. Risk for injury
   b. Pain
   c. Impaired physical mobility
   d. Knowledge deficit
5. Planning and implementation

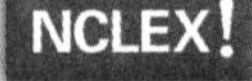

   a. Control localized bleeding through topical coagulants, pressure, elevation, and ice
   b. Control bleeding for significant bleeds through administration of the necessary factor; monitor factor levels as ordered
   c. Transfuse as ordered to help minimize disease complications
      1) Fresh whole blood is used primarily for severe bleeds into critical areas; it would take a large volume of whole blood to provide sufficient factor to control a bleed
      2) Fresh or fresh frozen plasma may be given
      3) Platelets are usually not administered because the child's platelet count is normal
   d. As indicated for mild hemophilia, administer desmopressin acetate (DDAVP) intravenously
   e. Many children now take factor prophylactically; if administered on a regular basis, the factor should be administered during the morning; because of the short half-life of the factor, factor levels should be highest when child is active

NCLEX!

   f. Take no rectal temperatures
   g. Manage pain utilizing analgesics as ordered
   h. If joint involved in the bleed, joint damage can be reduced via immobilization, elevation, and ice packs
   i. Physical therapy is used to prevent flexion contractures and to strengthen muscles and joints

NCLEX!

   j. Physical therapy is only initiated when bleeding is under control
   k. Provide opportunities for normal growth and development activities; as indicated, provide injury protection for activities
   l. Some children develop antibodies to the factor; these children will require higher doses of factor replacement in order to maintain a clot
6. Medications
   a. Factor VIII (8) and XI (11) are available
   b. Three forms of factor are available: intermediate, monoclonal, and recombinant; intermediate and monoclonal are extracted from plasma; recombinant forms are manufactured from human genes but do not include plasma

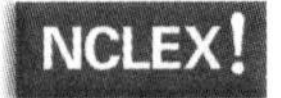

   c. DDAVP may be administered to children with mild Hemophilia A; it increases the level of factor VIII and the von Willebrand factor by releasing these factors from their storage sites

7. Child and family education
    a. Importance of wearing a Medic-Alert bracelet
    b. Injury prevention appropriate for the age
        1) Toddlers should wear clothes that contain extra padding to prevent injuries as they learn to walk
        2) Padding of furniture corners and providing a clean environment reduces falls and injuries
        3) Children and adolescents should avoid contact sports; however, non-contact athletics help maintain physical strength; swimming and golf are appropriate activities
    c. Signs and symptoms of internal bleeding and hemarthrosis

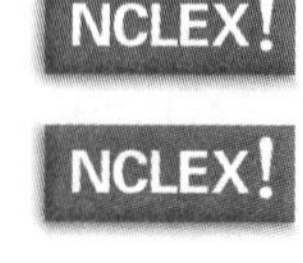

    d. Using a soft toothbrush and having regular dental checkups
    e. The importance of avoiding aspirin and aspirin-like medications that can affect platelet function; educate as to such over-the-counter products
    f. Medication administration techniques
        1) Factor may be stored in the refrigerator until needed
        2) Teach proper dilution of the factor; the diluent is provided with the factor; swirl the factor gently until completely mixed
        3) Teach IV administration; young child may have a subcutaneous port placed to aid in home infusion
        4) Use a plastic syringe, not glass
        5) Once factor is reconstituted, administer within 3 hours

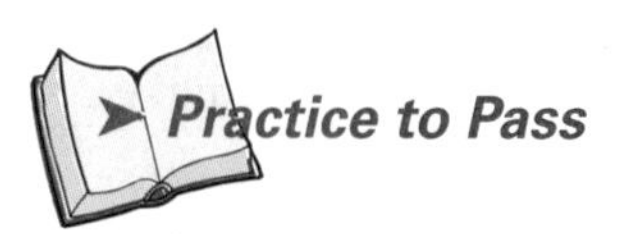

You are teaching the family of a 1-year-old newly diagnosed with hemophilia. The mother states she will continue to use ibuprofen for injuries and fever as previously instructed by her pediatrician. What would your best response be?

8. Evaluation
    a. Child will be free of pain and without joint deformities
    b. Child will demonstrate an age-appropriate level of independence
    c. Family and child will verbalize and demonstrate understanding of the disease, management, and sequelae

B. Sickle cell anemia

1. Description: a hereditary **hemoglobinopathy** primarily affecting African-Americans, although it may be seen in those of Mediterranean descent
2. Etiology and pathophysiology
    a. An autosomal recessive condition whereby normal hemoglobin is partially or completely replaced by the sickle-shaped, abnormal hemoglobin S (Hgb S)
    b. The sickle cell trait (carrying one gene for the disease) presents in 1 out of 12 African-Americans; the disease occurs in 1 out of 600 African-American infants
    c. When exposed to diminished levels of oxygen, the hemoglobin in the RBC develops a sickle or crescent shape; these cells are rigid and obstruct capillary blood flow, leading to congestion and tissue hypoxia; cyclically, this hypoxia causes additional sickling and extensive infarctions

d. Children with sickle cell disease have three types of problems (see also Box 14-1)

1) Vaso-occlusive crisis where stasis of blood causes ischemia and infarction; the seriousness of the sequelae depends upon the site of the occlusive crisis

2) Sequestration crisis is a potentially life-threatening crisis where the blood pools in the spleen; usually happens in the younger children

3) Aplastic crisis is the **anemia** associated with the increased destruction of the fragile red blood cell

NCLEX!

e. Hypoxia or low oxygen tension may trigger a crisis, as will any condition that increases the body's need for oxygen or alters oxygen transport; sickling of the RBCs can also be triggered by a fever or dehydration and emotional or physical stress

NCLEX!

f. Symptoms do not usually appear until 4 to 6 months of age as the sickling of cells is prevented secondary to the high levels of fetal hemoglobin

g. Those with sickle cell trait (carriers of the disease) rarely experience crises or symptoms, unless under conditions where there is abnormally low oxygen

3. Assessment

a. Newborns may be diagnosed via hemoglobin electrophoresis of cord blood

NCLEX!

b. The Sicklidex (sickle turbidity test) is a screening test used for children 6 years and older

c. Hemoglobin electrophoresis verifies the diagnosis

d. Obtain a detailed history as to crises, the precipitating events, medical management, and details of home management

e. Obtain current and accurate height and weight to asses for failure to thrive

Box 14-1

Types of Sickle Cell Crises

Vaso-occlusive Crises (Thrombotic)
Most common type of crisis, painful
Caused by stasis of blood with clumping of cells in the microcirculation, ischemia, and infarction
Signs include fever, pain, tissue engorgement

Splenic Sequestration
Life-threatening crisis; death can occur within hours
Caused by pooling of blood in the spleen
Signs include profound anemia, hypovolemia, and shock

Aplastic Crises
Diminished production and increased destruction of red blood cells
Triggered by viral infection or depletion of folic acid
Signs include profound anemia, pallor

Source: Ball, J. & Bindler, R. (1999). *Pediatric nursing: Caring for children* (2nd ed.). Stamford, CT: Appleton & Lange, p. 523.

f. Assess for any acute or chronic pain; if currently in crisis, also note any signs/symptoms of infection or inflammation

NCLEX!

g. An ill sickle cell client will necessitate a thorough multisystem assessment; fever must be considered an emergency and will require urgent treatment

4. Priority nursing diagnoses

a. Altered tissue perfusion

b. Risk for injury

c. Risk for infection

d. Pain

e. Knowledge deficit

5. Planning and implementation

NCLEX!

a. Assist hydration through intravenous fluids and oral intake

NCLEX!

b. Increase tissue perfusion through the administration of oxygen and blood products as ordered; this helps prevent further sickling

NCLEX!

c. Promote and encourage rest; schedule activities of daily living (ADLs) and play to maximize rest and comfort

d. Assist child and family to avoid emotional stress as much as possible

NCLEX!

e. Administer analgesics around the clock (ATC) when the child is in crisis; utilize patient-controlled analgesia if appropriate; position for comfort and to decrease stress upon painful joints

f. Assess for signs/symptoms of worsening anemia, shock, and altered neurological function

g. Provide emotional support during crisis, as well as on an ongoing basis when child is well and in the home setting

7. Child and family education

a. Necessity of following the plan of care as prescribed by the healthcare team

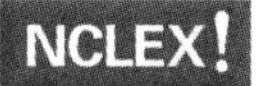

b. Signs and symptoms of impending crisis

c. Signs and symptoms of infection

d. Preventing hypoxia from physical and emotional stress

e. Providing adequate rest as well as avoiding heat and cold stress

8. Evaluation

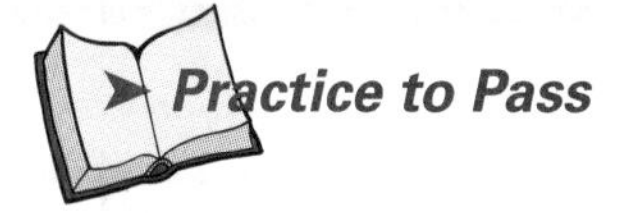

Sickle cell anemia may not be diagnosed until after infancy. Explain the reason for this.

a. Child will maintain adequate tissue perfusion as evidenced by oxygen saturation at level ordered by physician

b. Child experiences appropriate pain control and ability to resume age-appropriate activities

c. Child is without signs and symptoms of infection

d. Family and child demonstrate an understanding of disease process and treatment regimen

C. Thalassemia

1. Description

a. Another of the group of hereditary blood disorders of hemoglobin synthesis, characterized by mild to severe anemia

b. The most common type of these is β-thalassemia, also known as Cooley anemia; there are three types of β-thalassemia: thalassemia minor, thalassemia intermedia, and thalassemia major

1) Thalassemia minor is also known as thalassemia trait and produces mild anemia

2) Thalassemia intermedia produces severe anemia

NCLEX!

3) Thalassemia major produces anemia that requires transfusions; see Box 14-2 for transfusion procedures

2. Etiology and pathophysiology

a. The disorders are most commonly seen in those of Mediterranean descent; however, they may also be seen among the African, Asian, and Middle Eastern populations

b. The condition is autosomal-recessive and when both parents carry the gene, they have a 25 percent chance of passing the disorder to their child; if the child only acquires one gene for this disorder, the child will be a carrier

c. Thalassemia causes the synthesis of a defective hemoglobin; the RBC is fragile and has a shortened life span; this will lead to anemia and hypoxia

NCLEX!

d. The foremost consequences of thalassemia result from the chronic hypoxia and iron overload from the multiple blood supplements, which are part of supportive treatment

Box 14-2

Pediatric Transfusions

- The nurse should always follow agency policy regarding transfusing blood products.
- Wear gloves when handling blood products.
- Verify correct blood product and type, client name, identification number, and crossmatching before beginning to prevent potentially fatal error. Most agencies require identification of unit to be performed by two registered nurses.
- Review physician's order in relation to premedications and rate of infusion.
- Have intravenous site ready prior to blood arriving on unit. Blood administration should be started immediately upon its arrival on unit; blood should not be stored in the unit refrigerator.
- Check blood products—products that appear purplish or are bubbling should not be used because of risk of bacterial contamination.
- Obtain informed consent.
- Assemble administration equipment with appropriate blood filter. A separate blood filter and tubing is used for each unit. A Y set is usually recommended with saline used to prime the entire line including both Y legs.
- Start slowly. For the first 15 minutes, the blood is transfused slowly, and the child is monitored for transfusion reactions.
- Monitor vital signs before, during, and after the infusion. Usually vital signs are taken every 15 minutes × 4, then every 30 minutes throughout infusion, and 30 minutes after infusion is complete. Watch for other signs of reaction.

e. The body conserves iron from red cells which are aged and broken down; when blood is administered, the body will also retain the iron from the transfused cells; this leads to the excessive levels of iron in the body or **hemochromatosis;** hemochromatosis causes cellular damage resulting in long-term complications, which may include:

1) Splenomegaly
2) Cardiac complications
3) Gallbladder disease
4) Liver enlargement and cirrhosis
5) Growth retardation and endocrine complications
6) Jaundice and brown skin pigmentation
7) Skeletal changes including enlarged head, thickened cranial bones, enlarged maxilla, and malocclusion of the teeth

f. If untreated, the child may die at a young age

3. Assessment

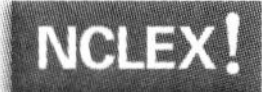

a. Thalassemia can be diagnosed early in infancy when the child presents with pallor, failure to thrive (FTT), hepatosplenamegaly, and severe anemia; see Box 14-3 for clinical manifestations of β-Thalassemia

Box 14-3

Clinical Manifestations of β-Thalassemia

Anemia
Hypochromic and microcytic changes
Folic acid deficiency
Frequent epistaxis

Skeletal Changes
Osteoporosis
Delayed growth
Susceptibility to pathologic fractures
Facial deformities: enlarged head, prominent forehead due to frontal and parietal bossing, prominent cheek bones, broadened and depressed bridge of nose, enlarged maxilla with protruding front teeth, eyes with mongolian slant and epicanthal fold

Heart
Chronic congestive heart failure
Myocardial fibrosis
Murmurs

Liver/Gallbladder
Hepatomegaly
Hepatic insufficiency

Spleen
Splenomegaly

Endocrine System
Delayed sexual maturation
Fibrotic pancreas, resulting in diabetes mellitus

Skin
Darkening of skin

Source: Ball, J. & Bindler, R. (1999). *Pediatric nursing: Caring for children* (2nd ed.). Stamford, CT: Appleton & Lange, p. 530.

b. There may also be signs and symptoms of chronic hypoxia such as lethargy, headache, bone pain, exercise intolerance, and anorexia

c. Diagnosis of thalassemia is made via hemoglobin electrophoresis that will demonstrate a decreased production of one hemoglobin chain; erythrocyte changes may be detected as early as 6 weeks of age

NCLEX!

d. Lab data will reveal a deceased hemoglobin, hematocrit, and reticulocyte count

e. A folic acid deficiency may be present

4. Priority nursing diagnoses

a. Body image disturbance

b. Risk for activity intolerance

c. Risk for injury

d. Pain

e. Knowledge deficit

5. Planning and implementation

NCLEX!

a. Administer blood products as ordered, observing for complications of multiple transfusions

NCLEX!

b. Assess for signs of iron overload (hemosiderosis) and hepatitis

NCLEX!

c. Observe for signs of infection and work to prevent infection through good handwashing, avoiding those with infection, proper rest, and nutrition

d. Administer folic acid as ordered

e. Work towards fracture prevention by encouraging and providing opportunities for physical activities that do not increase the risk of fractures

NCLEX!

f. Implement iron chelation therapy as ordered; iron chelation aids in the elimination of excessive iron

g. Provide support through opportunities for expression of feelings by child and family regarding the chronic life-threatening illness

h. Encourage child and family to allow child to live as normal a life as possible

i. Bone marrow transplantations may be offered to cure the disease

6. Child and family education

a. Nature of the disease and its medical management

b. Possible complications including iron overload as well as signs of infection

c. Activity restrictions designed to reduce the risk of fractures secondary to excessive iron stores

7. Evaluation

a. Child is without pain

b. Child exhibits no signs of infection

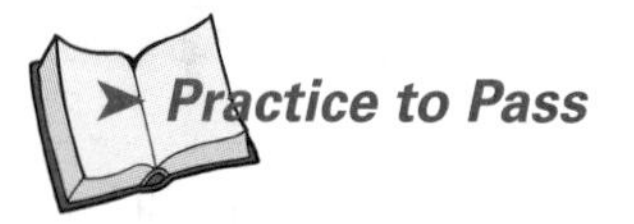

You are transfusing a child diagnosed with thalassemia major. You determine that a hemolytic reaction is occurring. What should be your first nursing action?

c. Child engages in age-appropriate activities and as normal a lifestyle as possible

d. Child demonstrates coping with body image changes

e. Family and child describe the disease process and medical plan of care

IV. Acquired Hematologic Health Problems

A. Disseminated intravascular coagulopathy (DIC)

1. Description

a. Disseminated intravascular coagulopathy occurs as a complication of another health problem; it is a secondary illness, not a primary one

b. It is an acquired life-threatening pathological process involving the abnormal simultaneous activation of the body's thrombin (clotting) mechanism and fibrinolytic system

2. Etiology and pathophysiology

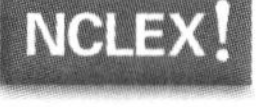

a. A complex process involving simultaneous excessive bleeding and clotting

b. Abnormal activation of the clotting system leads to extensive clot formation in the small vessels throughout the body; this process can lead to organ damage

c. Excess generation of thrombin occurs, leading to the abnormal deposition of fibrin strands through body tissues; these thromboses interfere with blood flow; tissue hypoxia occurs, which results in tissue necrosis

d. As the fibrin fragments circulate, they begin to interfere with aspects of the clotting mechanism; this includes platelet aggregation, with a resulting depletion of platelets, leading to hemorrhage and anemia (see Figure 14-1)

e. DIC may result from conditions causing cell or tissue damage; such damage can free up tissue thromboplastin, circulating endotoxins and immune complexes

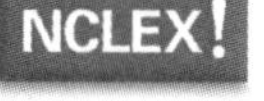

f. Primary conditions that can precipitate DIC include burns, cancer, hypoxia, liver disease, necrolyzing enterocolitis, sepsis, shock, trauma, and viruses

3. Assessment

NCLEX!

a. The onset of symptoms includes diffuse bleeding that may be seen as excessive bruising, hematuria, injection sites that do not stop oozing, and mild gastrointestinal bleeding

b. Assess progression which is indicated by petechiae, purpura, hypoxemia, renal failure, intercranial bleeding, ischemic pain, and progressive organ failure secondary to the ischemia

NCLEX!

c. Lab data will include low platelet count, deceased RBCs, prolonged prothrombin time (PT) and partial thromboplastin time (PTT), decreased fibrinogen levels, and increased levels of fibrin-fibrinogen split products

4. Priority nursing diagnoses

a. Altered tissue perfusion

b. Risk for injury

c. Anxiety

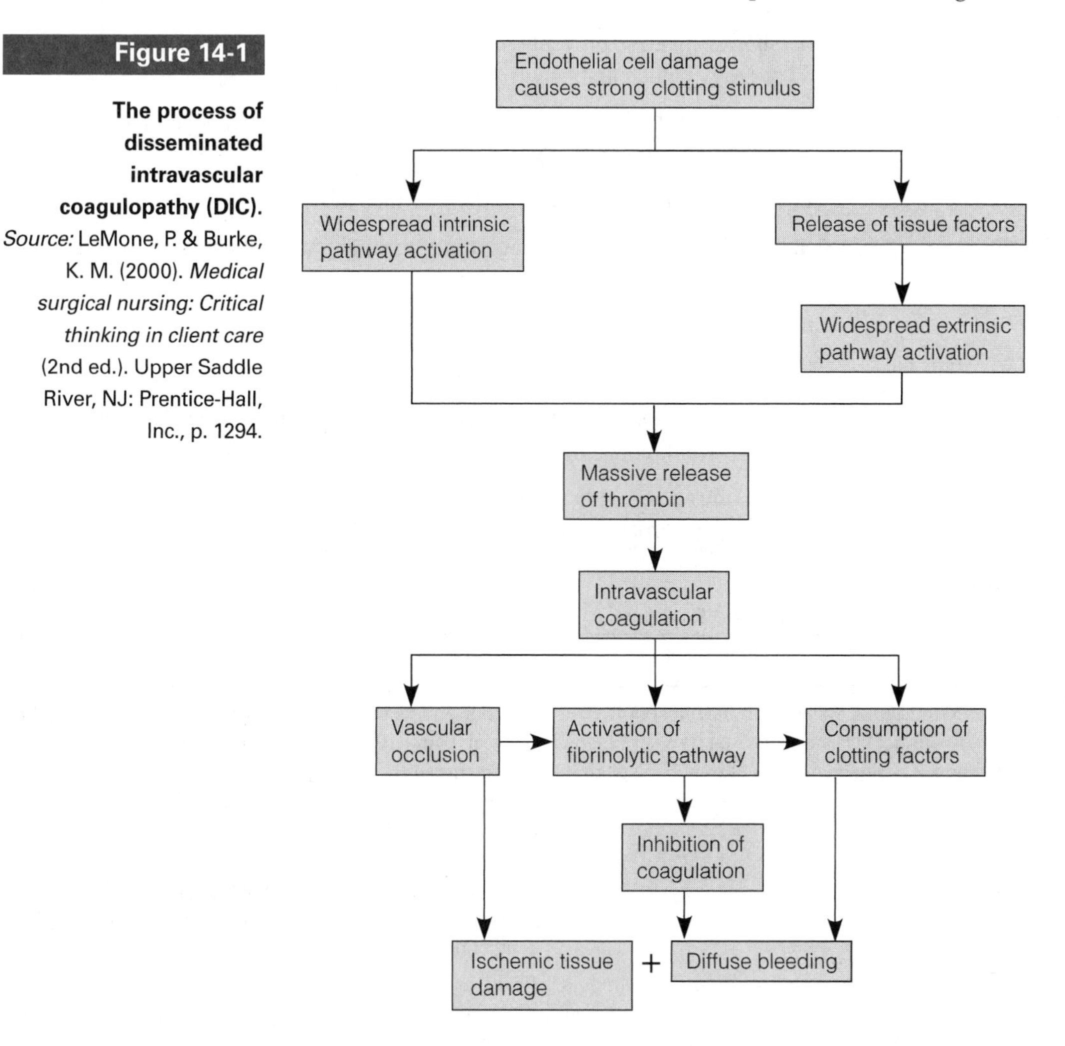

Figure 14-1

The process of disseminated intravascular coagulopathy (DIC). *Source:* LeMone, P. & Burke, K. M. (2000). *Medical surgical nursing: Critical thinking in client care* (2nd ed.). Upper Saddle River, NJ: Prentice-Hall, Inc., p. 1294.

5. Planning and implementation

a. Rigorous ongoing assessment of all body systems

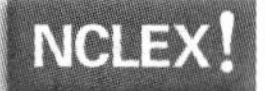

b. Monitor bleeding by assessing petechiae, ecchymoses, and oozing frequently

c. Ongoing evaluation of lab including CBC, PT, and PTT

d. Monitor arterial blood gases (ABGs) for indications of acidosis

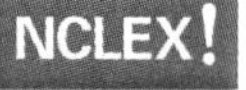

e. Take temperatures by the oral or axillary route, not rectal

f. Avoid trauma to delicate areas such as mucous membranes as much as possible

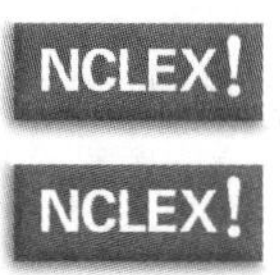

g. Minimize administration of parenteral medications and invasive procedures as much as possible

h. Areas of needle sticks such as injections or intravenous sites must be treated as an arterial stick and have pressure applied for at least 10 to 15 minutes; they must be observed every 15 minutes

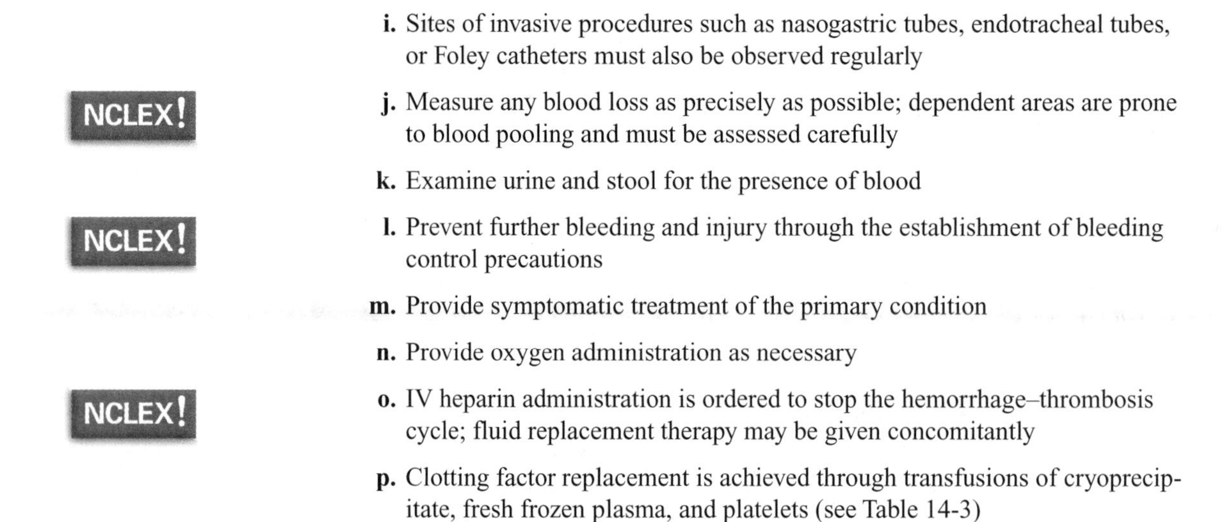

i. Sites of invasive procedures such as nasogastric tubes, endotracheal tubes, or Foley catheters must also be observed regularly

j. Measure any blood loss as precisely as possible; dependent areas are prone to blood pooling and must be assessed carefully

k. Examine urine and stool for the presence of blood

l. Prevent further bleeding and injury through the establishment of bleeding control precautions

m. Provide symptomatic treatment of the primary condition

n. Provide oxygen administration as necessary

o. IV heparin administration is ordered to stop the hemorrhage–thrombosis cycle; fluid replacement therapy may be given concomitantly

p. Clotting factor replacement is achieved through transfusions of cryoprecipitate, fresh frozen plasma, and platelets (see Table 14-3)

Table 14-3 Administration of Blood Products

Blood Product	Use	Comments
Whole blood	Used in trauma clients who have lost both cells and volume; occasionally used in other clients, although a blood component may be used in its place	Blood products must be kept refrigerated at a temperature between 0 and 10°C; normal refrigerators are inappropriate; the nurse should be prepared to administer the product as soon as it arrives on the unit and never store the blood product in the unit's refrigerator; if the length of administration exceeds the blood bank's recommendations, the blood bank can divide the unit; transfuse through blood filter; one unit usually raises Hct by 3 percent, Hgb by 1 g/dL; infuse only with 0.9 percent saline
Packed red blood cells	Often used in anemic clients who do not require volume expansion; packed cells are developed by removing the majority of the plasma from a unit of whole blood	Transfusion completed within 2 to 4 hours to prevent bacterial growth; leukocyte-poor red blood cells (filtered RBCs) may be used in clients with history of allergic reactions; these units have been exposed to an extra processing which removes the majority of white blood cells; 4-hour maximum infusion time; children with severe anemia are at risk for congestive heart failure if infused too rapidly
Platelets	Used for clients with thrombocytopenia	May be pooled from several donor units or from one donor; a leukocyte-reduction filter for platelets may be used; pretransfusion medications may include antihistamines or acetaminophen
Granulocytes	Usually only used for severely neutropenic client; sometimes used for neonates with sepsis	May be irradiated to reduce the risk of graft versus host disease; risk of cytomegalovirus with granulocytes transfusion; pretransfusion medication with antihistamine or acetaminophen recommended
Fresh frozen plasma (FFP)	Supplies clotting factors; may be used in severe liver disease or DIC	Half-life of plasma clotting factors short; must be fresh or fresh frozen to be of benefit; is transfused through a blood filter; may be given over 20 to 30 minutes
Factor VIII or IX	Concentrated forms of the specific factor; used for hemophiliacs type A and B; factor VIII may also be used for von Willebrand's Disease	Compatibility tests not required; quantity of factor varies for each vial; available in lyophilized concentrations, which can be kept in the home refrigerator until needed; reconstituted with diluent provided; various forms refer to level of purity; recombinant forms available

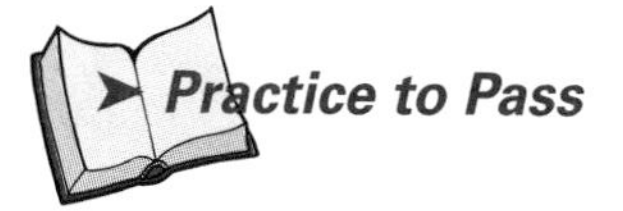

The client with disseminated intravascular coagulopathy (DIC) is to receive multiple doses of heparin SC. Discuss the safety issues involved in administering this drug.

q. Assess anticoagulant and transfusion therapy and relate any complications

r. Monitor carefully for transfusion reactions (see Table 14-4)

s. Assess for fluid overload as indicated by a slow bounding pulse and increasing central venous pressure

6. Medications

a. Heparin is often used to reduce the inappropriate utilization of the clotting factors

b. Heparin may be administered subcutaneously (SC) or intravenously (IV)

1) Subcutaneous heparin is given slowly with sites rotated; the injection site should not be massaged

2) Intravenous heparin may be given intermittently or continuously

c. Monitor PTT and platelet count

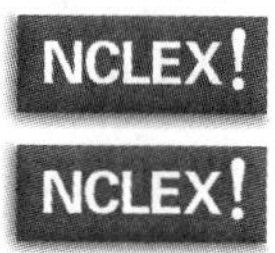

d. Protamine is a heparin antidote and should be available for emergency use

e. The child should avoid aspirin and nonsteroidal anti-inflammatory drugs

7. Child and family education

a. Teach the child and family about the condition, its cause, and treatment

NCLEX!

b. Explain to the child and family activities to reduce bleeding—using a soft toothbrush or gauze over the finger to "brush" teeth, maintaining a obstacle-free environment, handling the skin gently

c. Instruct the child and family about symptoms to be reported to the physician

8. Evaluation

a. Child maintains appropriate organ function

b. Bleeding from trauma is minimized

c. Family and child verbalize concerns as well as demonstrate effective coping mechanisms

Table 14-4 Transfusion Reactions

Reactions and Cause	Signs and Symptoms	Treatment
Hemolytic reaction—ABO incompatibility	Fever, pain at insertion site, hypotension, renal failure, tachycardia, oliguria, shock; positive Coombs' test	Stop blood transfusion, maintain IV line; notify physician; send remaining blood and tubing to lab; lab samples will be obtained from the client
Febrile nonhemolytic reaction—antigen-antibody reaction to something in donor blood	Fever, chills	Antipyretics; premedicate in future; use leukocyte-depleted products
Allergic reaction—client allergic to protein in donor blood	Rash, hives, respiratory distress, anaphylaxis	Pretreat with antihistamine
Viral transmission	Delayed fever	Treat symptomatically
Fluid volume overload—most frequently seen in severely anemic child	Signs and symptoms of congestive heart failure	Prevent by limiting speed of transfusion for the severely anemic child
Graft-versus-host disease—seen in the immunocompromised client	Fever, bone marrow suppression, and death	Prevention the key—provide irradiated red blood cells

B. Idiopathic thrombocytopenic purpura (ITP)

1. Description
   a. Also known as autoimmune thrombocytopenia purpura
   b. An autoimmune hematologic condition distinguished by increased destruction of platelets, despite normal platelet production in the bone marrow
   c. ITP is the most common bleeding disorder in children
2. Etiology and pathophysiology

NCLEX!

   a. ITP occurs most often in children ages 2 to 5
   b. ITP usually develops 1 to 3 weeks after a viral infection such as chicken pox, measles, or rubella
   c. ITP can manifest itself as acute and self-limiting or chronic, requiring treatment; the acute type accounts for approximately 80 percent of ITP cases
   d. As platelet destruction exceeds production, the total number of circulating platelets decreases (see Figure 14-2)
   e. Blood clotting is slowed, and uncontrolled bleeding may occur

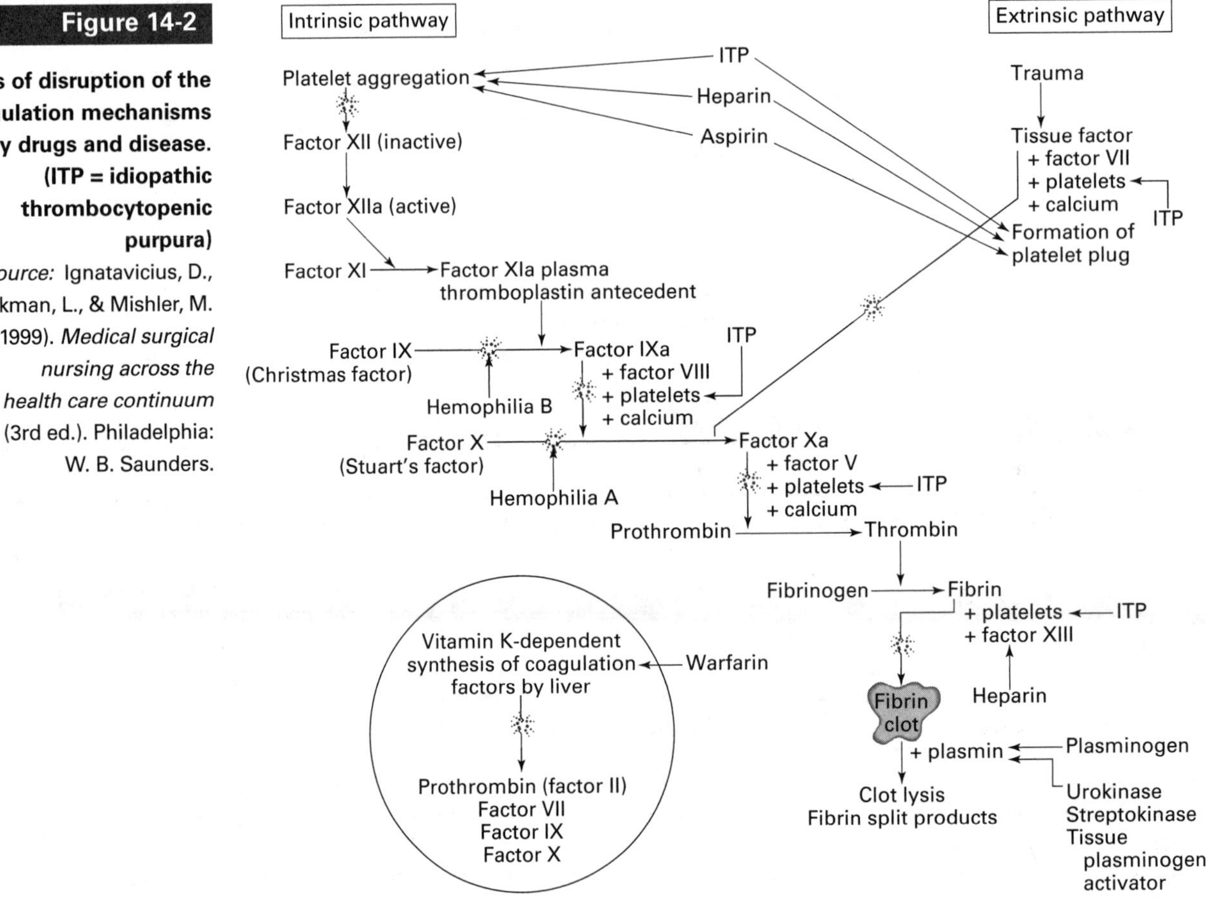

Figure 14-2

Sites of disruption of the coagulation mechanisms by drugs and disease. (ITP = idiopathic thrombocytopenic purpura)

Source: Ignatavicius, D., Workman, L., & Mishler, M. (1999). *Medical surgical nursing across the health care continuum* (3rd ed.). Philadelphia: W. B. Saunders.

3. Assessment

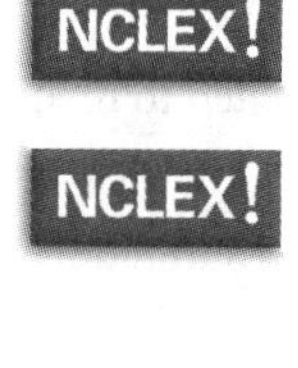

a. Petechiae and multiple ecchymoses are characteristic; mucous membranes and sclera are particularly affected with petechiae

b. Other symptoms include

1) Excessive bleeding, especially nosebleeds

2) Hematuria and bloody or tarry stools

c. History of recent medical events

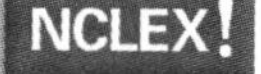

d. Lab data that shows decreased platelet count, as well as anti-platelet antibodies in the peripheral blood

e. Physical assessment must include thorough neurological assessment to rule out intracranial bleeds

f. Bone marrow aspiration is used to look for platelet precursors and rule out an oncologic disorder

4. Priority nursing diagnoses: Risk for infection; Risk for injury; Knowledge deficit

5. Planning and implementation

a. Assess frequently for bruising or active bleeding including mucous membrane, sclera, nosebleeds, hematuria, or bloody stools

b. Assess neurological status every shift and PRN

c. Closely monitor platelet counts

d. Monitor children who have undergone any invasive procedure closely

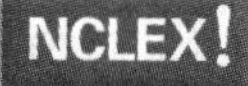

e. Use soft bristled toothbrush or toothettes on children with platelet counts less than 20,000 cells/mm^3

f. Avoid using rectal thermometers and aspirin-like products

g. If medications are not successful, a splenectomy may be attempted in the older child with 1 year of thrombocytopenia

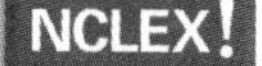

6. Medications

a. Steroids are ordered to reduce the inflammatory process

b. Intravenous immunoglobulins may also be used to reduce the autoimmune problem

7. Child and family education

a. The parents are instructed to obtain a Medic-Alert bracelet for the child

b. Teach the child and family ways to prevent bleeding episodes

c. Give instructions about means to control bleeding and when to seek emergency assistance

d. Teach the child and family safe administration of medications and potential side effects

e. Provide information to the child and parents about splenectomy and surgical care as appropriate

8. Evaluation

a. The child remains free of injury from bleeding episodes

b. The child and family identify safety precautions related to medication administration

c. The child and family demonstrate behaviors designed to reduce bruising/bleeding

C. Iron-deficiency anemia

1. Description

NCLEX!

a. Results from an inadequate supply of iron

b. The most common type of childhood anemia

2. Etiology and pathophysiology

a. The inadequate iron supply leads to smaller RBCs, a reduction in the number of RBCs and the quantity of hemoglobin, and a decrease in the oxygen-carrying capacity of the blood

b. Body stores of iron decrease and the severity of symptoms is directly related to the amount and duration of iron deficiency

c. Iron-deficiency anemia occurs as a result of blood loss or poor nutritional intake, or because of rapid growth with increased internal demands for blood production

NCLEX!

d. It is the most common nutritional-deficiency anemia in children

e. Premature or multiple-birth infants are at risk because of inadequate iron storage in the latter part of pregnancy

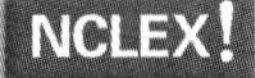

f. After the age of 6 months, infants who do not take appropriate solid food and are taking breast milk or formula without iron are at risk because of the depletion of neonatal iron stores

g. Chronic blood loss can be a cause of iron-deficiency anemia; clients at risk would include neonates who have experienced bleeding, hemophiliacs, those who have parasitic gastrointestinal problems, or females who have heavy menstrual bleeding (menorrhagia)

3. Assessment

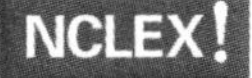

a. Classic symptoms include pallor, fatigue, and irritability, but the exact clinical signs will depend upon the severity of the anemia

b. Poor muscle development and growth retardation may occur; children with anemia may be at greater risk of infection

c. Nail-bed deformities, tachycardia, and systemic heart murmurs occur with prolonged anemia; growth retardation and/or developmental delay may also be seen

NCLEX!

d. Laboratory data from hemoglobin levels, mean corpuscular volume, and serum iron-binding capacity all indicate decreased iron content; microscopic analysis will reveal microcytic (small) and hypochromic (pale) red blood cells

e. Low iron stores are easiest identified by a decrease in serum ferritin

f. Nutritional intake can be assessed through a dietary history and analysis

4. Priority nursing diagnoses
   a. Knowledge deficit
   b. Altered nutrition, less than body requirements
   c. Activity intolerence
   d. Risk for altered growth and development
5. Planning and implementation
   a. Correct bleeding if it is the cause of the anemia

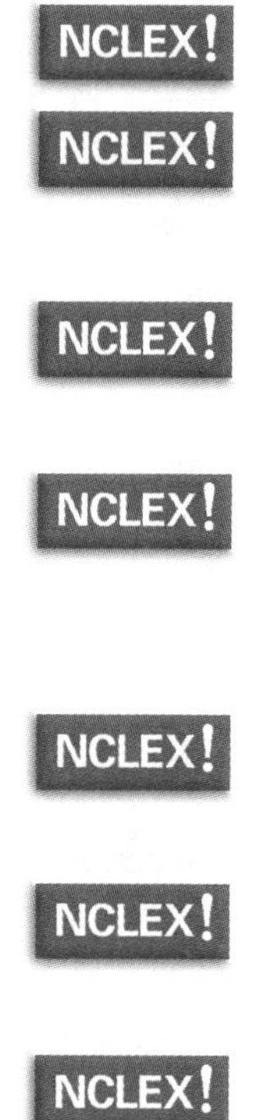

   b. Implement dietary modifications to provide a high-iron diet
   c. Promote rest, protect from infection; monitor cardiac functioning
   d. If packed cells are administered, administer slowly; rapid administration can overload the already-stressed heart leading to congestive heart failure
   e. Some infants drink large quantities of milk and refuse solid foods, limiting their iron intake; for these infants, it is often necessary to restrict their milk intake; milk intake should be limited to a maximum of 1 quart per day
   f. The child will also need protein and vitamin C in order to produce new cells; folic acid will help to convert the iron from ferritin to hemoglobin
6. Medications: oral iron supplements may be ordered; ferrous sulfate is the form preferred as it is better absorbed
   a. It is best absorbed on an empty stomach; iron may be taken with a vitamin C source such as orange juice to promote iron absorption; milk and antacids may inhibit absorption
   b. Oral iron preparations may temporarily stain teeth; liquid iron preparations should be taken through a straw to reduce contact with the teeth; the child should brush his or her teeth after administration
   c. Stools may be tarry and constipation may occur
7. Child and family education
   a. Teach appropriate oral iron supplement administration technique
   b. Instruct the child and family on dietary sources of iron
      1) For infants, iron-fortified formula and iron-fortified infant cereal
      2) Good sources of iron include organ meats, dried legumes, nuts, green vegetables, and iron-enriched flours
   c. Teach the family about side effects of iron, such as constipation; encourage high-fiber diet and fluid intake to minimize this risk
   d. Instruct the family to store the iron preparation where children can not reach it; iron supplement overdose could be fatal
   e. Provide the parents with information about conserving the child's energy and preventing trauma to blood cells to reduce red cell damage
8. Evaluation
   a. Child will demonstrate resolution of anemia with a return to normal lab values
   b. Family will verbalize an understanding as to the cause and treatment of iron deficiency anemia

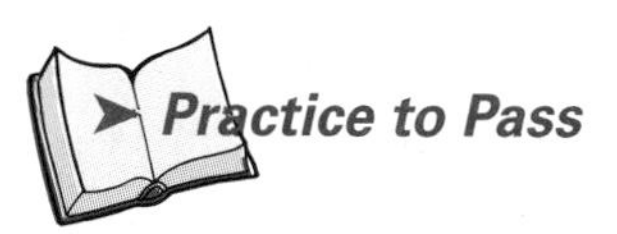

You are teaching the family of a 5-month-old with iron-deficiency anemia. In advising the family on how to minimize the side effects of the iron supplement, what administration guidelines will you give the family?

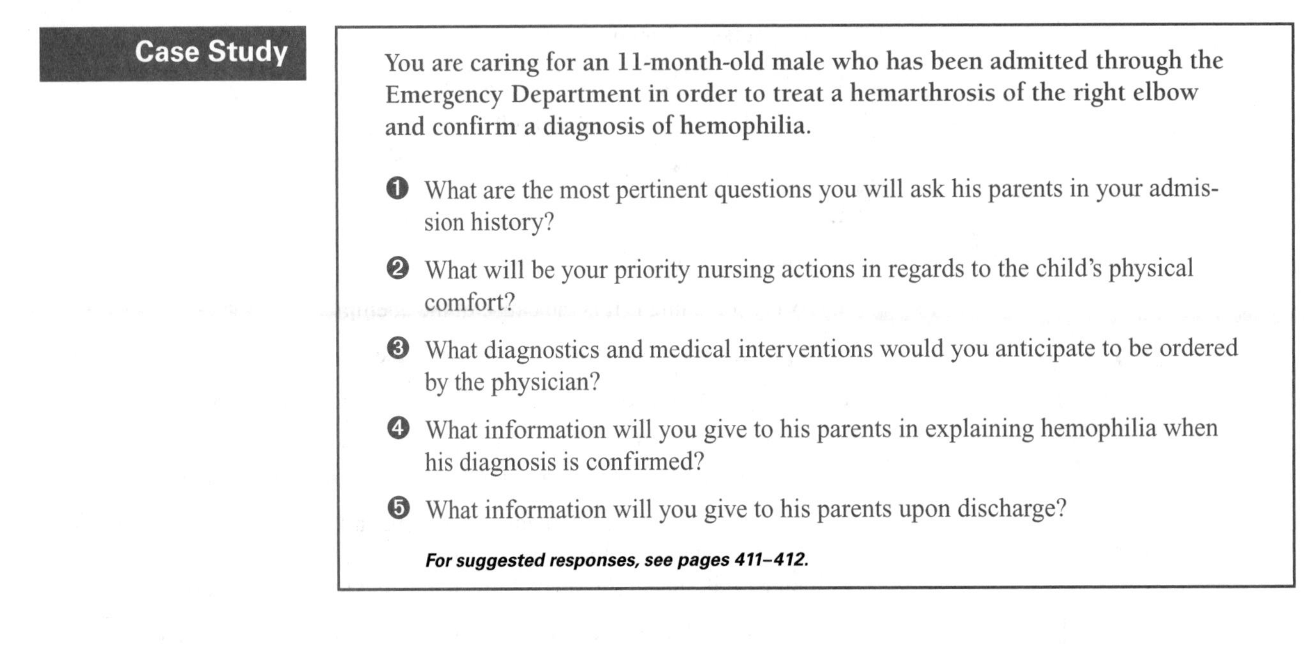

Case Study

You are caring for an 11-month-old male who has been admitted through the Emergency Department in order to treat a hemarthrosis of the right elbow and confirm a diagnosis of hemophilia.

❶ What are the most pertinent questions you will ask his parents in your admission history?

❷ What will be your priority nursing actions in regards to the child's physical comfort?

❸ What diagnostics and medical interventions would you anticipate to be ordered by the physician?

❹ What information will you give to his parents in explaining hemophilia when his diagnosis is confirmed?

❺ What information will you give to his parents upon discharge?

For suggested responses, see pages 411–412.

Posttest

1 A 2-year-old with hemophilia is being discharged, and the nurse is completing discharge teaching with his parents. Which of the following statements by the parents indicates they require further teaching regarding hemophilia?

(1) "It is good to know that his sister will not get hemophilia also."
(2) "If our son has a temperature, we will not give aspirin or ibuprofen, only acetaminophen."
(3) "We will get a Medic-Alert™ bracelet for our son as soon as we get home."
(4) "We will be sure to watch our son very closely to make sure he does not have another episode of bleeding."

2 The parents of a client with sickle cell anemia are asking for information about future pregnancies. Neither parent has sickle cell anemia. The nurse would provide them with the information that any future pregnancies will have a:

(1) 1 in 4 chance of producing a child with sickle cell trait.
(2) 1 in 4 chance of producing a child with sickle cell anemia.
(3) 1 in 2 chance of producing a child with neither sickle cell disease or trait.
(4) 1 in 2 chance of producing a child with sickle cell anemia.

3 The nurse is working with the family of an 8-month-old infant with severe nutritional anemia. In providing dietary recommendations, the nurse should instruct the family to:

(1) Switch the baby to cow's milk.
(2) Delay the introduction of table food in the diet.
(3) Restrict the amount of milk or formula in the baby's diet to 1 quart per day.
(4) Provide dietary iron sources such as peanuts and unsweetened chocolates.

4 A child is being admitted to the unit with thalassemia major. In preparing client assignments, the charge nurse would want to assign a nurse to this child who can:

(1) Teach dietary sources of iron.
(2) Administer blood transfusions.
(3) Work with a dying child.
(4) Monitor the child for bleeding tendencies.

5 The nurse is caring for a child who is being treated for extensive bleeding in the Emergency Department. The source and extent of bleeding are being determined as the nurse is trying to control the bleeding. Which of the following actions takes priority?

(1) Obtain the client's history.
(2) Talk with the family regarding the risk of HIV and hepatitis C with blood transfusions.
(3) Replace blood volume.
(4) Provide psychosocial support to the family.

6 The nurse is working with the family of a toddler who is being treated for iron-deficiency anemia. In teaching dietary considerations, the nurse will instruct the family to add sources of iron and:

(1) Vitamin D and thiamine.
(2) Calcium and riboflavin.
(3) Carbohydrates and vitamins.
(4) Folic acid and proteins.

7 The elementary school nurse is assessing and giving initial care to a hemophiliac who has a significant pain in his knee. The nurse suspects hemarthrosis. As the nurse waits for his family to pick up the child, the nurse would:

(1) Maintain joint mobility with passive range of motion exercises.
(2) Elevate the leg above his heart.
(3) Administer children's aspirin or ibuprofen for pain.
(4) Apply warm soaks to reduce the swelling.

8 The nurse has admitted a 2-year-old in vaso-occlusive crisis. As the nurse starts the initial assessment, the child insists upon lying in bed, on her side with her knees flexed to the abdomen. The nurse would want to further assess the child for the presence of:

(1) Stomach pain.
(2) Nausea.
(3) Constipation.
(4) Fear secondary to the impact of hospitalization.

9 The 10-year-old client in the Emergency Department has CBC results that include a hemoglobin of eight g/dL and hematocrit of 24 percent. The nursing activity with the highest priority is:

(1) Assessing and promoting skin integrity.
(2) Promoting hydration.
(3) Promoting nutrition.
(4) Conserving energy.

10 The nurse is caring for a child diagnosed with thalassemia major who is receiving her first chelation therapy. The parents ask the purpose of chelation therapy. The best response by the nurse is that chelation therapy is done to:

(1) Decrease the risk of hypoxia.
(2) Decrease the risk of bleeding.
(3) Eliminate excess iron.
(4) Prevent further sickling of RBCs.

See pages 374–375 for Answers and Rationales.

Answers and Rationales

Pretest

1 **Answer: 4** ***Rationale:*** A child diagnosed with thalassemia who will receive multiple transufsions throughout life will need chelation therapy for excessive iron stores. An iron supplement would be inappropriate in this child.
Cognitive Level: Analysis
Nursing Process: Evaluation; ***Test Plan:*** HPM

2 **Answer: 1** ***Rationale:*** Rectal temperatures can traumatize the fragile rectal mucosa leading to bleeding and should be avoided. The vital signs will need to be measured on a regular basis. An intravenous start kit is appropriate as the child will need plasma and blood products. A bedpan will be needed if the child is on bed rest.
Cognitive Level: Analysis
Nursing Process: Planning; ***Test Plan:*** SECE

3 **Answer: 3** ***Rationale:*** All of the injuries require nursing care; however, the child with the head injury has a potentially life-threatening injury and needs attention before the other three.
Cognitive Level: Analysis
Nursing Process: Analysis; ***Test Plan:*** PHYS

4 **Answer: 1** ***Rationale:*** RBCs sickle under conditions where low oxygen concentrations exist; therefore, administering oxygen will prevent additional sickling. The oxygen has no effect on the oxygen-carrying capacity of RBCs. It will not have an effect on development of respiratory complications. It will not decrease the potential for infection.
Cognitive Level: Analysis
Nursing Process: Implementation; ***Test Plan:*** PHYS

5 **Answer: 3** ***Rationale:*** Iron preparations should be taken through a straw in order to prevent staining the teeth. While it is generally best to give toddlers choices in the hospital setting, the other options are not appropriate as iron is best absorbed on an empty stomach.
Cognitive Level: Application
Nursing Process: Implementation; ***Test Plan:*** SECE

6 **Answer: 3** ***Rationale:*** In an acute care setting such as a hospital and with a potentially life-threatening disease such as DIC, the family may need help with coping with the stress they are feeling. This stress often interferes with communication. A patient response by the nurse with repetition of information will allow the family to absorb the information.
Cognitive Level: Application
Nursing Process: Analysis; ***Test Plan:*** HPM

7 **Answer: 2** ***Rationale:*** Factor VIII concentrate is a blood product. Fluid volume overload is an unlikely concern, as the factor will be given in a comparatively small volume of fluid. There is no greater a chance of emboli formation with administration of factor VIII than with any other IV preparation. Concern as to contracting AIDS from administration of a blood product is a long-term concern related to multiple administrations. It is not a concern during the actual administration of the factor.
Cognitive Level: Analysis
Nursing Process: Planning; ***Test Plan:*** PHYS

8 **Answer: 1** ***Rationale:*** As RBCs clump together, they block small blood vessels, which can lead to tissue ischemia, necrosis, and death. This is the chief cause of pain during a vaso-occlusive crisis. Blood sequestration, hepatosplenomegaly, and increased RBC destruction are not the primary causes of pain during a crisis.
Cognitive Level: Analysis
Nursing Process: Analysis; ***Test Plan:*** PHYS

9 **Answer: 3** ***Rationale:*** Anemia does occur easily infancy and infants have limited stores of iron. The first solid food offered to infants is often cereal, which is an excellent source of iron. All infants do not require iron supplements; it is preferable that the iron comes from dietary intake.
Cognitive Level: Application
Nursing Process: Planning; ***Test Plan:*** HPM

10 **Answer: 4** ***Rationale:*** Alterations in platelet function necessitate treating a break in the skin's integrity as you would an arterial stick—apply pressure for 5 minutes or more. The goal of treatment is to apply pressure long enough that the defective clotting mechanism will have time to form a clot. Steri-strips would not close the wound adequately, and restricting arm movement will not assist in the initial formation of a clot.
Cognitive Level: Application
Nursing Process: Implementation; ***Test Plan:*** PHYS

Posttest

1 **Answer: 4** ***Rationale:*** It is not possible for parents of a hemophiliac to prevent a bleeding episode, no matter how careful they are. The nurse should reinforce this information along with methods for decreasing the chance of an injury that will lead to a bleeding episode. The other statements all indicate an appropriate understanding of hemophilia.
Cognitive Level: Application
Nursing Process: Evaluation; ***Test Plan:*** HPM

2 **Answer: 2** ***Rationale:*** Sickle cell anemia is an autosomal recessive condition. Therefore, if both parents have the trait, each pregnancy carries a 25 percent risk that the child will have the disease.
Cognitive Level: Application
Nursing Process: Analysis; ***Test Plan:*** HPM

3 **Answer: 3** ***Rationale:*** Many infants with nutritional anemia rely primarily on the milk/formula for dietary intake and refuse solid foods. When the milk/formula is limited, the child will be more willing to take solid foods. Cow's milk is a poor source of iron. Peanuts and unsweetened chocolates are sources of iron but are not appropriate for a child this age.
Cognitive Level: Application
Nursing Process: Implementation; ***Test Plan:*** HPM

4 **Answer: 2** ***Rationale:*** Blood transfusions are utilized in order to maintain normal hemoglobin levels. This child has an excess of iron secondary to repeated transfusions and, thus, iron supplements will not be necessary. The other therapies are inappropriate for the child with thalassemia major.
Cognitive Level: Analysis
Nursing Process: Planning; ***Test Plan:*** SECE

5 Answer: 3 ***Rationale:*** Appropriate oxygenation is not possible when there is significant loss of blood volume. Replacing the blood volume is critical to saving the child's life, and it is imperative that replacement occurs prior to any of the listed nursing actions.
Cognitive Level: Application
Nursing Process: Planning; ***Test Plan:*** PHYS

6 Answer: 4 ***Rationale:*** Folic acid potentiates the removal of iron from ferritin, which makes it further available for heme production. The synthesis of albumin, blood proteins, fibrinogen, and hemoglobin is dependent upon the presence of proteins. None of the others are involved in building RBCs.
Cognitive Level: Application
Nursing Process: Implementation; ***Test Plan:*** HPM

7 Answer: 2 ***Rationale:*** Elevate the leg above the level of the heart to reduce bleeding. Aspirin or aspirin-like products such as ibuprofen interfere with the clotting mechanisms. During active bleeds, the joint should be immobilized. Warm soaks would promote bleeding; ice packs should be used instead.
Cognitive Level: Analysis
Nursing Process: Implementation; ***Test Plan:*** PHYS

8 Answer: 1 ***Rationale:*** Such positioning indicates the likelihood of abdominal pain. Nausea or constipation does not generally cause a child to self-position as described. Fear related to the hospitalization would be common in a child this age. However, if this were the case, it is more likely the child would seek refuge in the arms of one of her parents.
Cognitive Level: Analysis
Nursing Process: Assessment; ***Test Plan:*** PHYS

9 Answer: 4 ***Rationale:*** Such lab results indicate severe anemia. Fatigue results when the oxygen-carrying capacity of RBCs is impaired and cellular hypoxia is present. Fatigue can be diminished and oxygen depletion limited when the client's energy is conserved. There will be an increased oxygen requirement and increased fatigue with increased mobility. Increasing general hydration without transfusing RBCs will not positively affect the anemic state. Skin integrity is not a high priority at this point. Although improving nutrition is appropriate, the response would not be immediate. The priority activity would be conserving energy and reducing cardiac stress.
Cognitive Level: Analysis
Nursing Process: Planning; ***Test Plan:*** PHYS

10 Answer: 3 ***Rationale:*** Chelation therapy works to rid the body of excess iron storage that results from the frequent transfusions required to maintain adequate hemoglobin. Chelation will have no effect upon hypoxia or bleeding. Sickling of RBCs does not occur with thalassemia.
Cognitive Level: Application
Nursing Process: Implementation; ***Test Plan:*** HPM

References

Ball, J. & Bindler, R. (1999). *Pediatric nursing: Caring for children* (2nd ed.). Stamford, CT: Appleton & Lange, pp. 515–539.

Bowden, V. R., Dickey, S. B., and Greenberg, C. S. (1998). *Children and their families: The continuum of care.* Philadelphia: W. B. Saunders, pp. 460–461, 676, 1515–1605.

Hankins, J., Lonsway, R. A. W., Hedrick, C., & Perdue, M. B. (2001). *Infusion therapy in clinical practice* (2nd ed.). Philadelphia: W. B. Saunders Company, pp. 156–175.

Ignatavicius, D. D., Workman, M. L., & Mishler, M. A. (1999). *Medical surgical nursing across the health care continuum* (3rd ed.). Philadelphia: W. B. Saunders, pp. 951–988.

Lemone, P. & Burke, K. (2000). *Medical surgical nursing: Critical thinking in client care* (2nd ed.). Upper Saddle River, NJ: Prentice-Hall, Inc., pp. 1291–1297.

Monahan, F. & Neighbors, M. (1998). *Medical surgical nursing: Foundations for clinical practice.* (2nd ed.). Philadelphia: W. B. Saunders, p. 469.

Wilson, B. A., Shannon, M. T., & Stang, C. L. (2001). *Nursing drug guide 2001.* Upper Saddle River, NJ: Prentice-Hall, Inc., pp. 1199–1200.

CHAPTER 15

Special Considerations in Child Health

Joseann Helmes DeWitt, MSN, RN, C, CLNC

CHAPTER OUTLINE

OBJECTIVES

- Describe assessment findings and nursing management of a child with attention deficit hyperactivity disorder, autism, or mental retardation.
- Discuss the nursing management of the family suffering the loss of an infant to sudden infant death syndrome.
- Discuss assessment findings and nursing management of a child suffering from child abuse.
- Describe nursing management options for a child with the mental health problems of substance abuse or suicide risk.
- Describe nursing management of a child suffering from accidental poisoning.

[Media Link]

Use the CD-ROM enclosed with this text, or log onto the address given to access the free, interactive Companion Website created for this series. The CD-ROM and Companion Website accompanying this book offer additional practice opportunities and information—NCLEX Review, Case Studies, Glossary, In Depth with NCLEX, and more.

www.prenhall.com/hogan

Review at a Glance

art therapy *refers to the utilization of drawing as a form of therapeutic strategy; drawing exercises allow the child the opportunity to express feelings of fear, anger, and pain; art therapy is appropriate for all ages*

behavioral modification *a method utilized to alter inappropriate behaviors by reinforcing desirable behaviors, usually by stimulus or response conditioning (reward system); often used by parents of children with attention deficit hyperactivity disorder or mental retardation*

child abuse *the infliction of physical, psychological, or sexual harm on a child*

physical abuse *direct physical injury to a child as a result of hitting, striking, punching, kicking, shaking, biting, or burning*

play therapy *a method of therapeutic strategies through the use of toys, dolls, art, or other creative methods to allow the child an opportunity to reveal problems such as abuse; this method is appropriate for the preschool to school-aged child*

psychological abuse *the deliberate failure of the caregiver to provide emotional nurturance, affection, and attention, significantly impairing the child's self-esteem*

sexual abuse *sexual contact of a child resulting from fondling, rape, sodomy, intercourse, or exploitation through pornography*

suicide *the act of self-injury with the intention of the act resulting in death*

suicide attempt *the unsuccessful attempt of the act of suicide*

suicide ideation *thoughts about committing the act of suicide*

Pretest

1 After writing a suicide note, a 16-year-old swallows numerous anti-anxiety pills belonging to a friend. Which of the following factors would indicate to you that the teenager is at risk for a repeated attempt at suicide?

(1) She stated that she wishes she hadn't made such a "stupid mistake."
(2) Her grades have dropped over the past few weeks.
(3) Her father died recently.
(4) She lives with her mother and stepfather.

2 When performing a health screening on an adolescent in the health clinic, you would determine he is at a higher risk of suicide than other adolescents of his age based on which of the following facts that he discloses?

(1) He states that he sleeps late on the weekends.
(2) He states that he only has a small group of close friends.
(3) He states that he is a homosexual.
(4) He states that he often skips meals and does not worry about nutrition.

3 An 11-year-old female was discovered smoking cigarettes in the school bathroom. The school nurse should implement which of the following plans for this school-aged child?

(1) Assign the child to a peer-led program to teach the consequences of smoking.
(2) Recommend that the child attend a community-based smoking prevention program.
(3) Assign the child videos to view that demonstrate the effects of smoking.
(4) Assign the child to attend a session of health class that deals with smoking.

4 You are providing care to a toddler who has ingested an unknown amount of his grandfather's medication, which is described as "a white pill." The physician has ordered the administration of syrup of ipecac and activated charcoal. What action would you take?

(1) Question the order because syrup of ipecac and activated charcoal are not to be used together.
(2) Administer the ipecac, and after the child vomits, administer the activated charcoal.
(3) Administer the activated charcoal, then administer the syrup of ipecac.
(4) Insert a nasogastric tube for the administration of the syrup of ipecac and activated charcoal.

5 A child is brought to the Emergency Department with excessive drooling, edema of lips and tongue, swollen mucous membranes, and is hypotensive and tachycardic. Based on this initial assessment, you suspect that the child has ingested which of the following agents?

(1) A corrosive agent
(2) Aspirin
(3) Hydrocarbons
(4) Acetaminophen

6 You are the telephone triage nurse and have received a call from a mother who states that her 4-year-old son has ingested an unknown amount of aspirin. She administered 15 ml of syrup of ipecac 20 minutes ago, but the child has not vomited yet. You instruct the mother to take which of the following actions?

(1) Wait 15 more minutes, then if the child still has not vomited, take him to the Emergency Department.
(2) Take child to the Emergency Department immediately.
(3) Repeat the 15 mL of syrup of ipecac now, and immediately take the child to the Emergency Department.
(4) Repeat the syrup of ipecac, but increase the dose to 30 mL, and immediately take the child to the Emergency Department.

7 A 10-year-old child with mild mental retardation wants to join his younger brother's Cub Scout group. His parents are apprehensive about allowing him to join and ask you for advice. Your response will be based on the fact that children with mental retardation:

(1) Have the same need for socialization as children without mental retardation.
(2) Should not be encouraged to participate in clubs because of their developmental delay.
(3) Should participate in clubs especially created for children that are cognitively impaired.
(4) Do not have a need for socialization.

8 An 11-year-old child with attention deficit hyperactivity disorder (ADHD) being treated with methylphenidate (Ritalin) twice a day reports that he is having difficulty falling to sleep at night. Upon questioning him, you discover he is taking the medication in the morning before leaving for school and in the evening after supper. Based on the information provided, you would instruct him in which of the following?

(1) Continue taking the morning dose as previously, but take the evening dose earlier in the afternoon.
(2) Stop taking the medication until he can be evaluated by his physician.
(3) Take both doses of the medication in the morning before leaving for school.
(4) Reduce the evening dose of medication to half the prescribed dose.

9 The parents who have just experienced the death of an infant from sudden infant death syndrome (SIDS) request time alone with the infant. You should take which of the following actions?

(1) Discourage the parents from seeing the infant because it will be too painful.
(2) Allow the parents as much time alone with the infant as they need.
(3) Allow the parents to view the infant, but remain in the room with them.
(4) Deny the parents' request because they are emotionally distraught.

10 A 3-year-old child is brought to the Emergency Department for treatment of injuries the father stated were obtained when the child fell off of his tricycle. Upon assessment, numerous bruised areas, old and fresh, are noted on the child's back, buttocks, and shoulders. Radiologic examination reveals fractured ribs and a healed fractured humerus. Based on these findings, your next course of action would be which of the following?

(1) Report the child as a victim of child abuse immediately.
(2) Ask the father to provide further details of the incident, obtain a medical history of the child, and then interview the child separately.
(3) Ask the father if he has been physically abusive to the child.
(4) Ask the father if he believes the child's mother has been physically abusive to the child.

See page 396 for Answers and Rationales.

I. Congenital Health Problems

A. Attention deficit hyperactivity disorder (ADHD)

1. Definition: attention deficit hyperactivity disorder is defined as a persistence in hyperactivity, impulsiveness, or inattention that is observed more frequently than in other children at the same developmental level

2. Etiology and pathophysiology

a. The etiology is unknown, however, it is theorized that genetic and environmental factors can be attributed to ADHD; ADHD is associated with high blood lead level in childhood and prenatal exposure to alcohol

b. Occurs more frequently in males, is diagnosed when symptoms appear, generally around ages 3 to 4

3. Assessment

a. Easily distracted

b. Difficulty waiting turns

c. Excessive talking

d. Leaves uncompleted task to begin another

e. Does not appear to listen

f. Constant squirming or fidgeting in chair

g. Decreased attention span

h. Impulsiveness

i. Often loses things

4. Priority nursing diagnoses

a. Impaired verbal communication

b. Impaired social interaction

c. Ineffective family coping

d. Risk for caregiver strain

e. Risk for injury

f. Self-esteem disturbance

5. Planning and implementation

a. Assist with diagnostic procedures: MRI and psychological assessments

b. Help establish plan for promotion of optimal growth and development

1) Decrease excess stimulation (television, loud noises)

2) Provide quiet environment for learning

3) Promote self-esteem

4) Establish reward programs for completion of tasks

5) Provide parental support

c. Refer parent(s) to Children and Adults with Attention-Deficit Hyperactivity Disorder (CHADD) at www.chadd.org or 1-800-233-4050 and to the National Attention Deficit Disorder Association (ADDA) at www.add.org or 847-432-ADDA

NCLEX!

6. Medication therapy

a. Methylphenidate (Ritalin) enhances catecholamine effects which inhibit impulsiveness and hyperactivity; allows the child to concentrate better and benefit more from the school experience

b. Dextroamphetamine (Dexedrine) has demonstrated a positive effect on hyperactivity, allowing the child to concentrate on task

7. Child and family education

a. Teach safe medication administration of psychopharmacologic agents

b. Educate parents and teachers to provide structure and decrease classroom stimuli to enhance school performance

c. Educate the child and family about the disorder; provide the family with strategies to deal with the hyperactivity and inattentiveness

d. Provide information to the child and family about activities that serve to improve self-esteem

8. Evaluation: the parents identify safe and effective drug administration; the family identifies activities to decrease hyperactivity and promote learning; the child exhibits symptoms of positive self-esteem

B. Autism (sometimes referred to as autistic disorder)

1. Description

a. Autism is a developmental disorder of brain function characterized by deficits in intelligence and behavior

b. Involves abnormalities in behavior, interferes with the ability for social interactions, and impairs verbal communication

2. Etiology and pathophysiology

a. Seen more often in boys and occurs in 5 out of every 10,000 births

b. Etiology is unknown but may be linked genetically, and to biochemical imbalances and brain dysfunction

c. Most autistic children have cognitive impairment

NCLEX!

3. Assessment

a. Interview parent(s) regarding child's behavior

1) Disinterested in being held or cuddled, stiffens when being held

2) Avoids eye contact

3) Poor language development

4) Minimal facial responsiveness (doesn't smile)

5) Appears not to hear when being spoken to

6) Exhibits abnormal activities such as head-banging

7) Does not engage in social play with others

4. Priority nursing diagnoses

a. Impaired social interaction

b. Impaired verbal communication

c. Altered growth and development

d. Ineffective family coping

e. Caregiver role strain

f. Risk for injury

5. Planning and implementation

a. Decrease environmental stimuli (sounds and light)

NCLEX!

b. Maintain a safe environment, provide close supervision; self-abusive children need protective mechanisms in the least restrictive manner possible

c. Promote parental coping

NCLEX!

d. Maintain the hospitalized child's daily routine as much as possible to minimize stress

e. Encourage activities and specialized educational programs to child's ability to promote optimal growth and development

6. Child and family education

a. Teach the family protective items that reduce the child's risk of injury

b. Educate the parents about behavior modification methods

c. Refer parent(s) to the Autism Society of America at www.autism-society.org or 1-800-3AUTISM

7. Evaluation: the family identifies support systems within the community; the child demonstrates improved eye contact and ability to communicate; the child remains free from self-injury

C. Mental retardation (sometimes referred to as cognitive impairment)

1. Description

a. Mental retardation is defined as intelligence significantly below average, existing with limitation in adaptive skills

b. IQ scores used to denote mental retardation are generally below the 70 to 75 range; IQ is a computation of the individual's mental age divided by his or her chronologic age

2. Etiology and pathophysiology

a. Numerous causes, such as genetic (for example, Down Syndrome), prenatal (such as fetal alcohol syndrome and maternal infections), and postnatal factors (such as trauma, errors of metabolism, and hypoxia) are attributed to mental retardation

b. Mental retardation occurs more often in males than females

c. Severity of mental retardation

1) Mild retardation: an IQ between 50 and 70

2) Moderate retardation: an IQ between 35 and 50

3) Severe retardation: an IQ between 20 and 35

4) Profound retardation: an IQ below 20

3. Assessment

a. Prenatal and postnatal histories may provide clues to the presence of mental retardation; family history of genetic disorders should be investigated

NCLEX!

b. Delays in motor and language developmental milestones; these delays are often first recognized by the mother

c. Seizure disorders and other injuries may indicate trauma

d. Laboratory tests, including chromosomal analysis and blood levels for lead or enzymes, may be useful

e. The Denver Developmental Screening Test II provides information on developmental levels

NCLEX!

f. Neurologic exams may recognize soft neurologic signs such as a simian crease in the palms or abnormal hair swirls and low-set ears

4. Priority nursing diagnoses

a. Altered growth and development

b. Self-care deficit: toileting, hygiene

c. Impaired verbal communication

d. Ineffective family coping

e. Anticipatory grieving

5. Planning and implementation

NCLEX!

a. Early detection is essential; perform developmental screening to detect delays

b. Support parent(s) in choosing educational programs; depending on severity, child may be "mainstreamed" into public school classrooms, or attend special education classes

c. Parental support and guidance is needed, as they may experience shock and grief upon learning the diagnosis

d. When appropriate, perform a functional assessment to determine child's ability to provide self-care (toileting, feeding, dressing)

e. Encourage socialization (may participate in scouts, groups, or other activities, depending on the child's motor and developmental ability)

f. May require occupational and/or speech therapy

NCLEX!

g. Promote optimal growth and development, encourage promotion of self-esteem and self-care

h. Help parent(s) establish a behavior modification program if necessary

i. Help parent(s) identify any potential complications (cardiac, pulmonary, gastrointestinal, motor) and seek medical assistance when necessary

j. Educate parent(s) that child has the same needs for exercise and play as other children, and this should be tailored to the child's developmental age

6. Child and family education

a. Teach safety precautions to prevent injuries caused by developmental delays

b. Provide information that supports growth and development

c. Teach the parents to plan activities based on the child's mental age rather than the child's chronologic age

d. Refer parent(s) to American Association on Mental Retardation at www.aamr.org or 202-387-1968

7. Evaluation: the parents make positive statements about their child; family provides stimulation appropriate to the mental age of the child; the child displays evidence of a positive self-esteem

II. Acquired Health Problems

A. Sudden infant death syndrome (SIDS)

1. Definition: the sudden, unexplained death of an infant less than 1 year of age

2. Etiology and pathophysiology

a. Death remains unexplained even after autopsy

b. Most frequently occurs between ages 2 and 4 months

c. Occurs more commonly in males

d. Most often occurs in winter and spring

e. Child is discovered in crib after period of sleep; a change of position may have occurred, and there may be frothy, blood-tinged secretions around the mouth and nares

d. The syndrome is usually considered unpreventable

3. Assessment

a. Usually considered nonpredictable; however, risk factors are known

1) Prematurity

2) Infections

3) Brain stem defects

4) Use of soft bedding (infant suffocates by rebreathing CO_2)

5) Sleeping in prone position

6) Maternal smoking during pregnancy

7) Sibling with SIDS
8) Low birth weight
9) Increased incidence in winter
10) Increased incidence in lower socioeconomic groups

b. Infant is brought to the Emergency Department and death is confirmed; an autopsy will be ordered to determine cause of death

4. Priority nursing diagnoses

a. Ineffective coping related to death of child

b. Fear

c. Anxiety

5. Planning and implementation

NCLEX!

a. Nursing management of risk for SIDS includes education of the parents about risk factors and activities which can reduce risk factors

1) The child may be placed on an apnea monitor whenever the child is asleep
2) The parents need to be taught infant CPR

b. Nursing management of family experiencing loss of child from SIDS

1) Most often a nurse's first contact with suspected SIDS is in the Emergency Department after the infant is brought in for emergency resuscitation
2) Avoid questions that could imply parental negligence or involvement in the death
3) Provide emotional support for grieving family; seek assistance from social services, clergy, and/or others that have experience in helping families deal with the death of a child

NCLEX!

4) Parent(s) may verbally express feelings of anger and guilt; assure parent(s) that there is nothing that they could have done to prevent the infant's death
5) Allow parent(s) the opportunity to hold the child and say good-bye; infant should be presented cleaned and wrapped in a blanket
6) An autopsy will likely be necessary to verify the cause of death; this should be explained to the parent(s)
7) Assess sibling response to death and intervene with counseling as necessary; a sibling may feel guilty or responsible for the infant's death
8) Refer family to American SIDS Institute at www.sids.org or 1-800-232-SIDS

6. Child and family education

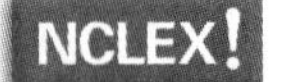

a. Educate parent(s) that the American Academy of Pediatrics recommends placing infants on their sides or backs, instead of prone, to sleep

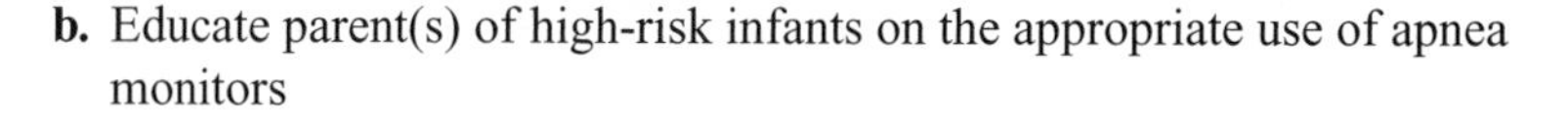

b. Educate parent(s) of high-risk infants on the appropriate use of apnea monitors

c. Provide information to parents of SIDS victims about what is known about the syndrome

7. Evaluation: all parents place their infants to sleep on their backs, not stomachs; parents of at-risk infants identify safety measures for using infant monitors; parents of at-risk infants demonstrate infant CPR correctly; parents of SIDS victims state that the child's death was unpreventable; the parents of SIDS victims participate in SIDS support groups

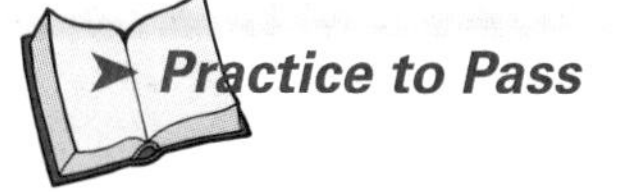

A 4-month-old infant is brought to the Emergency Department by the parents who found the infant dead in the crib when they woke up this morning. The initial cause of death is believed to be sudden infant death syndrome (SIDS). As the nurse who provided care to the infant and the family, what actions would you now take towards the parents?

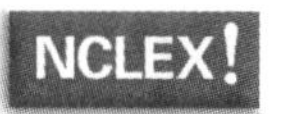

B. Child abuse

1. Description

a. Child abuse, sometimes referred to as child maltreatment, is the infliction of physical, psychological, or sexual abuse on a child

b. Physical abuse describes abuse that involves direct physical injury usually as a result of hitting, striking, punching, shaking, biting, or burning

c. Sexual abuse describes abuse that involves sexual contact as a result of fondling, rape, sodomy, intercourse, or exploitation through pornography

d. Psychological abuse, or emotional abuse, is characterized by the deliberate failure of the caregiver to provide emotional nurturance, affection, and attention, significantly impairing the child's self-esteem

e. Child neglect is the failure to provide basic needs such as physical, emotional, and educational needs

2. Etiology and pathophysiology; risk factors include:

a. Prematurity

b. Chronically ill child

c. Child is viewed as difficult

d. Unwanted child

e. Adult abuser characteristically has low self-esteem and a low tolerance for frustration, lives in social isolation, and has an inadequate understanding of normal growth and development

f. Incompatibility between parent(s)' and child's temperament

g. Parent abuses alcohol or drugs

3. Assessment

a. Physical assessment should include a thorough examination of entire body; assess for burns, scalds, scars, bruising, fractures, dislocated joints, vaginal tears or bleeding, and other signs of abuse

b. Height and weight to determine failure to thrive or other growth abnormalities

c. Assess child and family interaction

d. Assess for evidence of neglect (dirty, unkempt, withdraws from others)

e. Assess for delays in psychosocial, psychomotor, and cognitive development

f. Sexually abused child may exhibit bedwetting, frequent crying, excessive bathing, avoidance of family and peers

4. Priority nursing diagnoses

a. Altered growth and development

b. Fear related to physical harm

c. Risk for injury

d. Pain related to injuries

e. Impaired skin integrity related to injury

f. Altered health maintenance

5. Planning and implementation

a. Maintain a nonjudgmental and nonthreatening attitude during interactions with child and parent(s)

b. Document child and parent comments verbatim

NCLEX!

c. Be aware that the incompatibility between the *history* and the *injury* is the number-one criterion for suspecting child abuse

NCLEX!

d. Report all cases of suspected child abuse; healthcare professionals have a legal obligation to report suspected abuse

e. Do not inform parent(s) that child abuse is suspected

f. Child may be removed from home and placed in a safe environment to prevent further injury

g. If child remains in custody of family, assist them in identifying support systems and resources such as Parents Anonymous

NCLEX!

h. Acknowledge child's fears during hospitalization and provide a consistent caregiver to encourage establishment of trust and security

i. Refrain from stereotyping to decrease incidence of false-positive and false-negative accusations; there is no single predictor for who will commit child abuse

j. Be aware of the types of therapeutic strategies utilized by therapists

1) **Play therapy** utilizes toys, dolls, art, and other creative objects to allow the child an opportunity to reveal problems such as abuse; this strategy is used mostly for the preschool and school-aged child

2) **Art therapy** utilizes drawing exercises to allow expressions of feelings such as anger and pain; this strategy is appropriate for all ages

3) **Behavior modification** applies methods to alter inappropriate behavior by reinforcing desirable behaviors, usually by stimulus or response conditioning; an example is the use of the "reward system"

k. Refer family to the National Committee to Prevent Child Abuse (NCPCA) at www.childabuse.org or 1-877-224-8223 and to Parents Anonymous at www.parentsanonymous.org or 909-621-6184

6. Child and family education
    a. Teach the child that he or she can report abuse without fear of repercussions
    b. All families need to know where to seek help when overwhelmed by the situation
7. Evaluation: the child is maintained in a safe environment; the parents display appropriate parenting skills; the child remains free of injury

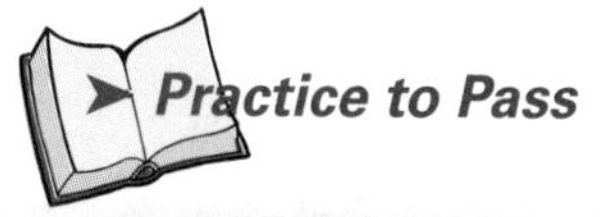

You are the school nurse treating a 6-year-old girl for an abrasion on the knee that she sustained while on the playground. As you are assessing the child, you note numerous areas on the upper legs that appear to be cigarette burns. What actions would you take?

C. Substance abuse

1. Definition: the voluntary use of a substance to obtain a state of euphoria or a state of calmness
2. Etiology and pathophysiology
    a. Most commonly abused substances
        1) Tobacco (cigarettes, chewing tobacco)
        2) Alcohol
        3) Marijuana
        4) Volatile substances (inhaled) such as spray paint and plastic cement
        5) Cocaine, narcotics, CNS depressants, and CNS stimulants
    b. Risk factors for substance abuse
        1) Parent who engages in substance abuse
        2) Peer association (wants to "fit in")
        3) School drop-out
        4) Problems with conduct
        5) Biologic factors
3. Assessment
    a. Physical, social, and psychological symptoms vary according to substance
        1) Cocaine produces euphoria, cardiovascular mainfestations, and seizures
        2) Central nervous system depressants have sedative effects such as drowsiness
        3) Central nervous system stimulants can lead to aggressive behavior, agitation, restlessness, paranoia, and boldness
        4) Narcotics use produces constricted pupils and respiratory depression
        5) Inhalants cause a feeling of euphoria or "high," loss of consciousness, respiratory arrest
    b. Assess for needle marks (tracks) on arms and legs
    c. Assess for behavioral changes
        1) Drop in school performance (grades, participation)
        2) Skipping school

3) Socializing with a "new" group of friends

4) No longer interested in activities previously enjoyed (sports activities, after-school functions)

5) Engaging in risk-taking behavior

6) Trouble resulting in intervention from law enforcement

4. Priority nursing diagnoses

a. Risk for injury

b. Risk for violence

c. Impaired social interaction

d. Self-esteem disturbance

5. Planning and implementation

a. Encourage participation in educational programs that increase substance abuse awareness

b. Treatment for acute drug toxicity or withdrawal is specific to the substance; gastric lavage or narcotic antagonists are most often utilized depending on the route of the substance involved

NCLEX!

c. Acute management includes maintaining patent airway, adequate tissue perfusion, and fluid volume status

NCLEX!

d. Treatment for chemical dependency/substance abuse often requires rehabilitation measures and involves a multidisciplinary approach

e. Encourage youth participation in prevention groups such as Students Against Driving Drunk (SADD)

f. Refer chemically dependent child to Alcoholics Anonymous or Ala-Teen at www.alcoholics-anonymous.org

Practice to Pass

A 16-year-old male is brought to the Emergency Department by a group of his friends who inform the nursing staff that "he took some drugs and now we can't get him to wake up." The adolescent is minimally responsive, pupils are constricted, and his respirations are 6 to 8 per minute. What immediate actions would you take?

6. Child and family education: educate parent(s) and teachers about the signs and symptoms of substance abuse

7. Evaluation: the child participates in substance abuse avoidance education program; the parents and teachers identify symptoms of substance abuse; symptoms of acute substance abuse are recognized and emergency treatment is provided

D. Suicide

1. Description

a. **Suicide** is defined as the act of self-injury, with the intention that the act result in death; the most common methods of suicide completion, in order, involve using firearms, hanging, and overdose

b. **Suicide attempt** is the intention to cause death but which is unsuccessful

2. Etiology and pathophysiology

a. The etiology of suicide is related to depression, poor self-concept, isolation, and family dysfunction

b. For adolescents between 15 and 19 years of age, suicide is the third-leading cause of death

c. For children between 5 and 14 years of age, suicide is the sixth-leading cause of death

d. The incidence of *completed* suicides is higher in males, but the incidence of suicide attempts is higher in females

e. Homosexual youths attempt suicide two to three times more often than heterosexual youths

f. Risk factors for suicide

1) Depression

2) Previous attempts at suicide (suicide gesture)

3) Family history of psychiatric disorders

4) Family violence

5) Substance abuse

NCLEX!

6) Homosexuality

7) Chronic illness

8) Overwhelming sense of guilt or shame

9) Frequent risk-taking behaviors

10) History of sexual abuse

3. Assessments of suicide risk

a. Makes specific statements about suicide

b. Gives away personal items

c. Sudden calmness (suicide decision has been made)

d. Any of the situations identified in risk factors (listed above)

e. **Suicide ideation:** thoughts about the act of suicide

4. Priority nursing diagnoses

a. Hopelessness related to fear and anxiety

b. Ineffective individual coping

c. Altered family processes

d. Risk for injury

e. Social isolation

5. Planning and implementation

a. Be supportive and nonjudgmental

b. Nurse's approach should be direct and clear; the nurse should be physically available to decrease child's sense of isolation

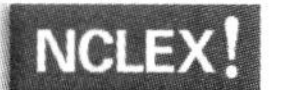

c. During hospitalization, take suicide precaution measures

d. Help child develop coping strategies

e. Help family develop coping strategies

Box 15-1

Assessment of Suicidality

SLAP

S Specificity: Is there a specific plan for suicide?
L Lethality: What is the intended method of suicide?
A Accessibility: Is the intended means of suicide available?
P Proximity: Is there a determined time to commit suicide?

Source: Wong, D., et al. (1999). *Whaley and Wong's nursing care of infants and children* (6th ed.). St. Louis: Mosby, p. 995.

f. Refer to mental health professional

g. Be aware that despair and hopelessness is not a normal part of adolescence

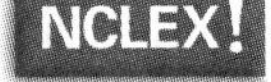

h. Assess the degree of suicidality (Box 15-1); it is important to note that all suicidal remarks should be taken seriously and should be further investigated

NCLEX!

i. Encourage "suicide contracts" with youths who are at risk or who have indicated a desire to commit suicide; the child signs an agreement to not attempt suicide for a specified period of time; these contracts are usually renewed daily

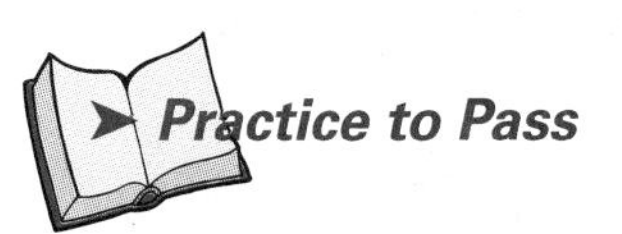

A 15-year-old female has been hospitalized numerous times for suicide attempts by swallowing various over-the-counter medications. You have provided care to her on several previous hospitalizations and are concerned because of the repeated attempts at suicide. What actions could you take to help this adolescent?

j. Community education: parents, teachers, healthcare providers, and children should be aware of warning signs of suicidal ideation; emphasize that most people attempting or completing suicide have revealed their thoughts about depression and/or suicide to someone—*the key is to listen and intervene*

k. Instruct parents to remove all firearms from the household, especially in presence of high-risk youths; firearms are the most commonly used method of suicide

l. Provide anticipatory guidance to parents and adolescents to help them obtain an understanding of normal adolescent growth and development

m. Refer parent(s) to the American Academy of Pediatrics: The Injury Prevention Program at www.aap.org or 1-800-433-9016

6. Child and family education: educate parent(s) and child about pharmacotherapeutic agents (antidepressants or antipsychotic medications) prescribed for the child

7. Evaluation: the child remains free of suicide attempts; the child and/or family identifies coping strategies

III. Accidents and Injuries Causing Health Problems

A. Accidental poisoning

1. Definition: accidental ingestion of poison or caustic substance

2. Etiology and pathophysiology

a. Most deaths from poisoning for young children occur during ages 1 to 4

b. Most deaths from poisoning for adolescents occur during ages 15 to 19

c. Risk factors for accidental poisoning

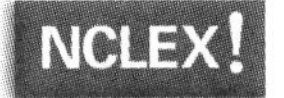

1) Curiosity related to developmental age

2) Lack of understanding of danger

3) Lack of parental or caregiver supervision

d. Most common agents of accidental poisoning

1) Acetaminophen (Tylenol)

2) Ibuprofen

3) Household plants

4) Cleaning solutions such as bleach

5) Cosmetic products (perfumes)

3. Assessments

a. Acetaminophen: assess for nausea, vomiting, diaphoresis; later signs involve the hepatic system, with jaundice, coagulation abnormalities, and pain in right upper quadrant

b. Aspirin: assess for nausea, vomiting, diaphoresis, tinnitus, seizures, oliguria, dehydration

NCLEX!

c. Corrosive agents: assess for drooling or inability to clear secretions, swollen mucous membranes, edema of tongue, lips, burning in mouth, throat, and stomach, and signs of shock

d. Hydrocarbons: assess for nausea, vomiting, weakness, pulmonary complications such as tachypnea and cyanosis, and alterations in sensorium

4. Priority nursing diagnoses

a. Risk for injury

b. Risk for ineffective airway clearance

c. Risk for impaired gas exchange

d. Risk for altered oral mucous membranes

e. Risk for decreased cardiac output

f. Risk for aspiration

5. Planning and implementation

a. Management is *specific to agent*

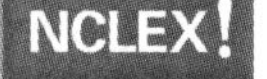

b. Treat the *child* first, not the poison

c. Maintain adequate respiratory and circulatory function

d. Be aware that condition may deteriorate rapidly

e. Keep child warm

f. Contact Poison Control Center for specific treatment of poisonings

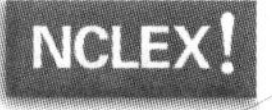

g. Refer to Table 15-1 for methods of treatment for poisonings

h. Refer parent(s) to the American Academy of Pediatrics: The Injury Prevention Program at www.aap.org or 1-800-433-9016

Table 15-1

Management of Poisonings in the Pediatric Population

Method of Treatment	Indications and Usage
Activated Charcoal The administration of a tasteless, odorless, black substance given to reduce systemic absorption of toxic agents	Given to reduce systemic absorption of toxic agents; may be mixed with sorbitol, water, or a saline cathartic. The child may drink the mixture through a straw, or it may be administered via nasogastric tube.
Antidotes The administration of an antidote specific to the agent of poisoning	Acetaminophen poisoning: *N*-acetylcysteine (Mucomyst) Carbon monoxide poisoning: oxygen Digoxin poisoning/toxicity: digoxin immune fab (Digibind) Benzodiazepine overdose: flumazenil (Romazicon) Opioid overdose: naloxone (Narcan) *Note:* Gastric decontamination, if indicated, is still required when administering antidotes
Cathartics The administration of cathartics is done to promote stimulation and evacuation of the bowel in order to decrease systemic absorption. Also administered to promote evacuation of activated charcoal	Sorbitol Magnesium sulfate Magnesium citrate These solutions are administered orally, or via a nasogastric tube.
Emetics The administration of substances to induce vomiting	Syrup of ipecac Ages 6 to 12 months: administer 10 mL and do not repeat. Ages 1 to 12 years: administer 15 mL and repeat once if has not vomited within 20 minutes. Over 12 years: administer 30 mL and repeat once if child has not vomited within 20 minutes *Note:* Do not induce vomiting in child with decreased level of consciousness or in absence of gag reflex; do not induce vomiting if caustic substance has been ingested.
Gastric Lavage The insertion of a nasogastric tube and subsequent irrigation and removal of gastric contents	Insert largest bore nasogastric tube possible; lavage with prescribed solution.

Practice to Pass

A 3-year-old male is brought to the Emergency Department by his father after the father returned home from work and discovered the toddler eating acetaminophen (Tylenol). The child is treated and has no complications from this episode. Upon review, you discover that the child was treated in the Emergency Department four months ago for a similar situation, except then the child consumed vitamins. As the nurse caring for this child, what actions should you take?

6. Child and family education
   a. Teach families safety measures related to poisoning prevention
      1) Safe storage of household chemicals
      2) The use of child-proof medication bottles and keeping medications away from young children; remind the family that toddlers get access to medications in mother's purse
   b. Encourage all families to keep the poison control center's phone number handy

7. Evaluation: parents identify interventions appropriate in an accidental poisoning; parents childproof child's environment; child remains free of accidental poisoning; accidental poisoning victim recovers without sequelae

Case Study

A 5-year-old female who is a victim of sexual abuse committed by her uncle is being admitted to your hospital unit for treatment of a urinary tract infection and labia lacerations.

1. As you admit the child to the unit, what will be your initial approach with her?
2. What measures can you take to promote a sense of security for the child?
3. The child tells you that she is "bad" because she told on her uncle. How would you respond?
4. The parents are arguing loudly in the child's hospital room. What actions would you take?
5. The child is exhibiting anger by throwing her breakfast tray and refusing to allow the nursing staff to assess her. What strategies could be initiated to support the child's well-being?

For suggested responses, see page 412.

Posttest

1 A 17-year-old male has informed his friends and family that he plans to commit suicide. As the school nurse, you further investigate this adolescent's comments. Your actions are based on which of the following?

(1) Most adolescents threaten to commit suicide.
(2) Threats of suicide should not be ignored.
(3) If he does not have a specific plan, then he is not serious.
(4) No intervention is required because he has made these threats in the past.

2 A 14-year-old who attempted suicide by overdosing on her mother's prescription Valium has just been admitted to the Emergency Department for treatment. In planning your care for this client, you would anticipate administering which of the following antidotes?

(1) Romazicon
(2) Narcan
(3) Digibind
(4) Oxygen

3 The parent of a 2-year-old child asks you what precautionary measures can be taken at home to help prevent accidental poisonings. You know that the parent requires further instructions when he makes which of the following comments?

(1) "I will have the poison control center phone number available at every phone."
(2) "I will lock up all medications, household cleaners, and other potentially poisonous substances."
(3) "I will check for poisonous houseplants and remove them from the home or place them out of my child's reach."
(4) "I will have syrup of ipecac available at home and administer it to my child if he swallows any type of poison."

4 **You are to administer activated charcoal to a child who has consumed numerous unidentified pills. Because the child has a decreased level of consciousness, your most appropriate action to administer the charcoal would be which of the following?**

(1) Administer the charcoal orally as long as the child has a gag reflex.
(2) Do not administer the charcoal because the child has a decreased level of consciousness.
(3) Insert a nasogastric tube and administer the activated charcoal as ordered.
(4) Question the order for activated charcoal until the pills have been identified.

5 **The parents of a small child report that he stiffens when being held and does not smile or make eye contact with them. Based on this initial information, what disorder might you suspect?**

(1) Autism
(2) Attention deficit hyperactivity disorder
(3) Mental retardation
(4) Down syndrome

6 **When performing a health screening on a 9-year-old male with mental retardation, you note that his weight is in the 98th percentile. When questioning the child and mother on his nutrition and exercise habits, the mother states that she does not allow her son to run and play because she is afraid he will be injured. Your teaching plan for the child and mother will be based on the fact that children with mental retardation:**

(1) Require a strict nutritional plan because they will not benefit from physical activities in the management of weight.
(2) Are unable to engage in exercise or play activities because of their lack of coordination.
(3) Have the same need for exercise and play as other children and it is beneficial to their health.
(4) Do not enjoy engaging in physical activities or participating in sports activities.

7 **The parents of a 7-year-old child with attention deficit hyperactivity disorder are appropriately utilizing a behavior modification plan when they implemented which of the following methods in order to encourage completion of tasks such as homework?**

(1) Punish him by taking away outside play privileges.
(2) Utilize a reward system for accomplishments.
(3) Allow him to choose what tasks he wants to complete.
(4) Increase his medication when he does not complete his tasks.

8 **When offering support to the family of a 5-month-old infant who died from sudden infant death syndrome (SIDS), it is important to recognize that the infant's older sibling may experience:**

(1) Lack of concern about where the infant is.
(2) Acceptance of the infant's death.
(3) Guilt that he or she may have caused the infant's death.
(4) An understanding that the infant is dead.

9 **A mother brings her 6-year-old daughter to the health clinic with concerns that the child is exhibiting unusual behaviors such as bedwetting and thumbsucking. In addition, her grades have dropped dramatically, and she is now taking baths up to six times a day. She has also been treated for a urinary tract infection numerous times over the past few months. Based on this initial information, you might suspect which of the following?**

(1) The child is experiencing school phobia.
(2) The child is trying to gain her mother's attention.
(3) The child needs psychological counseling.
(4) The child may be a victim of sexual abuse.

10 **In caring for an adolescent with suspected narcotic overdose, the nurse would monitor the adolescent for:**

(1) Constricted pupils and respiratory depression.
(2) Euphoria.
(3) Drowsiness.
(4) Aggressive behavior.

See page 397 for Answers and Rationales.

Answers and Rationales

Pretest

1 **Answer: 3** ***Rationale:*** Parental loss is a risk factor associated with suicide. A decline in grades is a symptom exhibited before her first suicide attempt, and without further investigation, there is no indication that there is a dysfunctional relationship between her and the mother or stepfather. Indicating remorse for the action is a positive step towards recovering.
Cognitive Level: Application
Nursing Process: Analysis; ***Test Plan:*** PSYC

2 **Answer: 3** ***Rationale:*** Homosexual adolescents are at an extremely higher risk of suicide that other adolescents their age, especially if the family does not offer support. Sleeping late on weekends and skipping meals without concern for nutrition is normal for adolescents, as is having a small group of close friends.
Cognitive Level: Analysis
Nursing Process: Assessment; ***Test Plan:*** PSYC

3 **Answer: 1** ***Rationale:*** Options 2, 3, and 4 are appropriate ongoing activities to promote substance abuse prevention; however, peer-led programs have proven to be the most successful when teaching children about the hazards of substance and tobacco use and abuse.
Cognitive Level: Application
Nursing Process: Implementation; ***Test Plan:*** HPM

4 **Answer: 2** ***Rationale:*** Option 1 is incorrect as ipecac is often given preceding the administration of activated charcoal. To reduce the risk of aspiration, activated charcoal should never be administered before syrup of ipecac (option 3), and there is no indication to insert a nasogastric tube. Administering the syrup of ipecac, waiting for the child to vomit, then administering the activated charcoal is the correct method.
Cognitive Level: Analysis
Nursing Process: Implementation; ***Test Plan:*** PHYS

5 **Answer: 1** ***Rationale:*** Corrosive agents cause the signs and symptoms listed. Indications of aspirin overdose are nausea, vomiting, diaphoresis, and seizures. Hydrocarbons cause nausea, vomiting, cyanosis, and altered sensorium, and acetaminophen causes nausea, vomiting, diaphoresis, and later, jaundice.
Cognitive Level: Analysis
Nursing Process: Assessment; ***Test Plan:*** PHYS

6 **Answer: 3** ***Rationale:*** 15 mL of syrup of ipecac can be repeated once for a 4-year-old child who has not vomited after 20 minutes. All children with accidental poisonings should be taken to the Emergency Department for evaluation and treatment even if vomiting has occurred.
Cognitive Level: Analysis
Nursing Process: Implementation; ***Test Plan:*** PHYS

7 **Answer: 1** ***Rationale:*** Children with mental retardation have the same need for socialization as others and should be encouraged to participate in clubs and activities with children of the same *developmental age*. There is no need to encourage participation only in clubs exclusive to children with cognitive impairment; this would limit the child's social interaction.
Cognitive Level: Application
Nursing Process: Implementation; ***Test Plan:*** HPM

8 **Answer: 1** ***Rationale:*** Ritalin is a central nervous system (CNS) stimulant, and if taken in the late evening, may cause insomnia. The medication should not be discontinued unless ordered by a physician, nor should the dosages be adjusted without the physician's instructions.
Cognitive Level: Application
Nursing Process: Implementation; ***Test Plan:*** PHYS

9 **Answer: 2** ***Rationale:*** Parents need the opportunity to hold their infant and to say goodbye in private for as long as they need. A peaceful, quiet, supportive environment should be provided. Options 1, 3, and 4 are incorrect as they do not demonstrate compassionate care for parents who have just experienced the death of a child.
Cognitive Level: Application
Nursing Process: Implementation; ***Test Plan:*** PSYC

10 **Answer: 2** ***Rationale:*** It is important to establish a thorough history and a detail of the incident before making assumptions of abuse. The child is safe from harm in the Emergency Department, allowing time to adequately assess the situation. You should not make premature assumptions (option 1), and if abuse is suspected, you should not inform the parent (options 3 and 4).
Cognitive Level: Analysis
Nursing Process: Assessment; ***Test Plan:*** PSYC

Posttest

1 **Answer: 2** ***Rationale:*** Threats of suicide should never be ignored. It is not normal for anyone to threaten to commit suicide, and the lack of a specific plan does not indicate the adolescent is not seriously contemplating suicide.
Cognitive Level: Analysis
Nursing Process: Implementation; ***Test Plan:*** PSYC

2 **Answer: 1** ***Rationale:*** Romazicon is the antidote for Valium. Narcan is the antagonist for opioids, Digibind is given for lanoxin overdose, and oxygen is administered for carbon monoxide poisoning.
Cognitive Level: Application
Nursing Process: Planning; ***Test Plan:*** PHYS

3 **Answer: 4** ***Rationale:*** Options 1, 2, and 3 are all appropriate responses. Syrup of ipecac should only be administered for specific types of poisoning because its use is contraindicated for corrosive agents, hydrocarbons, and some oral medications. Therefore, the parent must call the Poison Control Center or 911 and receive instructions to administer the syrup of ipecac.
Cognitive Level: Application
Nursing Process: Evaluation; ***Test Plan:*** SECE

4 **Answer: 3** ***Rationale:*** Activated charcoal is administered to decrease the systemic absorption of toxic agents and must be administered in a timely manner. Because of the risk for aspiration, oral solutions and medications should never be administered to those experiencing a decreased level of consciousness. Because the child has a decreased level of consciousness, inserting a nasogastric tube is the appropriate action to decrease the risk of vomiting and aspiration, which is a potential complication.
Cognitive Level: Analysis
Nursing Process: Implementation; ***Test Plan:*** PHYS

5 **Answer: 1** ***Rationale:*** Although a thorough evaluation and assessment is necessary to diagnose autism, it can be suspected based on the information provided. These symptoms are not normally associated with attention deficit hyperactivity disorder, mental retardation, or Down syndrome.
Cognitive Level: Analysis
Nursing Process: Assessment; ***Test Plan:*** PSYC

6 **Answer: 3** ***Rationale:*** Children with mental retardation need to exercise and play just as any other child does. Exercise and play is beneficial to the cardiovascular system, coordination, and weight control, as well as the promotion of socialization. Emphasize that activities should be appropriate to the child's physical and developmental maturity.
Cognitive Level: Application
Nursing Process: Assessment; ***Test Plan:*** HPM

7 **Answer: 2** ***Rationale:*** Rewarding positive behavior is generally an effective means of encouraging the completion of tasks. Punishment is usually reserved for undesirable behaviors (negative reinforcement), and the child needs to participate in play and exercise activities. The child should be involved in some decision-making processes but should not be allowed to choose the tasks he desires to complete. No adjustment in medications should be made without the instructions from the primary care provider.
Cognitive Level: Analysis
Nursing Process: Evaluation; ***Test Plan:*** PSYC

8 **Answer: 3** ***Rationale:*** It is not uncommon for older siblings to have bad thoughts or wishes toward a new sibling. They must be assured that their thoughts did not cause the infant's death. The understanding and acceptance of death depends on the child's developmental age. They will express feelings of concern about where the infant is, the loss of the infant, and the expression of parental grief.
Cognitive Level: Analysis
Nursing Process: Analysis; ***Test Plan:*** PSYC

9 **Answer: 4** ***Rationale:*** Regressive behavior such as thumb-sucking and bedwetting, in addition to a sudden decline in school performance, excessive bathing, nightmares, and recurrent urinary tract infections are signs of sexual abuse and must be investigated immediately. There is no indication of school phobia, nor that she lacks attention from her mother. The child may need psychological counseling, especially if sexual abuse is determined, but initially the abuse must be identified and appropriate interventions taken.
Cognitive Level: Analysis
Nursing Process: Assessment; ***Test Plan:*** PSYC

10 **Answer: 1** ***Rationale:*** Side effects of narcotic ingestion are constricted pupils and respiratory depression. Euphoria is a symptom of cocaine and inhalant abuse; drowsiness is a side effect of central nervous system depressants; aggressive behavior is a side effect of central nervous system stimulants.
Cognitive Level: Analysis
Nursing Process: Assessment; ***Test Plan:*** PHYS

References

Ball, J. & Bindler, R. (1999). *Pediatric nursing: Caring for children* (2nd ed). Stamford, CT: Appleton & Lange, pp. 414–416, 652–657, 958–1000.

Wong, D., Hockenberry-Eaton, M., Wilson, D., Winkelstein, M., Ahmann, E., & DiVito-Thomas, P. (1999). *Whaley and Wong's nursing care of infants and children* (6th ed.). St. Louis: Mosby, pp. 622–658, 740–770, 870–875, 975–995, 1073–1091.

Web sites

American Academy of Pediatrics: The Injury Prevention Program at www.aap.org

American Association on Mental Retardation at www.aamr.org

American SIDS Institute at www.sids.org

Autism Society of America at www.autism-society.org

Children and Adults with Attention-deficit Hyperactivity Disorder (CHADD) at www.chadd.org

National Attention Deficit Disorder at www.add.org

National Committee to Prevent Child Abuse (NCPCA) at www.childabuse.org

Parents Anonymous at www.parentsanonymous.org

Appendix

➤ Practice to Pass Suggested Answers

Chapter 1

Page 11: *Solution*—With normal motor development, a 10-month-old infant can:
- Stand while holding onto furniture.
- Sit down by falling down.
- Cruise around furniture.
- Crawl.
- Use pincer grasp.
- Say dada and mama.
- Develop object permanence.

Page 13: *Solution*—Safety precautions to be discussed will include:
- Continue proper use of car seat in automobile.
- Supervision of indoor and outdoor play activities.
- Risk for accidental poisonings: sources and use of syrup of ipecac.
- Avoid food such as cherries, hard candy, small pieces of hot dogs that can be aspirated by the young child.
- Water safety.
- Risks for burns, falls, and suffocation.

Page 14: *Solution*—The child will need to have received:
- Diptheria, tetanus, and acellular pertussis (DtaP) #5
- Inactivated poliovirus vaccine (IPV) #4
- Measles, mumps, and rubella (MMR) #2
- Hepatitis A—in selected areas (4 to 18 years)

Page 16: *Solution*—The nurse will want to discuss with the parents these facts:

- Temper tantrums during toddlerhood are common. Children may display outbursts of negative behaviors such as screaming, yelling, crying.
- Toddlers will have mood swings; fluctuate between pleasant temperament and displays of being difficult.
- Toddlers are striving to become more independent at this age, not as dependant on the parent(s). They seek autonomy within the environment.
- Common displays of negativism are observed in this age group.

Page 21: *Solution*—Activities to decrease anxiety include:
- Allow child to manipulate or play with equipment.
- Provide simple explanations: use visual aids such as dolls, pictures.
- Allow parent to be present with child.
- Use EMLA with IV starts and venipunctures.
- Avoid medical terminology.
- Use distraction during procedure.
- Use therapeutic play to facilitate expression of fear and feelings.
- Allow child choices that are realistic.
- Tell child it's OK to cry as long as he/she remains still.

Page 22: *Solution*—The nurse will be aware that a 15-year-old:
- Has a good understanding of illness related to death.
- Views death as irreversible.
- Perceives death as something that happens to old people, not "me."
- Common reactions: feelings of sadness, loneliness.

Chapter 2

Page 30: *Solution*—The nurse should have the environment at a comfortable temperature and free of distractions. Sitting at eye level with the informant will put the individual at ease. Demonstrate a nonjudgmental attitude. The nurse should explain simply and directly the reasons for needing particular information, directing questions to the child as appropriate based on age and developmental level.

Page 33: *Solution*—Some questions the nurse might ask include asking about the family's identification with a particular religious/ethnic group and what special religious or cultural traditions are practiced in the home—food choices and preparation for example. Other questions might include asking about languages spoken in the home or if there are any cultural or religious healers the family relies on at times of illness.

Page 40: *Solution*—To ensure an adequate examination of a toddler, the nurse should first allow the child to become familiar with the nurse's presence. In addition, allow the child to touch or hold equipment. The nurse should approach the child by first examining a doll or stuffed animal the child might have. Tell, rather than ask, the child what needs to be done and have the child participate if possible, lift arms for example. The child may sit on the parent's lap for much of the exam if that feels reassuring to the child.

Page 49: *Solution*—A 7-year-old who is otherwise healthy and has not had a recent hemoglobin or hematocrit level should be screened. If the child lives in a high-risk environment, a lead-level test would be appropriate. A family history of elevated cholesterol or triglycerides in a parent may indicate a desirability of checking those levels in a child to get baseline levels.

Page 52: *Solution*—The Denver II is used to assess a child's motor and social development. It is not a test of intelligence nor does it predict future academic ability. It is also not intended to diagnose specific developmental problems. The Denver II is part of a routine screening done on many children.

Chapter 3

Page 63: *Solution*—After the health care provider has explained the procedure to the parents, the nurse should teach the parents about:

a. Admission procedures to the day-surgery area
b. Any necessary lab tests ordered prior to anesthesia
c. Preoperative medications for sedation (if prescribed)
d. What will happen in the period before transport to the operating room
e. What will happen when the child and family are reunited following the procedure in the post anesthesia care area.

The child, if age and developmental level permit, should be taught similar developmentally appropriate content to encourage cooperative behavior.

Postoperative teaching should include information about:

a. How to relieve pain (use of acetaminophen or other analgesic as prescribed)
b. How to administer medications prescribed (oral analgesics and ear drops are frequently prescribed)
c. How to prevent water from entering the child's ear during bathing or swimming activities; often ear plugs are recommended if the healthcare provider cautions against activity that might allow water to enter the ear and the tube

The child's caregivers should be taught to promptly report signs and symptoms of ear infection, such as fever and purulent ear drainage to the health care provider. They should be taught that tubes commonly extrude and fall out, and they should notify the physician if they note a tube visible in the ear canal. Information should be provided about how to resume the child's diet and activity, and when to see the health care provider for postoperative follow-up appointments.

Page 64: *Solution*—The child is no longer considered contagious after receiving antibiotic therapy for 24 hours. The nurse will need to emphasize that the child will continue the antibacterial eye drops or ointment as prescribed, usually 7 to 10 days.

Page 66: *Solution*—The nurse can perform the cover-uncover test and the corneal light reflex test as follows:

1. Cover-uncover test: Ask the client to fix his or her gaze straight ahead, focusing on a distant object. Cover one eye with an opaque card. As the eye is covered, observe the uncovered eye for movement. Remove the card while observing the eye just uncovered for movement. This is a screening test for deviation in eye alignment and eye muscle weakness. Eye muscle weakness is seen as movement of the "lazy eye" when it attempts to refocus during the cover test.
2. Corneal light reflex test (Hirschberg test): This test is done to assess parallel symmetry of the eyes. The examiner shines a penlight directly onto the corneas of both eyes, holding the penlight about 12 inches away from the client's nasal bridge while the client focuses on a distant object. The examiner should see the light reflected at the same spot in both eyes. An asymmetric light reflex indicates a deviation in the alignment of the client's eyes.

Page 68: *Solution*—Because symptoms of pain and fever usually subside within 24 to 48 hours of antibiotic therapy, the child or family may have stopped the medication because the child experienced relief of symptoms. The nurse must research what antibiotic was prescribed to the child six days ago. If a 10-day course of antibiotic was prescribed, the antibiotic therapy is not finished, and the health care provider must be consulted because the infection is not eradicated until all of the prescribed medication is taken. If it is discovered that the antibiotics were not completed, it is important that the nurse reteach medication administration, including appropriate administration and side effects. The nurse should stress the need to complete the full course of antibiotics even though the child may feel better after a short period of time.

The nurse should assess the child's vital signs, including temperature, and assess the child's pharynx using a tongue blade and light source. The nurse could also assess the child's ears through otoscopic examination. The nurse should refer the child to the health care provider and supply all data collected in the nursing assessment.

Page 70: *Solution*—Humidify the air in the home, especially in the child's room during the night and during the winter. Discourage the child from picking at or forcefully blowing the nose. Encourage the child to blow the nose gently and release sneezes through the mouth. Encourage keeping the external nasal septum soft and moist by applying a layer of petroleum jelly twice per day.

Chapter 4

Page 79: *Solution*—A bronchoscopy is performed under general anesthesia. The child must be kept NPO until swallow and gag reflexes have returned. Reassure the mother that vital signs and respiratory effort are normal. Advise the mother that the child should be fully awake before being fed to guard against vomiting and aspiration. Encourage her to hold and cuddle the child. Listen to her concerns; encourage and answer all questions.

Page 84: *Solution*—The treatment of pulmonary infection in children with cystic fibrosis is a priority. Pathogens are unusually difficult to clear and the risk of chronic colonization with resistant organisms increases if antibiotic therapy is not aggressive. Although life expectancy for children with cystic fibrosis has increased, pulmonary infections continue to pose the greatest threat to survival. In this situation, the socialization needs of a child with a chronic illness are also important. The nurse could consider having the child attend the puppet show while his antibiotics are being administered via infusion pump. If there is sufficient time, perhaps the medication could be completed before the activity. The nurse could also ascertain the duration for the activity.

Page 87: *Solution*—BPD is a chronic pulmonary disease that primarily affects premature infants who received prolonged mechanical ventilation and oxygen therapy at birth. Full-term infants may be affected also. Respiratory distress or failure, requiring oxygen and ventilation for a minimum of 3 days, can contribute to development of BPD.

Page 92: *Solution*—Epiglottitis is a medical emergency. Laryngospasm, increased edema, and complete airway obstruction can occur rapidly if there is any manipulation or irritation of the mouth and throat. Airway obstruction can also occur as a result of anxiety and crying. For these reasons, a child with epiglottitis is kept as calm and quiet as possible. Parental presence reassures the child and decreases distress. The mother of this child should be encouraged to remain with her child and you can offer to telephone the husband. If there is a portable telephone available, it can be brought to the mother.

Page 97: *Solution*—Peanut butter is a common food to be aspirated by young children. The thick consistency easily occludes a child's airway and is difficult to remove. This dad needs safety information regarding appropriate snack foods and the danger of aspiration in a small child. Peanut butter, if offered, must be spread in a thin layer on a cracker and never fed from a spoon. Counsel this dad that aspiration is the leading cause of death in small children.

Chapter 5

Page 111: *Solution*—

1. The child should increase activity gradually.
2. Observe for signs of wound infection, fever, flu-like symptoms, an increased respiratory rate, and dyspnea.
3. The child may return to school in about 3 weeks.
4. The child should be monitored for signs of infective endocarditis (sudden onset of high fever and heart failure).

Page 112: *Solution*—

1. Following cardiac catheterization, it is important to limit activity for 24 hours to avoid disturbing the insertion site.
2. The child is instructed on intake of fluids. Maintaining hydration is important because the contrast medium used during the procedure has a diuretic affect.
3. The parents are instructed to monitor for temperature elevation, which is an early sign of infection.

Page 116: *Solution*—Transposition of great vessels is a condition whereby the two main arteries leaving the heart are reversed. The aorta, which is supposed to leave the left ventricle and take oxygenated blood to the body, actually leaves the right ventricle and directs blood back to the body without receiving oxygenation. The pulmonary artery, which is supposed to leave the right ventricle and take blood to the lungs, actually leaves the left ventricle and directs blood back to the lungs for reoxygenation. In effect, there are two closed systems. Families need to understand that the infant will need palliative surgery in order to survive. A medication called Prostaglandin 1 will be given to maintain an open ductus arteriosus that allows for mixing of the blood and provides a small amount of oxygen to the rest of the body.

Page 119: *Solution*—Rheumatic fever is an inflammation of collagen tissue. The cardiac muscle has much of this connective tissue within it. Increased activity can aggravate the inflammation and ultimately lead to damaged heart valves. If there is no evidence of cardiac involvement, activity can resume as normal; however, caution needs to be taken at the first sign of cardiac pathology.

Page 120: *Solution*—The child needs to be seen by a physician to identify the exact cause. Kawasaki's disease is one possibility. Kawasaki's is not communicated person to person, so isolation techniques are not needed. Laboratory data will help rule out a staphylococcal infection or other similar infections. Cardiac complications are serious complications of this condition, and hospitalization is usually required during the acute period.

Chapter 6

Page 133: *Solution*—One-third of children with cerebral palsy also have some degree of mental retardation and 50 percent have seizures. Many also have mobility challenges, feeding problems, and vision, hearing, and developmental delays. It is obvious that to address this requires a multidisciplinary team approach. The parent must be the core of this team since a high degree of coordination must take place. For optimal development to be fostered, all the therapy regimens must be maintained at home and supported by the family. Family-centered care recognizes the pivotal role the family plays in the health of children.

Page 137: *Solution*—There are clear differences in what a parent would be instructed to watch for as signs of shunt malfunction based on the physical development of the child. For an infant whose cranial suture lines have not fused and fontanels are still open, assess for increased head circumference, high-pitched cry, bulging fontanel, irritability when awake, and seizures. Toddlers and older children usually present with vomiting, irritability, and headache. As the condition persists, the child may exhibit setting-sun eyes, seizures, papilledema, decreased level of consciousness, and change in vital signs (increased blood pressure and widening pulse pressure). Older children may have difficulty with balance or coordination. All children can present with lethargy and Cheyne-Stokes respiratory pattern.

Page 139: *Solution*—Client education should focus on:

1. Parental understanding of what a seizure is and what triggers it for their child.
2. The basic "first aid" or safety measures to take when their child has a seizure.
3. The names of medications, a medication schedule, and potential side effect of the medications. Instructions specific to the administration of the medication should be included, such as Dilantin chewable tablets should not be swallowed whole.
4. Who to call with questions. Referrals to support organizations allow the parents to talk to someone about their feelings and emotions.
5. The need to inform people (teachers, daycare workers, baby-sitters, etc.) who will have frequent contact with their child on the nature of the disease as well first aid measures.

These are just a few of the possible approaches to ensure that the parents have a realistic understanding of the health problem, and the knowledge, skills, and adequate resources to cope to deal with seizures.

Page 149: *Solution*—The major cause of injuries in young children is falls—from changing tables, beds, sofas, etc. Initially a young infant lacks the ability to turn over. A caregiver who is not alert to the possibility of the child doing this places the child at risk for a fall. Young children are curious and want to explore their environment. If gates are not put up, they are at risk to fall down stairs. Child abuse or shaken baby syndrome is a possible cause of head injury in infants under one year of age. The brain is highly vascular and the dura is more likely to shear from shaking. Adolescents and older children often think of themselves as invincible and disregard both safety devices, such as use of seatbelts and bike helmets, and speed limits. Many head injuries result from motor vehicle accidents (MVAs) and bicycle, skateboard, snowboard, and skiing accidents, especially where the child did not wear a protective helmet. Teenagers may also be injured in alcohol- or drug-related MVAs and sports injuries.

Page 152: *Solution*—Glasgow scores are indicated in square brackets, [ ]. A child with a minor head injury might present with transient confusion [4] but no loss of consciousness, spontaneous opening of the eyes [4], and will obey a command [6]. This child has a high score indicating good prognosis.

A child with a major head injury might present with loss of consciousness, some moaning but not oriented to time, person, and place [2], eyes open to pain [2], and the only motor response is to painful stimulation [4]. This child's score is much lower, reflecting the severity of symptoms. The prognosis would be less positive for this child.

Chapter 7

Page 162: *Solution*—

1. The renal system is responsible for the formation and excretion of urine. If this function were impaired, the client may present with decreased urinary output (oliguria) or absent urinary output (anuria).
2. The renal system regulates fluid and electrolyte balance within the body. If this function were impaired, the client may present with signs and symptoms edema, dehydration, hyper-/hypokalemia, hyper-/hyponatremia, or hyper/hypocalcemia. Elevated blood pressure may also be present.
3. The renal system regulates acid–base balance within the body. If this function were impaired, the client may present with signs and symptoms of metabolic acidosis or alkalosis.
4. The renal system regulates blood pressure. If this function were impaired, the client may present with hypertension or hypotension.
5. The renal system stimulates the production of red blood cells in bone marrow. If this function were impaired, the client may present with signs and symptoms of anemia.
6. The renal system regulates calcium metabolism in the body. If this function were impaired, the client may present with signs and symptoms of bone disorders.

Page 167: *Solution*—Infants: Clean-catch urine specimens are obtained with the application of a urine collection bag. The infant cannot voluntarily void and thus depends on a nurse or parent to apply and remove the collection device.

Toddlers: Clean-catch urine specimens are obtained with the application of a urine collection bag. The toddler cannot voluntarily void and depends on a nurse or parent to apply and remove the collection device.

School-age children: School-age children are able to void voluntarily. Instructions regarding correct specimen collection technique must be given to the parent if they are assisting in the collection process. The school-age child needs assistance with specimen collection.

Adolescents: Adolescents may collect their own specimens after instruction in correct specimen collection technique. Adolescents require privacy and may feel uncomfortable with this procedure.

Page 172: *Solution*—Discharge instructions should include demonstration and return demonstration of ostomy care and catheter care if applicable. Instructions should include monitoring for changes in urinary output, signs and symptoms of infection, and dehydration. If an appliance is present, instructions regarding skin care and odor management are necessary. Instructions are also provided in writing. A contact number for help should be provided. Community resources are also made available at the time of discharge.

Page 174: *Solution*—Nursing measures specific to caring for children with acute glomerulonephritis include prevention measures, (prompt and thorough treatment of all group A beta-hemolytic streptococcal infections) and management of hypertension (medication administration, dietary salt restrictions, frequent blood pressure monitoring). Nursing measures specific to caring for children with nephrotic syndrome include parent education regarding signs and symptoms, treatment regimes, disease chronicity, and behavioral changes in the child that may manifest due to distorted body image secondary to massive edema and weight gain. How do they differ? Acute glomerulonephritis can be prevented; nephrotic syndrome cannot. Client education regarding treatment of strep infections can prevent acute glomerulonephritis; client education cannot prevent nephrotic syndrome. Distortions in body image do not usually occur with acute glomerulonephritis. Acute glomerulonephritis is not chronic in nature; coping skills and treatment regimes are necessary long-term for clients with nephrotic syndrome.

Page 180: *Solution*—The three types of renal replacement therapy are hemodialysis, peritoneal dialysis, and kidney transplantation.

- Hemodialysis: an advantage is better clearance of toxins from the bloodstream, while a disadvantage is disruption of family with travel to dialysis center three times a week or increased risk for infection related to needed vascular access.
- Peritoneal dialysis: an advantage is it that is continuous and easy to learn to do at home; a disadvantage is that the client is at risk for peritonitis or that clearance of toxins is not as effective as with hemodialysis.
- Renal transplantation: an advantage is that this regime provides for optimal return to homeostasis and provides for optimal growth and development of the child; a disadvantage is that organ procurement can be difficult or that immunosuppression can result from medications used to prevent organ rejection.

Chapter 8

Page 194: *Solution*—The nurse should explain that some of the signs and symptoms of congenital hypothyroidism will not be obvious at birth. If the screening is not done immediately, and the baby has the disease, he/she could suffer from irreversible brain damage. Other complications include lethargy, decreased peristalsis, scaly skin, poor feeding, thick tongue, and anorexia. The mother needs to be aware that state law mandates all infants be tested. If the mother continues to refuse the testing, the nurse should report the situation to the child's pediatrician or to the birth hospital for follow-up.

Page 195: *Solution*—Since adolescents like to possess control over their bodies and their life situations, it is imperative that the teenager is involved in this decision. As a school nurse, you could offer an opportunity for rest periods during study hall and recreational time at school. The nurse might want to seek a physician's release from physical education class. Other options might include a half-day school schedule or pursuing a GED diploma.

Page 198: *Solution*—Because children with PKU lack the pigment melanin, their skin is fair-colored and extremely sensitive. These children should actually avoid the sunlight, but when exposed, they should have a sunscreen with SPF 60 or higher for protection.

Page 206: *Solution*—By drawing up the regular (clear) insulin first, the liklihood of contamination of the regular insulin is reduced, resulting in less dose variance. That same regular insulin may be used alone at times for sudden high glucose levels. If it were contaminated with NPH, the rapid action of the regular insulin would be impaired.

Chapter 9

Page 228: *Solution*—The nursing care for the child with Legg-Calve-Perthes disease and for the adolescent with slipped capitol femoral epiphysis is very similar. Both clients should be on bedrest until the hip is surgically repaired or medical management is begun. With both clients, the nurse will assess neurovascular status of the lower extremities. Both clients will need pain assessments and appropriate pain management. Both clients will require age-appropriate diversional activities, as both will not feel ill and will have plenty of energy. The difference in care lies in client and family teaching, as the disease process is different and the treatment may be different. If a child with Legg-Calve-Perthes disease is treated medically with a containment device, the discharge teaching must include information about the care of and wearing of the device and reinforcing compliance with wearing the device for the long length of treatment. Discharge teaching for the child with either condition who had surgical containment or repair will include activity restrictions according to the surgeon, and need for followup care.

Page 230: *Solution*—

- Respiratory care is a priority for a postop client following a spinal fusion. Logrolling by two people must be done every 2 hours to mobilize respiratory secretions. This client must also engage in respiratory exercises such as deep-breathing, coughing, and incentive spirometry every 2 hours. The nurse carefully assesses respiratory status.
- A second priority for this postop client is pain management. Spinal surgery for scoliosis is very painful; pain assessments must be done frequently and pain medication is given frequently; PCA pain management is often used. The client's pain must be under control in order to participate in the needed respiratory care.
- Other priorities of care include assessing neurological function of the lower extremities every hour for the first 24 hours postop and then every 4 hours; maintaining a nasogastric tube for decompression, along with NPO status and frequent assessments of bowel sounds; and maintaining antiembolism stockings to prevent venous stasis.

Page 231: *Solution*—By the time a male client with Duchenne's muscular dystrophy reaches 15 years of age, his muscles are usually quite weak. The client is usually confined to a wheelchair, as the child is unable to walk independently. The cough reflex becomes weak and ineffective by this time and pneumonia develops easily. The main priority of care is centered on his respiratory status with administration of intravenous antibiotics, aggressive turning, coughing, and respiratory exercises. To maintain his level of muscle strength and use, physical therapy should become quickly involved, as short periods of bedrest can lead to further muscle wasting and weakness.

Page 236: *Solution*—Bryant's traction is used to treat developmental dysplasia of the hip and fracture of the femur in children less than 3 years of age and weighing less than 35 pounds. Bryant's traction is skin traction that involves having the hips at 90-degree flexion, with both legs straight up in the air, and the buttocks just off the bed. The care of this child includes neurovascular checks of the extremities. The nurse ensures that the weights on the traction are the ordered weight and hang freely and safely. The bandages on the legs that hold the skin traction in place need to be checked to ensure they are not too loose or too tight. Good skin care must be maintained as well as assessments of elimination patterns. A normally energetic and busy toddler will not take to bedrest lightly, and appropriate diversional activities must be employed quickly and often.

Page 237: *Solution*—Immediately following cast application, the nurse must carefully assess neurovascular status of the involved extremity and compare it with the uninvolved extremity. Circulation to the affected extremity must be checked every 15 minutes for the first hour, hourly for 24 hours, and every 4 hours after that. Assess for color, warmth, presence of distal pulses, and sensations of numbness and tingling. Assess for pain. If the nurse's assessment revealed signs of impaired neurovascular function (pallor, pulselessness, severe pain in the casted part of the extremity, tingling sensation, severe swelling not relieved by elevation), the physician should be notified, as the constricting cast can lead to neurologic damage.

Chapter 10

Page 249: *Solution*—Some comfort measures the nurse could suggest include giving the child tepid baths followed by a gentle massage of nonaffected areas with nonperfumed lotion. Keeping the child in cotton garments with tags removed helps reduce itching. Put cotton mittens or socks on the child's hands to prevent scratching. Do not allow the child to get so warm that he or she begins to perspire.

Page 252: *Solution*—Lice and nits can survive on human hosts, so the environment must be deloused. All clothing the child has worn in the last week should be washed in hot water and dried in a hot dryer for at least 20 minutes. All bedding should be similarly washed and dried. Things that cannot be washed and dried (blankets or stuffed toys, for example) should be placed in plastic bags for about 2 weeks. Discard or soak all combs, brushes, and hair ornaments. Thoroughly vacuum all furniture, carpets, and floors. Check all members of the household for the presence of lice or nits.

Page 254: *Solution*—Scabies presents with intense pruritus, but impetigo is painless. Because scabies causes intense itching, the nurse can frequently see scratch marks that may almost obscure the small papules or vesicles at the end of a scabies mite burrow. Scabies is often found on particular body areas such as hands, feet, finger webs, or body creases. Impetigo typically presents on the face, arms, or legs.

Page 256: *Solution*—The nurse will ask about recent episodes of otitis media or sinusitis. It is also important to ask about any insect bites or scratches the child had in the recent past. The nurse will want to know when redness was first noticed and what treatment has been attempted at home. The nurse will get baseline vital signs. The site will be examined for the extent of redness, edema, and tenderness.

Page 258: *Solution*—A second-degree burn has bright pink or red skin that may have blisters. It may also appear moist if blisters have ruptured. The skin will blanch on pressure. The child will experience intense pain at the site.

Chapter 11

Page 269: *Solution*—The body in response to any antigen produces a nonspecific immunity. It is the earliest response and is therefore not specific to any one antigen. This response includes protective barriers such as interferon, inflammation, and phagocytosis. Once the body has responded to an antigen in a nonspecific way, the body produces specific immunity in the form of an antibody. These antibodies match with the antigen in a key/lock manner. The antibody is specific to the antigen and will not attack other antigens.

Page 269: *Solution*—The patient and family need explanations of each of the tests. The patient needs to know that a bone marrow aspiration is painful and that analgesics will be given. WBC and differential involves a needle stick and blood aspiration. Allergy testing may involve blood aspiration and/or skin pricks with various allergens.

Page 270: *Solution*—Referring to the most recent Recommended Childhood Immunization Schedule, United States, for the American Academy of Pediatrics will ensure current knowledge of immunization schedules. These standards change periodically and nurses must ensure they are practicing by the most current standards.

Page 274: *Solution*—The child and family may need to evaluate the home setting for potential allergens. Carpets, bedding, and other upholstery may need to be taken up and changed. If it is impossible to change the entire house, the family should begin these changes in the child's bedroom. Because the child spends long hours at night sleeping in the bedroom, this room plays an important role in the child's allergic reaction. Laundry and cleaning procedures may need adapted to allow for more frequent cleaning. The family will be taught to store out-of-season clothes out of the child's room. All clothing should be stored in drawers or closets and these devices should be kept closed to decrease dust collection. The bedroom should be used as a room for sleeping, so toys should be removed from the room as much as possible in an attempt to reduce dust-collecting items. In addition, stuffed toys should be limited as they hold dust. Fresh flowers should not be kept in the home as they will hold dust and molds. Pets may need to find a new home, kept outdoors, or restricted from the child's bedroom. If the pets are kept in the home, they need to be washed frequently to reduce dander. If the allergy is to foods, the family will learn to read ingredient lists before purchasing an item as it might contain the allergen.

Page 282: *Solution*—The first stage: The incubation period is the time period between exposure to the organism and the development of the first general symptoms. During this period, the organism is growing in numbers and in strength. It is not strong enough to cause disease symptoms at this time. Toward the end of this period, it may be communicable.

The second stage: The prodromal stage is when the organism has sufficient strength to cause generalized symptoms of illness. It is difficult to diagnose the organism but the patient is exhibiting symptoms. This is a communicable stage.

The third stage: This is the active stage. During this time, the specific symptoms of the disease are exhibited. It is possible to spread the disease through body fluids. The patient is communicable while there is an elevated temperature or secretion of body fluids.

The fourth stage: This is recovery stage. The infectious disease has abated and the body is rebuilding its stores. Immunity is diminished, and the patient is vulnerable to becoming ill if exposed.

Chapter 12

Page 293: *Solution*—This behavior would be very predictable given the life-threatening nature of this disease process. The family-centered goals would be that the parents will understand all tests and therapies and that they will be able to express their concerns freely. They would then continue to participate appropriately in the care of their child.

Page 297: *Solution*—This child is immunocompromised because of chemotherapy and is at risk for infection. His developmental tasks include increasing mental abilities and increasing independence. It would be appropriate to reason with this child and allow independence in the minimum of oral hygiene and perineal care.

Page 301: *Solution*—This tumor is intrarenal and is often accompanied by increased renin production with increasing blood pressure. The finding is expected.

Page 303: *Solution*—Encourage the parents to answer the child's questions honestly and simply. The parents should utilize their religious beliefs in the discussion with the child. The child will often have concerns about abandonment and separation. The parents should assure the child that he or she will not be alone. If the parents' religious beliefs involve an afterlife, the parents might refer to a relative who has gone before and is waiting for the child. Children of this age often view illness as a punishment and may feel that they have done something wrong. Assure the child that this is not the case. Preschool children still are preoperational and have magical thinking so they are less concerned with the scientific answer and are more concerned with feelings.

Page 304: *Solution*—It is not unusual for family members to be at different stages of bereavement. This puts tremendous strain on relationships. Parents need to understand there is no wrong way to grieve. As nurses, we must also recognize there is no schedule for grieving. Questions that the parents ask should be answered honestly and simply. When the father expresses anger at the nurses, it should not be taken personally but be recognized for what it is—a symptom of grief. A clergyperson can be offered, but the nurse should not abandon the parents to the clergy. Physical comfort can be offered by those who have developed a relationship with the parents, including medical personnel. Physical presence is important, and the nurse must be careful not to avoid contact because of personal discomfort. The nurse should listen attentively to the parents. Use the child's name when talking with the parents. Don't offer platitudes.

Chapter 13

Page 316: *Solution*—Your teaching includes feeding the infant in an upright position, feeding the infant slowly, and burping frequently. Also included in the discussion would be using an enlarged nipple, stimulating the suck by rubbing the nipple on the lower lip, and allowing the infant to rest after each swallow to allow for complete swallowing. You may also suggest using alternate feeding devices such as an elongated nipple or breast shield. Initial postoperative feeding instructions include refraining from the use of straws, pacifier, and spoons. No oral temperatures are taken in the immediate postoperative period.

Page 318: *Solution*—Ideally, you want to inform the client and family about preoperative and postoperative care. Therefore, you would inform the client and family that it is necessary to remain NPO prior to surgery and that feeding resumes within 4 to 6 hours postoperatively. Explain the purpose of intravenous therapy and strict I & O monitoring. Another important aspect of care to include is the necessity of the nasogastric tube to decompress the stomach. Briefly, you would discuss the pattern of resuming feeding with small frequent feedings of clear liquids, moving to full strength formula as tolerated.

Page 325: *Solution*—Routine pre- and postoperative care should be discussed, including remaining NPO, nasogastric tube placement, strict I & O and vital sign monitoring. However, the major topic for discussion is the placement of a temporary colostomy. Older children need to be emotionally prepared and educated, as will the caregiver of an infant. A colostomy represents a change in body image so misconceptions and concerns need to be addressed. Verbal explanation, drawings, and dolls can be effective methods for teaching this procedure.

Page 330: *Solution*—Signs and symptoms of appendicitis typically include generalized abdominal pain that gradually increases and localizes in the right lower quadrant at McBurney's point, nausea, vomiting, fever, chills, anorexia, diarrhea or acute constipation, and an elevated white blood cell (WBC) count.

Page 343: *Solution*—Evaluating the client's hydration status is the highest priority. You want to establish if there has been any weight loss, assess level of consciousness, blood pressure, pulse, skin turgor, mucous membranes, urine output, fontanels, skin color, and capillary refill. A complete and thorough history is also vital in determining the causative factor and will assist in the prescribed treatment plan.

Chapter 14

Page 358: *Solution*—Although the pediatrician previously recommended ibuprofen, it, like aspirin, can increase the risk of continued bleeding related to the effect on platelet function. Therefore, acetaminophen is now the OTC medication of choice for injuries and fever, unless otherwise indicated by the physician.

Page 360: *Solution*—Children affected with sickle cell anemia are usually asymptomatic until approximately 4–6 months of age because the sickling of red blood cells is inhibited by high levels of fetal hemoglobin. The level of fetal hemoglobin may mask the results of the hemoglobin electrophoresis test that is done on the infant's cord blood. After 6 months of age, the sickle-turbidity test (Sicledex) can be used for quick screening purposes. The results are then verified with hemoglobin electrophoresis.

Page 364: *Solution*—If you suspect a reaction of any type to a blood transfusion, no matter how mild, you should always first stop the transfusion. Keep the line open with normal saline and notify the physician.

Page 367: *Solution*—

- After verifying physician's orders and checking the medication, dose, and route, the nurse would also identify the patient.
- Subcutaneous heparin administration is an invasive procedure that can cause problems with bleeding.
- The subcutaneous sites should be rotated.
- The injection is given slowly and the site is not massaged after administration. Pressure is applied to the injection site for 10 to 15 minutes. The site is observed for at least 15 minutes after the injection.
- Protamine is an antidote for heparin and should be available.
- The nurse would monitor PTT and platelet count.

Page 371: *Solution*—The liquid iron preparations are to be given with a straw to minimize the possibility of staining the teeth. Giving the iron with a citrus juice can lessen the bad taste. Such juice will also help improve absorption. Constipation can be a problem with iron preparations. Instruct the family to encourage increased fluid intake and to have the child eat foods with a high fiber content such fruits and grains.

Chapter 15

Page 386: *Solution*—Maintaining a compassionate and caring attitude during this time of grief is essential. You should provide the parents with a quiet, supportive environment. The parents will be experiencing shock and overwhelming grief over the death of a child. The parents should be encouraged to hold the infant and to say goodbye. The infant should be cleaned and wrapped in a blanket. Support services should be available to offer grief counseling, and you should also be available to help the parents contact the family members, clergy or rabbi, and funeral home.

Page 388: *Solution*—Begin by asking the child non-threatening questions. Avoid questions such as "Did someone burn you with a cigarette?" Ask the child to tell you what the areas on her legs are and how they got there. More information can be obtained by asking the child open-ended questions. If abuse is suspected or reported, you must notify authorities immediately to protect the child from further injury.

Page 389: *Solution*—The symptoms of constricted pupils, respiratory depression, and difficulty arousing suggest the ingestion of an opiate such as morphine. Initially, Narcan, an opiate antagonist, may be ordered to reverse the symptoms of respiratory depression. Support the airway since there is a strong potential for respiratory arrest, and monitor vital signs. Upon stabilization, the adolescent should be referred for counseling and further evaluated for substance abuse.

Page 391: *Solution*—The adolescent needs intense therapy and counseling to help her to develop problem-solving skills. She may require in-patient psychiatric treatment; therefore, you should request the adolescent be evaluated by a counselor, therapist, or psychologist to determine the best method of intervention for her. While she is hospitalized, it is important to maintain a nonjudgmental attitude. Establishing a strong nurse–client relationship, which includes trust, with the adolescent may provide you with the opportunity to help her develop problem-solving skills. During the hospitalization, maintain all precautionary measures for the suicidal adolescent.

Page 393: *Solution*—Obtain a full detailed history of the current incident and compare with the past incident for similarities. The family made need counseling on the developmental issues and safety measures for the 3-year-old child or there may be signs parental neglect. It is recommended that social services make a home visit to evaluate the environment and safety measures being taken to prevent this type of incident from recurring.

➤ *Case Study Suggested Answers*

Chapter 1

1. The primary growth and development expectations for a 6-month-old include that the infant:
   - Doubles birth weight.
   - Grows 1 in. (2.5 cm) monthly for first 6 months.
   - Rolls from back to abdomen.
   - Holds own bottle.
   - Has taste preferences.
   - Erupts lateral incisors.
   - Begins to eat solid foods.
   - Begins to fear strangers.
2. Common behaviors at this age include that:
   - The child is able to discriminate between familiar and unfamiliar persons.
   - The child begins to fear strangers. Infants will show signs of fear and distress such as crying, clinging to the parent, pulling away from strangers.
3. Recommended immunizations at this age include:
   - Diptheria–tetanus–acellular pertussis (DTaP) #3.
   - Haemophilus influenzae type B (Hib) #3.
   - Inactivated poliovirus vaccine (IPV) #3 (6 to 18 months).
   - Heptavalent conjugant pneumococcal vaccine (PCV) #3.
   - Hepatitis B #3 (6 to 18 months).
4. Appropriate toys would include:
   - Soft balls.
   - Teething rings.
   - Large blocks.
   - Toys that child can manipulate.
5. Anticipatory guidance would include the following points:
   - Developmental milestones for the first year.
   - Safety: car seat facing the rear in the middle of the back seat of the car should be use for infants up to 20 lb (9 kg).
   - Infant becoming more mobile—never leave unattended on table, bed, bathtub, near stairs, balconies, or open windows.
   - Avoid bottles at bedtime—can contribute to dental caries.
   - Review injury prevention: sources of aspiration, poisonings, suffocation, falls, and accidental burns.
   - Introduction of solids into the diet: cereals, vegetables, fruits, and meats.

Chapter 2

1. Establishing the reason for the visit enables the nurse to focus questions in greater depth in specific parts of the review of systems, family history, and/or developmental areas. It also lets the nurse know that parts of the assessment might have to have greater depth of questioning.
2. The nurse should sit in a comfortable position on the same level as the parent. Keep the environment free of distractions and focus on the parent by listening attentively and asking questions that clarify data as needed. Explain what information is needed and why, as well as what will be done during the exam. Always ask if the parent has any questions or concerns as the history taking and the exam proceed.
3. The nurse should allow the child to "warm up" to the nurse. Direct questions and attention to the parent first. Ask questions of the child and display an interest in objects pertaining to the child. When proceeding with the examination, allow the child to help with undressing and to touch equipment first or to try it on the nurse. Explain to the child in understandable terms what will be done and what is expected. The nurse must not lie or deceive the child about anything that may be uncomfortable.
4. The nurse can ask the parent about what the child ate in the last 24 hours and if that was a typical day. The nurse can ask questions that ascertain how frequent representative foods from each section of the food pyramid are eaten as well as specific cultural or religious practices that determine the family's diet. The child's height and weight should be plotted on growth curves to see where they fall with respect to each other and to national percentiles. Assess the abdomen to see if it is gently rounded. Results from hemoglobin and hematocrit levels may indicate if the child is iron deficient.
5. It would be appropriate for the nurse to check hemoglobin and hematocrit if they have not been recently checked or if results are not available. Unless other familial or environmental risk factors or health problems are evident, further lab testing is not indicated.

Chapter 3

1. A complete health history should be taken, because the child will likely be undergoing general anesthesia. Information about the child's primary problem (chief complaint) should be obtained, as well as any concurrent illnesses. Information about current medications should be included. The history of the illness that preceded the need for surgery should be detailed. Past medical history, including allergies to medication, food, and environment should be elicited. The child's birth history and past medical and health history should be documented. A review of body systems should be completed. The nurse should inquire about familial and hereditary diseases and any difficulties with anesthesia (such as malignant hyperthermia) should be recorded. The health status of family members, including parents, siblings, and extended family should be explored during the health history interview.
2. One of the most important tests is evaluation of bleeding and clotting function. A complete blood count (CBC), which includes platelet count, may be ordered. Prothrombin time (PT) and partial thromboplastin time (PTT) are

commonly ordered lab tests. The child's blood chemistry may also be analyzed prior to anesthesia and the tonsillectomy.

3. After the surgical procedure is explained by the health care provider, the nurse should reinforce the teaching about the procedure. The nurse should explain events related to the operation, such as admission procedures and preoperative lab procedures. Teaching should be provided about preoperative medications for sedation (if prescribed), what will happen in the period before transport to the operating room, and what will happen when the child and family are reunited following the procedure in the post anesthesia care area.
4. The child, if age and developmental level permit, should be taught similar, developmentally appropriate content to encourage cooperative behavior. Special attention should be given to explaining the sight, sounds, smells, touches, and tastes that the child will experience in the operating room and when the child wakes up from anesthesia. A tour of the day surgery area, including operating room and post-anesthesia care areas should be provided.
5. A complete physical assessment is indicated for the child undergoing surgery. The nurse should make certain the child shows no current symptoms of illness. A child of this age should have the oral cavity checked for any loose teeth.

Chapter 4

1. Peak expiratory flow is a pulmonary function test that measures the amount of air that can be exhaled forcibly. It monitors asthma and acts as a signal of an asthma episode. To use the peak flow meter, move the pointer to zero, take a deep breath and blow out hard and fast into the meter. Repeat three times and record the highest value. Peak flow should be done every day and values below a child's "personal best" indicate that an acute episode may be imminent.
2. Exercise is recommended for children with asthma to enhance self-esteem and encourage endurance. Physical education activities that do not require prolonged endurance are usually not a problem for children with asthma. Exercise-induced bronchospasm can be prevented by prophylactic treatment with inhaled cromolyn sodium before strenuous exertion.
3. Keep records of peak flow readings to establish a "personal best." A reading that is 50 to 80 percent below personal best is a caution. Other subtle signs may be increased nonproductive cough and episodes of shortness of breath.
4. A spacer deposits medication deeper into the airways and avoids large droplets of steroids on the oral mucosa, thereby minimizing the risk of oral yeast infections. A spacer is also useful for parents of infants and small children who are unable to manipulate the MDI. The spacer prevents the loss of medication.
5. The overall goal of asthma education is to prevent asthmatic episodes, improve respiratory capacity, and facilitate optimal psychologic and social development of the child and family.

Chapter 5

1. The nurse needs to assess parents' level of understanding of the condition. Second, the nurse needs to know how they cope in times of crisis and should help the parents to identify their coping strategies. Third, the family needs to have an emergency plan to respond to an acute cyanotic spell. The family needs to be knowledgeable about the medications that are ordered and be able to administer the medications effectively.
2. Assess for increasing cyanosis and note the activity that precipitated it, irritability (which may be a sign of hunger, pain, or air hunger) and fever, fatigue, and malaise (which can be signs of infective endocarditis).
3. Maintain venous access for infant receiving continuous infusion of prostaglandin E1. Have intubation and resuscitation equipment available. In the event of an acute cyanotic spell, place the child in knee-chest position and administer oxygen. Assess for postoperative bleeding. Assess cardiac performance.
4. The nurse should ensure that the parents are knowledgeable about:
   - Signs of infective endocarditis.
   - Acute cyanotic spells.
   - Promoting as normal activity and as possible.
   - Administering medications.
   - How to observe for abnormal delays in growth and development.
5. Parents should be knowledgeable about cardiopulmonary resuscitation. They must be able to recognize and respond to an acute cyanotic spell (assist the child to the knee-chest position and administer oxygen). Emergency numbers need to be easily visible at the telephone, including 911 and the number of the client's physician. Discuss that being prepared for an emergency is a good idea; however, they need to relax and enjoy their child in as near-normal a way as possible.

Chapter 6

1. The physical parameters the nurse should monitor include:
   - Vital signs, especially temperature for fever.
   - Behaviors such as suck, cry, posture, muscle tone.
   - Bulging fontanel and other indicators of increased intracranial pressure.
   - Hydration status: mucous membranes, urine $\geq$ to 1 cc/kg/hr, weight daily on same scale.
2. Nursing interventions that would have priority during the first 48 hours include:
   - Monitoring respiratory status, heart rate, and blood pressure.
   - Provide an environment that minimizes ICP elevation: head of bed should be at 30-degree angle, maintain head in neutral position, quiet environment.
   - Administer antibiotic therapy as soon as prescribed.
   - Maintain IV fluids as prescribed.

- Administer antipyretics as needed for temperature elevation.

3. The usual medical treatment for meningitis is based on diagnosis from the results of a lumbar puncture. Cerebrospinal fluid is cultured to determine the causative organism and appropriate intravenous antibiotic therapy is initiated. Fluid status and serum sodium levels are closely monitored during the early period because clients with this diagnosis are at risk for developing syndrome of inappropriate antidiuretic hormone.
4. There are numerous developmental implications for this family. This infant is in a sensitive bonding period with her parents. Since she has an older sibling who also needs the attention of the parents, this poses the dilemma to the family of how to handle visitation. Parents will have some stress since they lack extended family in the geographical proximity; however, that does not rule out that they may have many friends and neighbors who can help out with babysitting when one of them cannot be home. The separation of family members because of the hospitalization could be more stressful for the preschooler than the hospitalized infant because of the preschooler's age-appropriate separation anxiety.
5. In planning for discharge, specific areas of support for or teaching with the family include:
   - When to return for follow-up visit.
   - Resources in the community if indicated. Fifty percent of children with meningitis suffer some degree of neurological sequelae. This infant could develop deafness and then require referral to hearing and speech specialists.

Chapter 7

1. Dietary management for children with ESRD focuses on maximizing calories for growth while limiting demands on the kidney and minimizing fluid and electrolyte disturbances. Sodium-, potassium- and phosphate-restricted diets may be necessary. Daily fluid restrictions may also be necessary.
2. Renal transplantation is considered to be the optimal renal replacement choice for children. Transplantation provides for a normalization of physiology and the potential for normal growth and development.
3. Complications of hemodialysis are hypotension, rapid changes in fluid and electrolyte balance, and disequilibrium syndrome. Hemodialysis provides for more efficient clearance of toxins than peritoneal dialysis. Hemodialysis significantly lowers the BUN and creatinine levels in the bloodstream more quickly than does peritoneal dialysis.
4. Peritoneal dialysis is more widely used in the treatment of children with ESRD because it is a continuous process, can be done at home, and is an easier process for family or child to learn and implement. It is also is less disruptive to the family social structure than hemodialysis.
5. Children with ESRD suffer body image disturbance related to small size and their perception of being and looking different than other children. Because their condition is chronic, they have altered health maintenance, which impacts their social and psychological growth. Psychosocial concerns for the child undergoing hemodialysis are care and maintenance of a vascular access site and travel to a hemodialysis center three times a week. Psychosocial concerns for the child undergoing peritoneal dialysis include caregiver role strain related to daily dialysis treatments and potential for frequent peritonitis resulting in hospitalization. Psychosocial concerns for renal transplantation include immunosuppressive therapy management and the potential for transplant rejection. Also, a living, related donor contributes to a higher kidney survival rate than does a cadaver kidney.

Chapter 8

1. It is necessary to obtain all necessary information regarding the teenager's present condition. Appropriate questions include:
   - How long has she been ill?
   - Is she able to keep fluids down?
   - What types and how much fluid has she taken?
   - Does she have fever?
   - What were her last four blood glucose results?
   - Is she urinating?
   - Are there any ketones in her urine?
   - Is she eating anything more than toast?
2. Continue to give insulin, but the teenager might need to use the sliding scale utilizing regular insulin only. Test blood glucose every 3 to 4 hours and administer insulin as needed. Check urinary ketones also.
3. The teenager would benefit from calorie-free liquids to clear ketones in the urine, if necessary. Simple carbohydrates are allowed for nutrition, especially if the teenager has a poor appetite. Encourage frequent blood testing.
4. If ketones are present in the urine:
   - Encourage calorie-free fluid intake
   - Encourage rest
   - Discourage exercise at this time
5. Notify the doctor or nurse practitioner for the following complications:
   - Moderate to high urinary ketones
   - Hyperglycemia
   - Acetone or fruity breath
   - Lethargy
   - Deep, rapid respirations

Chapter 9

1. The assessment findings in a newborn with developmental dysplasia of the hip (DDH) include a positive Ortolani or Barlow's sign. The nurse will also find limited abduction of the hips, asymmetry of the thigh and gluteal folds, and unequal knee and leg lengths. A wide perineum will be found in the infant with bilateral disease.

2. The exact cause of DDH is not known, though certain factors are known to increase the risk of it. Family history increases the risk tenfold. Prenatal conditions affecting the development of DDH, such as the frank breech position and maternal hormones of relaxin and estrogen, may cause laxity of the hip joint and capsule and lead to joint instability. Twinning or large infant size are additional conditions associated with DDH.
3. The priorities of care for this newborn include teaching the parents about the care of this infant, along with helping the parents deal with their feelings of their newborn having a deformity.
4. DDH is treated by keeping the hip in abduction by way of an abduction device. For infants less than 3 months, the most common treatment is use of a Pavlik harness, which is an adjustable chest halter that abducts the legs. Soft plastic stirrups hold the hips flexed, abducted, and externally rotated.
5. Teaching that should be completed with the parents of an infant who will be wearing a Pavlik harness includes proper application, the need for sponge bath, and assessing skin under the straps daily for irritation or redness. A t-shirt and knee socks should be worn under the brace to prevent skin irritation and the diaper should be placed under the straps and changed without taking the harness off. The harness is worn 23 hours a day, and the hips and buttocks should be supported carefully when not in the harness. The nurse should also discuss the necessary modification of the car seat and strollers, and modification of positioning for nursing and eating. Parents need to ensure the child has adequate stimulation with toys and activities at appropriate eye level and should encourage activities that stimulate upper extremities.
6. Early detection and treatment enable the majority of children with DDH to attain normal hip function.

Chapter 10

1. The nurse saw a small area of papules and vesicles on skin that was otherwise clear. The child said they did not itch.
2. Impetigo is highly contagious, and the child could infect many of his classmates by holding hands or playing on the playground or sharing books.
3. The nurse will explain that the mother needs to seek medical attention for her child as this is a bacterial infection that requires antibiotics. The mother should gently wash the infected area with antibacterial soap and warm water and remove crusts. The antibiotic ointment that is prescribed should be applied to the site as directed for the full duration of therapy, a week to 10 days. The child's fingernails should be cut short and he should be reminded not to scratch or pick at the lesions. The child and all family members should wash hands frequently with antibacterial soap.
4. The primary goal is to prevent the spread of impetigo to other areas on the child and to other individuals.
5. The child should be able to return to school after using topical antibiotics for 48 hours.

Chapter 11

1. CBC with differential. Dependent on the differential results, the physician may begin treatment or may decide to do allergy testing. Frequently the physician will begin the allergy testing with the skin or scratch test. This test allows a quick evaluation of many possible allergens (antigens) with results within 30 minutes. There is a small risk of anaphylaxis from this type of testing. Based on the scratch tests results, the physician may order a RAST to further evaluate allergens. The RAST test is more specific and carries no risk of anaphylaxis.
2. The nurse will ask questions relative to recent exposures to communicable diseases. The nurse would want information about the risk of exposure, such as whether the child attends a preschool or kindergarten or if anyone else in the family been sick. The nurse will question if the child has a history of allergies, including food allergies, skin allergies, and insect sting/bite allergies. The nurse would also be interested if there is a family history of allergies as the tendency towards allergies runs in families. Finally, the nurse will question the history of present illness looking for onset, prodromal symptoms as well as precipitating events.
3. Priority nursing diagnosis for this child would include:
   - Hyperthermia, related to infectious disease process.
   - Risk for fluid volume deficit related to increased insensible fluid loss and possible refusal to drink adequate liquids.
   - Knowledge deficit (parents) of infectious disease process (no etiology required for knowledge deficit diagnoses).
4. Nursing interventions appropriate for the child would include:
   - Monitoring the child's temperature and intervening as appropriate. If the child is hyperthermic, the nurse needs to reduce the temperature. Antipyretics would be administered as appropriate. The nurse would teach the parents to use acetaminophen (Tylenol) instead of aspirin. Studies have shown that in viral infections, the use of aspirin increases the risk of Reye syndrome. The nurse would also want to teach the use of a tepid bath, increased fluid intake, and minimal clothing to allow heat dissipation.
   - Blood and body fluid precautions. All patients should be have the same precautions applied to their care. This is for the safety of the patients and the health care workers. If admitted to the hospital and while in the clinic, the child should be isolated from other children until the cause of the fever and potential rash is known.
   - The nurse would also provide information to the family about the potential rash. Antihistamines may be used if the child is itching. The child's nails should be kept short to decrease the risk of impaired skin integrity. Oatmeal (Aveeno) baths may make the child more comfortable.

5. Recovery will have occurred when:
   - Body temperature returns to normal parameters.
   - Body fluid secretions decrease.
   - Skin lesions decrease.

Chapter 12

1. It is essential to do a complete physical assessment as a comparison for changes that may occur during therapy. The child will have an increased risk for infection and injury subsequent to chemotherapy. The client will also need to be monitored for such side effects as nausea and vomiting, so baseline nutrition information and all other physical assessments are needed for accurate evaluation of response to interventions.
2. It would be important to look at the child's usual behaviors and coping abilities to evaluate response to treatment.
3. The priority of therapeutic medical management is to induce remission. Nursing management will focus on providing information so the family can learn about the disease and its treatment and providing emotional support to the child and family. Treatment for this illness lasts 2 1/2 to 3 years, so goals need to be appropriate for this chronic, life-threatening cancer.
4. Initial information must include the reason for central venous line, while addressing the fear related to the unknown, pain and threat to life. In addition, each test, treatment, and side effect must be discussed in a timely way. It is essential to allow time for questions. Families often need to have information repeated, until they become more comfortable in the situation.
5. The planned vacation will have to be postponed. The parents may be using denial to cope or they may have a knowledge deficit about the length of treatment. It is very likely that this trip will be possible at another time in the treatment.

Chapter 13

1. It is imperative to complete a thorough pain assessment. Ask the client to point to the painful area and to describe the pain. Note the onset, location, and intensity of pain. Determine if there are precipitating factors or if any relief measures have been attempted. In addition to a thorough pain assessment, a complete history and head-to-toe assessment should be obtained. Vital signs and weight should be assessed for variances from the normal. Assessment of the abdomen includes observation, auscultation and palpation, taking note of guarding, abdominal distention, rigidity, activity of bowel sounds, and rebound tenderness.
2. Orders should include frequent vital signs, keeping the client NPO, initiating IV therapy, intermittent antibiotics, strict I & O, apply cold packs as needed for comfort, and acetaminophen (Tylenol) every 4 hours as needed for fever.
3. Let the client assume a position of comfort, usually side-lying with knees bent. Administer analgesics if ordered and apply cold packs as needed to minimize discomfort. Demonstrate how to splint the abdomen for coughing and moving.
4. Many times this is the first hospitalization for a family, so anxiety and apprehension is to be expected. Providing emotional support is an important aspect of care that cannot be overlooked. Good preoperative teaching can reduce anxiety. Answering questions thoroughly and reviewing the plan of care is extremely beneficial. When interacting with children always remember the child's developmental level.
5. The postoperative care for a nonruptured appendix includes frequent vital signs, monitoring I & O, maintaining NPO status until bowel function returns, administering antibiotics if ordered, and maintaining IV fluids. Other orders include turning, coughing, and deep-breathing, early ambulation, and management of pain. Monitoring the incision site and changing sterile dressings may be included. Postoperative care is short in duration; many times the client is discharged within 24 hours of surgery. Postoperative care of the child with a ruptured appendix is more complex and longer in duration. The postoperative orders would include the same orders as for the nonruptured appendix with the addition of intermittent IV antibiotics for at least a 7-day regimen and maintaining a nasogastric tube to low intermittent wall suction until bowel function returns. The client who has experienced a perforated appendix may have a drain in place or large abdominal dressing, so care for these would also be included. The incision must be monitored, and temperature control measures will be ordered.

Chapter 14

1. In the complete medical history, including birth information, be sure to ask about any previous bleeding episodes, no mater how minor. Specifically, inquire as to any history of hemophilia or other bleeding conditions among other family members. Ask the parents as to any previous episodes of joint pain or swelling as well as a change in joint/extremity appearance. Check to see if there have been urinary problems such as hematuria or flank pain. Previously undiscovered cerebral bleeding may have caused peripheral neuropathies or neurologic impairment. Question the parents as to change in motor function/capabilities as well as cognitive abilities.
2. Pain and bleeding control with hemarthrosis will be managed through immobilization and elevation of the limb as well as ice pack. Oral or IV analgesics will also be administered per physician's preference. Analgesics that contain aspirin, aspirin like substances, NSAIDs, or other medication that might affect platelet function are to be avoided.
3. Bleeding control is the first order of medical management. This will be accomplished through the administration of the missing factor. Laboratory tests including prothrombin time (PT), partial thromboplastin time (PTT), complete blood count (CBC), and fibrinogen levels will be monitored to assess the child's status. X-rays and/or a CT scan might be

done to assess the degree of joint involvement or damage. Factor will be administered for a mild or major bleeding episode or if the child is in a life-threatening situation. If the child's situation were to include surface bleeding, a topical hemostatic agent might be applied to control capillary bleeding. Pain management will be handled as discussed above.

4. Hemophilia is a genetic disorder with an X-linked recessive trait. This means that it will result almost solely in carrier families and affected males. The disorder results from a deficiency in specific clotting factors. The missing factor will guide the treatment regimen. Classic hemophilia or hemophilia A is caused by a deficiency of factor VIII. Approximately 80% of hemophiliacs have hemophilia A. The occurrence rate is approximately 1 in 5,000 male births. Hemophilia B, also known as Christmas disease, results from a deficiency in factor IX. Approximately 15% of those with hemophilia have hemophilia B. Females with hemophilia trait do not often manifest the disease. However, they may experience prolonged bleeding time with dental work, surgery, or trauma. Males will have bleeding tendencies ranging from mild to severe. The presence of a child with hemophilia means there are implications for future childbearing, both for the parents as well as any of their children. Other family members may also bee affected. Genetic testing and counseling are imperative.
5. Explain to the family that although the child may require hospitalization for diagnosis and management or with the first bleeding episode, most care can be managed in the home and outpatient clinic. Parents and child will need a good understanding of the origin of bleeding to understand the disease process and plan their lives accordingly. A medical identification bracelet is imperative for the child to wear at all times. The family must recognize that acetaminophen is to be used for fever and pain as opposed to aspirin or aspirin-like medications, including ibuprofen. The family needs to understand which situations and injuries can cause bleeding to occur. The family must learn how to identify internal bleeding and how to respond to all bleeding episodes, minor or not. It is particularly important for the family to recognize that abdominal pain, joint pain, and obvious bleeding are implications for an urgent infusion of factor. If the child is to receive factor in the home setting, the family will require instruction as to preparation and administration. If administration is to be on a regular basis, have the family verbalize the schedule and the principle that missing a scheduled infusion may lead to a bleeding episode. Assist the family to notify school officials and work with the appropriate personnel to handle any problems as they arise. Assist the family to plan for as normal a life as possible for the child at home and school. Overprotection should be avoided. However, the family should recognize that contact sports are not appropriate, but the child can engage in swimming. Certain other activities such as hiking, bicycling, roller blading, and so on can be done also with certain precautionary measures. Assist the family to schedule regular clinic visits and to coordinate with their regular pediatrician and dentist. If not already done, encourage the family to seek testing and genetic counseling for appropriate members. Lastly, place family in contact with appropriate support groups and social services.

Chapter 15

1. Begin by not having any physical contact with the child. She has been traumatized by someone she trusted, so establishing a nurse–client relationship will be more difficult. Maintain eye contact with the child by sitting in a chair or squatting down beside the child. Inform her of everything you are going to do. Ask her if she has any questions and answer them truthfully. Remember that the abused child has the same developmental and physical needs as any other child.
2. Maintain consistent care providers, and encourage a parent to stay with the child. Never attempt any type of invasive procedure or any other act that could be threatening to the child without fully explaining what is to be done, and always be truthful when answering questions. Encourage the child to participate in the routine playroom activities on the hospital unit.
3. The comment from the child is likely because the uncle told her she would be in trouble if she told anyone, a common ploy by sexual abusers of children. Assure the child that she did nothing wrong, and praise her for coming forward with the truth. It is important to allow the child to vent her feelings. The child will need counseling as a result of the abuse.
4. The parents should be asked to step into the hall or given a private area, if needed, until they can speak calmly in front of the child. When a child is the victim of sexual abuse, the parents feel guilt and anger, especially if the abuse is committed by a close friend or family member, as in this case. One parent may blame the other, and if interventions are not taken, the marriage could deteriorate from this incident. Consult social services, a counselor, or the available support services for parents of abused children to intervene and offer support through this traumatic event.
5. Therapeutic communication is essential during this crisis. Encourage the child to verbalize her feelings of anger, pain, and fear. Therapeutic strategies utilized by therapists such as art therapy and play therapy may be beneficial for the release of these feelings. Assure that the child is receiving appropriate counseling.

Credits

Chapter 1

Box 1-1 From *Pediatric Nursing: Caring for Children*, by Jane Ball and Ruth Bindler, © 1999, Edition 2, Page 61, Chart 2-14, Appleton & Lange, A Simon & Schuster Company.

Box 1-2 From *Pediatric Nursing: Caring for Children*, by Jane Ball and Ruth Bindler, © 1999, Edition 2, Page 58, Chart 2-12, Appleton & Lange, A Simon & Schuster Company.

Fig. 1-1 From Centers for Disease Control, Atlanta, GA.

Chapter 2

Fig. 2-1 Art; © Prentice Hall Health, Upper Saddle River, New Jersey.

Fig. 2-2 Art / Precision Graphics; From *Maternal-Newborn Nursing: A Family and Community Approach*, by Sally B. Olds, Marcia L. London, Patricia Wieland Ladewig, © 2000 by Prentice-Hall, Inc., Upper Saddle River, New Jersey, Page 717, Fig. 25-14.

Fig. 2-3 Art; Reprinted with permission. From Denver Developmental Materials Inc., Denver, CO. in *Pediatric Nursing: Caring for Children*, by Jane Ball and Ruth Bindler, © 1999, Edition 2, Page 215 and 217, Fig. 5-5 and 5-6, Appleton & Lange, A Simon & Schuster Company.

Chapter 3

Fig. 3-1 Art; From *Pediatric Nursing: Caring for Children*, by Jane Ball and Ruth Bindler, © 1999, Edition 2, Page 713, Fig. 17-1, Appleton & Lange, A Simon & Schuster Company.

Fig. 3-2 Art; © Prentice Hall Health, Upper Saddle River, New Jersey.

Chapter 4

Fig. 4-1 Art; *Pediatric Nursing: Caring for Children*, by Jane Ball and Ruth Bindler, © 1999, Edition 2, Page 439, Fig. 11-12, Appleton & Lange, A Simon & Schuster Company.

Chapter 5

Fig. 5-1 Art; From *Pediatric Nursing: Caring for Children*, by Jane Ball and Ruth Bindler, © 1999, Edition 2, Page 480, Art from Chart 12-3, Appleton & Lange, A Simon & Schuster Company.

Fig. 5-2 Art; *Pediatric Nursing: Caring for Children*, by Jane Ball and Ruth Bindler, © 1999, Edition 2, Page 481, Art from Chart 12-3, Appleton & Lange, A Simon & Schuster Company.

Fig. 5-3 Art; *Pediatric Nursing: Caring for Children*, by Jane Ball and Ruth Bindler, © 1999, Edition 2, Page 483, Art from Chart 12-4, Appleton & Lange, A Simon & Schuster Company.

Fig. 5-4 Art; *Pediatric Nursing: Caring for Children*, by Jane Ball and Ruth Bindler, © 1999, Edition 2, Page 490, Art from Chart 12-9, Appleton & Lange, A Simon & Schuster Company.

Fig. 5-5 Art; *Pediatric Nursing: Caring for Children*, by Jane Ball and Ruth Bindler, © 1999, Edition 2, Page 491, Art from Chart 12-9, Appleton & Lange, A Simon & Schuster Company.

Chapter 6

Fig. 6-1 Art, A&B; © Prentice Hall Health, Upper Saddle River, New Jersey.

Fig. 6-2 Art; From *Pediatric Nursing: Caring for Children*, by Jane Ball and Ruth Bindler, © 1999, Edition 2, Page 783, Fig. 18-11 A&B, Appleton & Lange, A Simon & Schuster Company.

Fig. 6-3 Art; From *Pediatric Nursing: Caring for Children*, by Jane Ball and Ruth Bindler, © 1999, Edition 2, Page 787, Fig. 18-13, Appleton & Lange, A Simon & Schuster Company.

Table 6-1 From *Medical Surgical Nursing: Critical Thinking in Client Care*, by LeMone, Priscilla and Burke, Karen M., © 2000, Edition 2, Page 1683, Table 39-4, Prentice-Hall, Inc., Upper Saddle River, New Jersey.

Chapter 7

Fig. 7-1 Art; © Prentice Hall Health, Upper Saddle River, New Jersey.

Fig. 7-2 Art; From *Pediatric Nursing: Caring for Children*, by Jane Ball and Ruth Bindler, © 1999, Edition 2, Page 665, Fig. 16-5 A&B, Appleton & Lange, A Simon & Schuster Company.

Fig. 7-3 Art; © Prentice Hall Health, Upper Saddle River, New Jersey.

Chapter 8

Fig. 8-1 Art, From J. Black, E. Matassarian-Jacobs, *Medical Surgical Nursing: Clinical Management for Continuity of Care*, Edition 5,

Page 1958, Philadelphia: W. B. Saunders, 1997. Reprinted with permission.

Fig. 8-2 Art, From *Pediatric Nursing: Caring for Children*, by Jane Ball and Ruth Bindler, © 1999, Edition 2, Page 892, Fig. 20-9, Appleton & Lange, A Simon & Schuster Company.

Table 8-1 From *Pediatric Nursing: Caring for Children*, by Jane Ball and Ruth Bindler, © 1999, Edition 2, Page 886, Chart 20-6, Appleton & Lange, A Simon & Schuster Company.

Chapter 9

Fig. 9-1 Art, From *Pediatric Nursing: Caring for Children*, by Jane Ball and Ruth Bindler, © 1999, Edition 2, Page 827, Fig. 19-7 "A", Appleton & Lange, A Simon & Schuster Company.

Fig. 9-2 Art, From *Pediatric Nursing: Caring for Children*, by Jane Ball and Ruth Bindler, © 1999, Edition 2, Page 855, Fig. 19-18, Appleton & Lange, A Simon & Schuster Company.

Fig. 9-3 Chart with Art, From *Pediatric Nursing: Caring for Children*, by Jane Ball and Ruth Bindler, © 1999, Edition 2, Page 854, Chart 19-13, Appleton & Lange, A Simon & Schuster Company.

Chapter 10

Fig. 10-1 Art, From *Pediatric Nursing: Caring for Children*, by Jane Ball and Ruth Bindler, © 1999, Edition 2, Page 909, Fig. 21-1, Appleton & Lange, A Simon & Schuster Company.

Chapter 11

Box 11-1 Table, From *Pediatric Nursing: Caring for Children*, by Jane Ball and Ruth Bindler, © 1999, Edition 2, Page 346, Chart 9-4, Appleton & Lange, A Simon & Schuster Company.

Chapter 12

Fig. 12-1 Art, From *Pediatric Nursing: Caring for Children*, by Jane Ball and Ruth Bindler, © 1999, Edition 2, Page 549, Fig. 14-5, Appleton & Lange, A Simon & Schuster Company.

Fig. 12-2 Art, From *Pediatric Nursing: Caring for Children*, by Jane Ball and Ruth Bindler, © 1999, Edition 2, Page 565, Fig. 14-13, Appleton & Lange, A Simon & Schuster Company.

Chapter 13

Fig. 13-1 Art A & B; © Prentice Hall Health, Upper Saddle River, New Jersey.

Fig. 13-2 Art, From *Pediatric Nursing: Caring for Children*, by Jane Ball and Ruth Bindler, © 1999, Edition 2, Page 607, Fig. 15-5, Appleton & Lange, A Simon & Schuster Company.

Fig. 13-3 Art, From *Pediatric Nursing: Caring for Children*, by Jane Ball and Ruth Bindler, © 1999, Edition 2, Page 618, Fig. 15-10, Appleton & Lange, A Simon & Schuster Company.

Table 13-1 From *Pediatric Nursing: Caring for Children*, by Jane Ball and Ruth Bindler, © 1999, Edition 2, Page 610, Chart 15-2, Appleton & Lange, A Simon & Schuster Company.

Table 13-4 From *Pediatric Nursing: Caring for Children*, by Jane Ball and Ruth Bindler, © 1999, Edition 2, Page 325, Chart 8-15, Appleton & Lange, A Simon & Schuster Company.

Table 13-5 From *Pediatric Nursing: Caring for Children*, by Jane Ball and Ruth Bindler, © 1999, Edition 2, Page 294, Chart 8-3, Appleton & Lange, A Simon & Schuster Company.

Chapter 14

Fig. 14-1 Art, From *Medical Surgical Nursing: Critical Thinking in Client Care*, by LeMone, Priscilla and Burke, Karen M., © 2000, Edition 2, Page 1294, Fig. 31-10, Prentice-Hall, Inc., Upper Saddle River, New Jersey. Nea Hanscomb—Artist.

Fig. 14-2 Art, From Ignatavicius, D, Workman, L, Mishler, M, *Medical Surgical Nursing Across the Health Care Continuum*, Edition 3, W. B. Saunders, 1999.

Table 14-1 Adapted from *Handbook of Pediatrics,* by G. B. Merenstein, D. W. Kaplan, & A. A. Rosenberg, © 1997, Edition 18, Pages 986–989.

Table 14-2 From *Pediatric Nursing: Caring for Children*, by Jane Ball and Ruth Bindler, © 1999, Edition 2, Page 518, Table 13-2, Appleton & Lange, A Simon & Schuster Company.

Table 14-3 From *Pediatric Nursing: Caring for Children*, by Jane Ball and Ruth Bindler, © 1999, Edition 2, Page 530, Table 13-7, Appleton & Lange, A Simon & Schuster Company.

Box 14-1 From *Pediatric Nursing: Caring for Children,* by Jane Ball and Ruth Binder, © 1999, Edition 2, Page 523, Table 13-5, Appleton & Lange, A Simon & Schuster Company.

Index

O

P